Food Science and Nutrition

Food Science and Nutrition

Edited by
Keegan Mason

Larsen & Keller
www.larsen-keller.com

Food Science and Nutrition
Edited by Keegan Mason
ISBN: 978-1-63549-201-9 (Hardback)

Larsen & Keller
Published by Larsen and Keller Education,
5 Penn Plaza,
19th Floor,
New York, NY 10001, USA

Cataloging-in-Publication Data

Food science and nutrition / edited by Keegan Mason.
p. cm.
Includes bibliographical references and index.
ISBN 978-1-63549-201-9
1. Food. 2. Nutrition. I. Mason, Keegan.
TX353 .F66 2017
641.3--dc23

Printed and bound in China.

For more information regarding Larsen and Keller Education and its products, please visit the publisher's website www.larsen-keller.com

Table of Contents

Preface

Food science is a field, which studies the nature, causes of deterioration, processing and other important characteristics of food, so as to make it more consumer friendly. The book provides detailed information about the biochemical, physical and chemical processes of food and how they are used by engineers to make it more nutritious and better for people. The topics included in this text are of utmost significance and bound to provide incredible insights to readers. It is a complete source of knowledge on the present status of this important field. It will also serve as a reference guide for students and academicians.

Given below is the chapter wise description of the book:

Chapter 1- Nutrition sustains the growth, reproduction and health of an organism. The basic focus of nutrition is to reduce or prevent diseases with a healthy diet. A healthy diet is necessary for the growth an organism and this also includes preparation of food and storage methods. The chapter on nutrition offers an insightful focus, keeping in mind the complex subject matter.

Chapter 2- Nutrition has a number of branches and some of these are nutrigenomics, sports nutrition and nutrition and pregnancy. Nutrigenomics is the study of food and its constituents on gene expression whereas the plan prescribed by a doctor to a woman before, during and after pregnancy is known as nutrition and pregnancy. The following text strategically encompasses and incorporates the major branches of nutrition.

Chapter 3- Nutrients are constituents found in food items that are consumed by an organism to survive and to grow. Macronutrients provide an organism with the energy it requires, and also provides the necessary co-factors for metabolism. This section will provide an integrated understanding of nutrients.

Chapter 4- The food industry has progressed over the years; only hunter- gatherers and the farmers who survive on what they grow are considered to be separate from this industry. Some of the topics covered in this chapter are food fortification, food grading, food processing, food packaging, food coloring and food technology. This following content is an overview of the subject matter incorporating all the major aspects of the food industry.

Chapter 5- Dietary supplements are consumed in order to provide nutrients to an individual. Fiber supplements, iron supplements and spirulina are some of the aspects dealt within this text. This chapter elucidates the crucial theories of food supplements.

Chapter 6- Energy bars contain cereals and high-energy food items. They are used as energy sources for particular events like marathons, 100-meter races, and other events. Energy drinks, energy gels and sports drinks are also discussed in the following section. The section serves as a source to comprehend all the numerous energy bars and drinks.

Chapter 7- The significant aspects of nutrition and food sciences are examined in this chapter. The study of the interactions of biological and non-biological components of food items is known as food chemistry. Other facets elucidated are food engineering, food microbiology, molecular gastronomy and malnutrition. The topics discussed in the text are of great importance to broaden the existing knowledge on nutrition and food science.

Indeed, my job was extremely crucial and challenging as I had to ensure that every chapter is informative and structured in a student-friendly manner. I am thankful for the support provided by my family and colleagues during the completion of this book.

Editor

1

Introduction to Nutrition and Food Science

Nutrition sustains the growth, reproduction and health of an organism. The basic focus of nutrition is to reduce or prevent diseases with a healthy diet. A healthy diet is necessary for the growth an organism and this also includes preparation of food and storage methods. The chapter on nutrition offers an insightful focus, keeping in mind the complex subject matter.

Nutrition

Nutrition is the science that interprets the interaction of nutrients and other substances in food in relation to maintenance, growth, reproduction, health and disease of an organism. It includes food intake, absorption, assimilation, biosynthesis, catabolism and excretion.

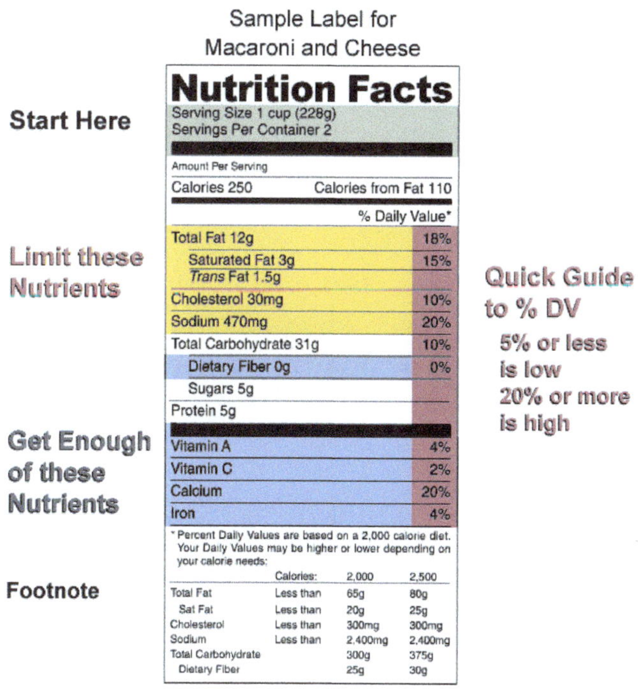

The "Nutrition Facts" table displayed on packaged food labels in the United States and Canada indicates the amounts of nutrients recommended by the US Food and Drug Administration to limit or consume according to the Daily Value

The diet of an organism is what it eats, which is largely determined by the availability, the processing and palatability of foods. A healthy diet includes preparation of food and storage methods that preserve nutrients from oxidation, heat or leaching, and that reduce risk of food-born illnesses.

Registered dietitian nutritionists (RDs or RDNs) are health professionals qualified to provide safe, evidence-based dietary advice which includes a review of what is eaten, a thorough review of nutritional health, and a personalized nutritional treatment plan. They also provide preventive and therapeutic programs at work places, schools and similar institutions. Certified Clinical Nutritionists or CCNs, are trained health professionals who also offer dietary advice on the role of nutrition in chronic disease, including possible prevention or remediation by addressing nutritional deficiencies before resorting to drugs. Government regulation especially in terms of licensing, is currently less universal for the CCN than that of RD or RDN. Another advanced Nutrition Professional is a Certified Nutrition Specialist or CNS. These Board Certified Nutritionists typically specialize in obesity and chronic disease. In order to become board certified, potential CNS candidate must pass an examination, much like Registered Dieticians. This exam covers specific domains within the health sphere including; Clinical Intervention and Human Health.

A poor diet may cause health problems, causing deficiency diseases such as blindness, anemia, scurvy, preterm birth, stillbirth and cretinism; health-threatening conditions like obesity and metabolic syndrome; and such common chronic systemic diseases as cardiovascular disease, diabetes, and osteoporosis. A poor diet can cause the wasting of kwashiorkor in acute cases, and the stunting of marasmus in chronic cases of malnutrition.

History

Antiquity

The first recorded dietary advice, carved into a Babylonian stone tablet in about 2500 BC, cautioned those with pain inside to avoid eating onions for three days. Scurvy, later found to be a vitamin C deficiency, was first described in 1500 BC in the Ebers Papyrus.

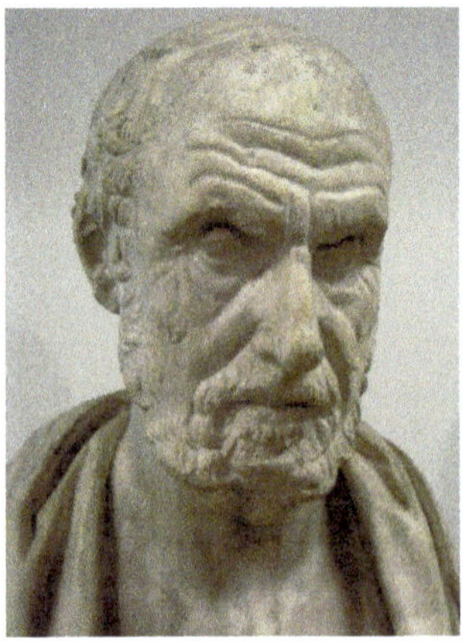

Hippocrates lived about 400 BC, and Galen and the understanding of nutrition followed him for centuries.

According to Walter Gratzer, the study of nutrition probably began during the 6th century BC. In China, the concept of *Qi* developed, a spirit or "wind" similar to what Western Europeans later called *pneuma*. Food was classified into "hot" (for example, meats, blood, ginger, and hot spices) and "cold" (green vegetables) in China, India, Malaya, and Persia. *Humours* developed perhaps first in China alongside *qi*. Ho the Physician concluded that diseases are caused by deficiencies of elements (Wu Xing: fire, water, earth, wood, and metal), and he classified diseases as well as prescribed diets. About the same time in Italy, Alcmaeon of Croton (a Greek) wrote of the importance of equilibrium between what goes in and what goes out, and warned that imbalance would result in disease marked by obesity or emaciation.

The first recorded nutritional experiment with human subjects is found in the Bible's Book of Daniel. Daniel and his friends were captured by the king of Babylon during an invasion of Israel. Selected as court servants, they were to share in the king's fine foods and wine. But they objected, preferring vegetables (pulses) and water in accordance with their Jewish dietary restrictions. The king's chief steward reluctantly agreed to a trial. Daniel and his friends received their diet for ten days and were then compared to the king's men. Appearing healthier, they were allowed to continue with their diet.

Around 475 BC, Anaxagoras stated that food is absorbed by the human body and, therefore, contains "homeomerics" (generative components), suggesting the existence of nutrients. Around 400 BC, Hippocrates, who recognized and was concerned with obesity, which may have been common in southern Europe at the time, said, "Let food be your medicine and medicine be your food." The works that are still attributed to him, *Corpus Hippocraticum*, called for moderation and emphasized exercise.

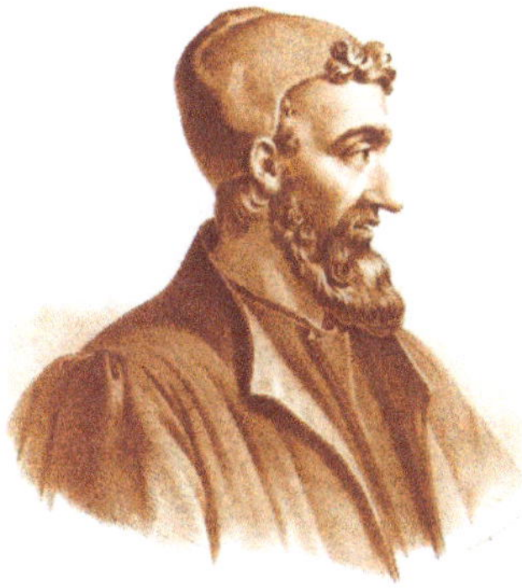

Followed for a millennium and a half, Galen (1st century) created the first coherent (although mistaken) theory of nutrition.

Salt, pepper and other spices were prescribed for various ailments in various preparations for example mixed with vinegar. In the 2nd century BC, Cato the Elder believed that cabbage (or the urine of cabbage-eaters) could cure digestive diseases, ulcers, warts, and intoxication. Living about the turn of the millennium, Aulus Celsus, an ancient Roman doctor, believed in "strong" and "weak" foods (bread for example was strong, as were older animals and vegetables).

Galen to Lind

One mustn't overlook the doctrines of Galen: In use from his life in the 1st century AD until the 17th century, it was heresy to disagree with him for 1500 years. Galen was physician to gladiators in Pergamon, and in Rome, physician to Marcus Aurelius and the three emperors who succeeded him. Most of Galen's teachings were gathered and enhanced in the late 11th century by Benedictine monks at the School of Salerno in *Regimen sanitatis Salernitanum*, which still had users in the 17th century. Galen believed in the bodily *humours* of Hippocrates, and he taught that *pneuma* is the source of life. Four elements (earth, air, fire and water) combine into "complexion", which combines into states (the four temperaments: sanguine, phlegmatic, choleric, and melancholic). The states are made up of pairs of attributes (hot and moist, cold and moist, hot and dry, and cold and dry), which are made of four humours: blood, phlegm, green (or yellow) bile, and black bile (the bodily form of the elements). Galen thought that for a person to have gout, kidney stones, or arthritis was scandalous, which Gratzer likens to Samuel Butler's *Erehwon* (1872) where sickness is a crime.

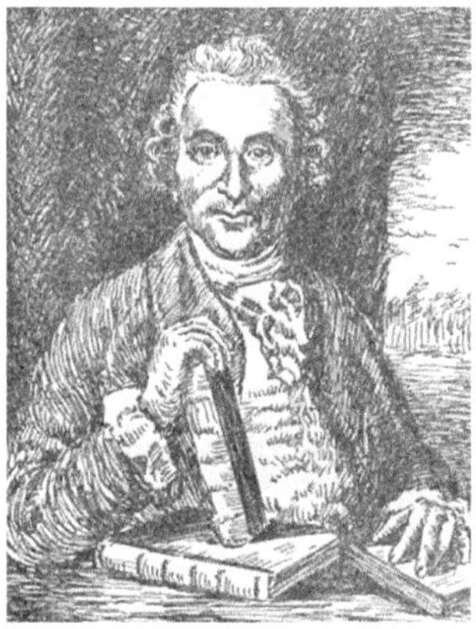

James Lind conducted in 1747 the first controlled clinical trial in modern times, and in 1753 published *Treatise on Scurvy*.

In the 1500s, Paracelsus was probably the first to criticize Galen publicly. Also in the 16th century, scientist and artist Leonardo da Vinci compared metabolism to a burning candle. Leonardo did not publish his works on this subject, but he was not afraid of thinking for himself and he definitely disagreed with Galen. Ultimately, 16th century works of Andreas Vesalius, sometimes called the father of modern medicine, overturned Galen's ideas. He was followed by piercing thought amalgamated with the era's mysticism and religion sometimes fueled by the mechanics of Newton and Galileo. Jan Baptist van Helmont, who discovered several gases such as carbon dioxide, performed the first quantitative experiment. Robert Boyle advanced chemistry. Sanctorius measured body weight. Physician Herman Boerhaave modeled the digestive process. Physiologist Albrecht von Haller worked out the difference between nerves and muscles.

Sometimes overlooked during his life, James Lind, a physician in the British navy, performed the first scientific nutrition experiment in 1747. Lind discovered that lime juice saved sailors that had been at sea for years from scurvy, a deadly and painful bleeding disorder. Between 1500 and 1800, an estimated two million sailors had died of scurvy. The discovery was ignored for forty years, after which British sailors became known as "limeys." The essential vitamin C within citrus fruits would not be identified by scientists until 1932.

Lavoisier and Modern Science

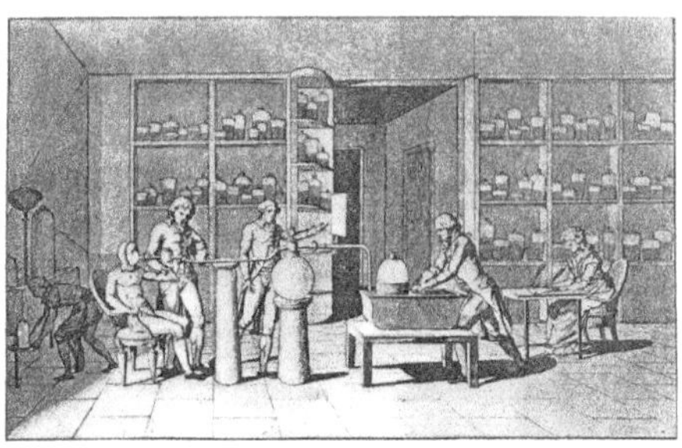

By containing his assistant, Armand Seguin, inside a rubber suit fitted with a tube sealed to his mouth with putty, Antoine Lavoisier first measured basal metabolic rate. Drawing by Madame Lavoisier (seated at right).

Around 1770, Antoine Lavoisier discovered the details of metabolism, demonstrating that the oxidation of food is the source of body heat. Called the most fundamental chemical discovery of the 18th century, Lavoisier discovered the principle of conservation of mass. His ideas made the phlogiston theory of combustion obsolete.

In 1790, George Fordyce recognized calcium as necessary for the survival of fowl. In the early 19th century, the elements carbon, nitrogen, hydrogen, and oxygen were recognized as the primary components of food, and methods to measure their proportions were developed.

In 1816, François Magendie discovered that dogs fed only carbohydrates (sugar), fat (olive oil), and water died evidently of starvation, but dogs also fed protein survived, identifying protein as an essential dietary component. William Prout in 1827 was the first person to divide foods into carbohydrates, fat, and protein. During the 19th century, Jean-Baptiste Dumas and Justus von Liebig quarrelled over their shared belief that animals get their protein directly from plants (animal and plant protein are the same and that humans do not create organic compounds). With a reputation as the leading organic chemist of his day but with no credentials in animal physiology, Liebig grew rich making food extracts like beef bouillon and infant formula that were later found to be of questionable nutritious value. In the 1860s, Claude Bernard discovered that body fat can be synthesized from carbohydrate and protein, showing that the energy in blood glucose can be stored as fat or as glycogen.

In the early 1880s, Kanehiro Takaki observed that Japanese sailors (whose diets consisted almost entirely of white rice) developed beriberi (or endemic neuritis, a disease causing heart problems and paralysis), but British sailors and Japanese naval officers did not. Adding various types of vegetables and meats to the diets of Japanese sailors prevented the disease, (not because of the increased protein as Takaki supposed but because it introduced a few parts per million of thiamine to the diet, later understood as a cure).

In 1896, Eugen Baumann observed iodine in thyroid glands. In 1897, Christiaan Eijkman worked with natives of Java, who also suffered from beriberi. Eijkman observed that chickens fed the native diet of white rice developed the symptoms of beriberi but remained healthy when fed unprocessed brown rice with the outer bran intact. Eijkman cured the natives by feeding them brown rice, discovering that food can cure disease. Over two decades later, nutritionists learned that the outer rice bran contains vitamin B1, also known as thiamine.

From 1900 to The Present

In the early 20th century, Carl von Voit and Max Rubner independently measured caloric energy expenditure in different species of animals, applying principles of physics in nutrition. In 1906, Edith G. Willcock and Frederick Hopkins showed that the amino acid tryptophan aids the well-being of mice but it did not assure their growth. In the middle of twelve years of attempts to isolate them, Hopkins said in a 1906 lecture that "unsuspected dietetic factors," other than calories, protein, and minerals, are needed to prevent deficiency diseases. In 1907, Stephen M. Babcock and Edwin B. Hart conducted the single-grain experiment, which took nearly four years to complete.

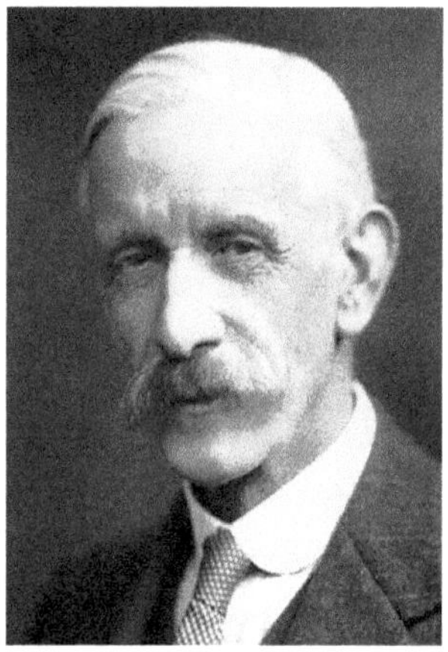

Frederick Hopkins discovered vitamins, for which he shared a Nobel prize with Eijkman.

Vitamin	Year Isolated
Thiamin	1926
Vitamin C	1926
Vitamin A	1939
Vitamin D	1931
Vitamin E	1936
Niacin	1937
Biotin	1939
Vitamin K	1939
Pantothenic acid	1939
Folate	1939
Riboflavin	1933
Vitamin B6	1936

Oxford University closed down its nutrition department after World War II because the subject seemed to have been completed between 1912 and 1944.

In 1912, Casimir Funk coined the term vitamin, a vital factor in the diet, from the words "vital" and "amine," because these unknown substances preventing scurvy, beriberi, and pellagra, were thought then to be derived from ammonia. The vitamins were studied in the first half of the 20th century.

In 1913, Elmer McCollum and Marguerite Davis discovered the first vitamin, fat-soluble vitamin A, then water-soluble vitamin B (in 1915; now known to be a complex of several water-soluble vitamins) and named vitamin C as the then-unknown substance preventing scurvy. Lafayette Mendel and Thomas Osborne also performed pioneering work on vitamins A and B. In 1919, Sir Edward Mellanby incorrectly identified rickets as a vitamin A deficiency because he could cure it in dogs with cod liver oil. In 1922, McCollum destroyed the vitamin A in cod liver oil, but found that it still cured rickets. Also in 1922, H.M. Evans and L.S. Bishop discover vitamin E as essential for rat pregnancy, originally calling it "food factor X" until 1925.

In 1925, Hart discovered that trace amounts of copper are necessary for iron absorption. In 1927, Adolf Otto Reinhold Windaus synthesized vitamin D, and was awarded the Nobel Prize in Chemistry in 1928. In 1928, Albert Szent-Györgyi isolated ascorbic acid, and in 1932 proved that it is vitamin C by preventing scurvy. In 1935, he synthesized it, and in 1937, he won a Nobel Prize for his efforts. Szent-Györgyi concurrently elucidated much of the citric acid cycle.

In the 1930s, William Cumming Rose identified essential amino acids, necessary protein components that the body cannot synthesize. In 1935, Underwood and Marston independently discovered the necessity of cobalt. In 1936, Eugene Floyd DuBois showed that work and school performance are related to caloric intake. In 1938, Erhard Fernholz discovered the chemical structure of vitamin E and then he tragically disappeared. It was synthesised the same year by Paul Karrer.

In 1940, rationing in the United Kingdom during and after World War II took place according to nutritional principles drawn up by Elsie Widdowson and others. In 1941, the first Recommended Dietary Allowances (RDAs) were established by the National Research Council.

In 1992, The U.S. Department of Agriculture introduced the Food Guide Pyramid. In 2002, a Natural Justice study showed a relation between nutrition and violent behavior. In 2005, one inconclusive study found that obesity could be caused by adenovirus in addition to bad nutrition.

World leaders are looking at alternatives like genetically modified foods to tackle the problem of world hunger and food shortages.

Nutrients

The list of nutrients that people are known to require is, in the words of Marion Nestle, "almost certainly incomplete". As of 2014, nutrients are thought to be of two types: macro-nutrients which are needed in relatively large amounts, and micronutrients which are needed in smaller quantities. A type of carbohydrate, dietary fiber, i.e. non-digestible material such as cellulose, is required, for both mechanical and biochemical reasons, although the exact reasons remain unclear. Other micronutrients include antioxidants and phytochemicals, which are said to influence (or protect) some body systems. Their necessity is not as well established as in the case of, for instance, vitamins.

Most foods contain a mix of some or all of the nutrient types, together with other substances, such as toxins of various sorts. Some nutrients can be stored internally (e.g., the fat-soluble vitamins), while others are required more or less continuously. Poor health can be caused by a lack of required nutrients or, in extreme cases, too much of a required nutrient. For example, both salt and water (both absolutely required) will cause illness or even death in excessive amounts.

Macronutrients

The macronutrients are carbohydrates, fiber, fats, protein, and water. The macronutrients (excluding fiber and water) provide structural material (amino acids from which proteins are built, and lipids from which cell membranes and some signaling molecules are built) and energy. Some of the structural material can be used to generate energy internally, and in either case it is measured in Joules or kilocalories (often called "Calories" and written with a capital *C* to distinguish them from little 'c' calories). Carbohydrates and proteins provide 17 kJ approximately (4 kcal) of energy per gram, while fats provide 37 kJ (9 kcal) per gram, though the net energy from either depends on such factors as absorption and digestive effort, which vary substantially from instance to instance. Vitamins, minerals, fiber, and water do not provide energy, but are required for other reasons.

Molecules of carbohydrates and fats consist of carbon, hydrogen, and oxygen atoms. Carbohydrates range from simple monosaccharides (glucose, fructose, galactose) to complex polysaccharides (starch). Fats are triglycerides, made of assorted fatty acid monomers bound to a glycerol backbone. Some fatty acids, but not all, are essential in the diet: they cannot be synthesized in the body. Protein molecules contain nitrogen atoms in addition to carbon, oxygen, and hydrogen. The fundamental components of protein are nitrogen-containing amino acids, some of which are essential in the sense that humans cannot make them internally. Some of the amino acids are convertible (with the expenditure of energy) to glucose and can be used for energy production, just as ordinary glucose, in a process known as gluconeogenesis. By breaking down existing protein, the carbon skeleton of the various amino acids can be metabolized to intermediates in cellular respiration; the remaining ammonia is discarded primarily as urea in urine. This occurs normally only during prolonged starvation.

Carbohydrates

Carbohydrates may be classified as monosaccharides, disaccharides, or polysaccharides depending on the number of monomer (sugar) units they contain. They constitute a large part of foods such as rice, noodles, bread, and other grain-based products. Monosaccharides, disaccharides, and polysaccharides contain one, two, and three or more sugar units, respectively. Polysaccharides are often referred to as *complex* carbohydrates because they are typically long, multiple branched chains of sugar units.

Traditionally, simple carbohydrates are believed to be absorbed quickly, and therefore to raise blood-glucose levels more rapidly than complex carbohydrates. This, however, is not accurate. Some simple carbohydrates (e.g., fructose) follow different metabolic pathways (e.g., fructolysis) that result in only a partial catabolism to glucose, while, in essence, many complex carbohydrates may be digested at the same rate as simple carbohydrates. Glucose stimulates the production of insulin through food entering the bloodstream, which is grasped by the beta cells in the pancreas.

Fiber

Dietary fiber is a carbohydrate that is incompletely absorbed in humans and in some animals. Like all carbohydrates, when it is metabolized it can produce four Calories (kilocalories) of energy per gram. However, in most circumstances it accounts for less than that because of its limited absorption and digestibility. Dietary fiber consists mainly of cellulose, a large carbohydrate polymer which is indigestible as humans do not have the required enzymes to disassemble it. There are two subcategories: soluble and insoluble fiber. Whole grains, fruits (especially plums, prunes, and figs), and vegetables are good sources of dietary fiber. There are many health benefits of a high-fiber diet. Dietary fiber helps reduce the chance of gastrointestinal problems such as constipation and diarrhea by increasing the weight and size of stool and softening it. Insoluble fiber, found in whole wheat flour, nuts and vegetables, especially stimulates peristalsis – the rhythmic muscular contractions of the intestines, which move digesta along the digestive tract. Soluble fiber, found in oats, peas, beans, and many fruits, dissolves in water in the intestinal tract to produce a gel that slows the movement of food through the intestines. This may help lower blood glucose levels because it can slow the absorption of sugar. Additionally, fiber, perhaps especially that from whole grains, is thought to possibly help lessen insulin spikes, and therefore reduce the risk of type 2 diabetes. The link between increased fiber consumption and a decreased risk of colorectal cancer is still uncertain.

Fat

A molecule of dietary fat typically consists of several fatty acids (containing long chains of carbon and hydrogen atoms), bonded to a glycerol. They are typically found as triglycerides (three fatty acids attached to one glycerol backbone). Fats may be classified as saturated or unsaturated depending on the detailed structure of the fatty acids involved. Saturated fats have all of the carbon atoms in their fatty acid chains bonded to hydrogen atoms, whereas unsaturated fats have some of these carbon atoms double-bonded, so their molecules have relatively fewer hydrogen atoms than a saturated fatty acid of the same length. Unsaturated fats may be further classified as monounsaturated (one double-bond) or polyunsaturated (many double-bonds). Furthermore, depending on the location of the double-bond in the fatty acid chain, unsaturated fatty acids are classified as omega-3 or omega-6 fatty acids. Trans fats are a type of unsaturated fat with *trans*-isomer bonds; these are rare in nature and in foods from natural sources; they are typically created in an industrial process called (partial) hydrogenation. There are nine kilocalories in each gram of fat. Fatty acids such as conjugated linoleic acid, catalpic acid, eleostearic acid and punicic acid, in addition to providing energy, represent potent immune modulatory molecules.

Saturated fats (typically from animal sources) have been a staple in many world cultures for millennia. Unsaturated fats (e. g., vegetable oil) are considered healthier, while trans fats are to be avoided. Saturated and some trans fats are typically solid at room temperature (such as butter or lard), while unsaturated fats are typically liquids (such as olive oil or flaxseed oil). Trans fats are very rare in nature, and have been shown to be highly detrimental to human health, but have properties useful in the food processing industry, such as rancidity resistance.

Essential Fatty Acids

Most fatty acids are non-essential, meaning the body can produce them as needed, generally from other fatty acids and always by expending energy to do so. However, in humans, at least two fatty acids are essential and must be included in the diet. An appropriate balance of essential fatty acids—omega-3 and omega-6 fatty acids—seems also important for health, although definitive experimental demonstration has been elusive. Both of these "omega" long-chain polyunsaturated fatty acids are substrates for a class of eicosanoids known as prostaglandins, which have roles throughout the human body. They are hormones, in some respects. The omega-3 eicosapentaenoic acid (EPA), which can be made in the human body from the omega-3 essential fatty acid alpha-linolenic acid (ALA), or taken in through marine food sources, serves as a building block for series 3 prostaglandins (e.g., weakly inflammatory PGE3). The omega-6 dihomo-gamma-linolenic acid (DGLA) serves as a building block for series 1 prostaglandins (e.g. anti-inflammatory PGE1), whereas arachidonic acid (AA) serves as a building block for series 2 prostaglandins (e.g. pro-inflammatory PGE 2). Both DGLA and AA can be made from the omega-6 linoleic acid (LA) in the human body, or can be taken in directly through food. An appropriately balanced intake of omega-3 and omega-6 partly determines the relative production of different prostaglandins, which is one reason why a balance between omega-3 and omega-6 is believed important for cardiovascular health. In industrialized societies, people typically consume large amounts of processed vegetable oils, which have reduced amounts of the essential fatty acids along with too much of omega-6 fatty acids relative to omega-3 fatty acids.

The conversion rate of omega-6 DGLA to AA largely determines the production of the prostaglandins PGE1 and PGE2. Omega-3 EPA prevents AA from being released from membranes, thereby skewing prostaglandin balance away from pro-inflammatory PGE2 (made from AA) toward anti-inflammatory PGE1 (made from DGLA). Moreover, the conversion (desaturation) of DGLA to AA is controlled by the enzyme delta-5-desaturase, which in turn is controlled by hormones such as insulin (up-regulation) and glucagon (down-regulation). The amount and type of carbohydrates consumed, along with some types of amino acid, can influence processes involving insulin, glucagon, and other hormones; therefore, the ratio of omega-3 versus omega-6 has wide effects on general health, and specific effects on immune function and inflammation, and mitosis (i.e., cell division).

Protein

Proteins are structural materials in much of the animal body (e.g. muscles, skin, and hair). They also form the enzymes that control chemical reactions throughout the body. Each protein molecule is composed of amino acids, which are characterized by inclusion of nitrogen and sometimes sulphur (these components are responsible for the distinctive smell of burning protein, such as the keratin in hair). The body requires amino acids to produce new proteins (protein retention) and to replace damaged proteins (maintenance). As there is no protein or amino acid storage provision, amino acids must be present in the diet. Excess amino acids are discarded, typically in the urine. For all animals, some amino acids are *essential* (an animal cannot produce them internally) and some are *non-essential* (the animal can produce them from other nitrogen-containing compounds). About twenty amino acids are found in the human body, and about ten of these are essential and, therefore, must be included in the diet. A diet that contains adequate amounts of amino acids (especially those that are essential) is particularly important in some situations: during early development and maturation, pregnancy, lactation, or injury (a burn, for instance). A *complete* protein source contains all the essential amino acids; an *incomplete* protein source lacks one or more of the essential amino acids.

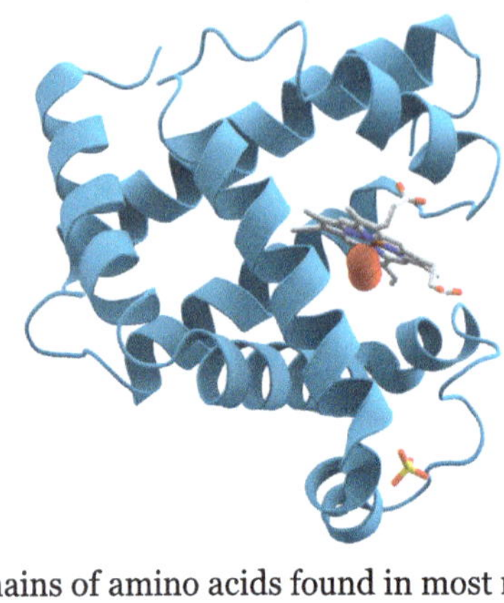

Proteins are chains of amino acids found in most nutritional foods.

It is possible with protein combinations of two incomplete protein sources (e.g., rice and beans) to make a complete protein source, and characteristic combinations are the basis of distinct cultural cooking traditions. However, complementary sources of protein do not need to be eaten at the same meal to be used together by the body. Excess amino acids from protein can be converted into glucose and used for fuel through a process called gluconeogenesis. The amino acids remaining after such conversion are discarded.

Water

Water is excreted from the body in multiple forms; including urine and feces, sweating, and by water vapour in the exhaled breath. Therefore, it is necessary to adequately rehydrate to replace lost fluids.

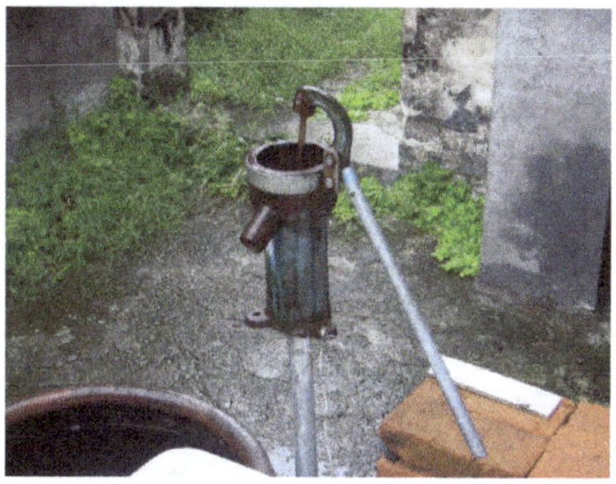

A manual water pump in China

Early recommendations for the quantity of water required for maintenance of good health suggested that 6–8 glasses of water daily is the minimum to maintain proper hydration. However the notion that a person should consume eight glasses of water per day cannot be traced to a credible scientific source. The original water intake recommendation in 1945 by the Food and Nutrition Board of the National Research Council read: "An ordinary standard for diverse persons is 1 milliliter for each calorie of food. Most of this quantity is contained in prepared foods." More recent comparisons of well-known recommendations on fluid intake have revealed large discrepancies in the volumes of water we need to consume for good health. Therefore, to help standardize guidelines, recommendations for water consumption are included in two recent European Food Safety Authority (EFSA) documents (2010): (i) Food-based dietary guidelines and (ii) Dietary reference values for water or adequate daily intakes (ADI). These specifications were provided by calculating adequate intakes from measured intakes in populations of individuals with "desirable osmolarity values of urine and desirable water volumes per energy unit consumed." For healthful hydration, the current EFSA guidelines recommend total water intakes of 2.0 L/day for adult females and 2.5 L/day for adult males. These reference values include water from drinking water, other beverages, and from food. About 80% of our daily water requirement comes from the beverages we drink, with the remaining 20% coming from food. Water content varies depending on the type of food consumed, with fruit and vegetables containing more than cereals, for example. These values are estimated using country-specific food balance sheets published by the Food and Agriculture Organisation of the United Nations. Other guidelines for nutrition also have implications for the beverages we consume for healthy hydration- for example, the World Health Organization (WHO) recommend that added sugars should represent no more than 10% of total energy intake.

The EFSA panel also determined intakes for different populations. Recommended intake volumes in the elderly are the same as for adults as despite lower energy consumption, the water requirement of this group is increased due to a reduction in renal concentrating capacity. Pregnant and breastfeeding women require additional fluids to stay hydrated. The EFSA panel proposes that pregnant women should consume the same volume of water as non-pregnant women, plus an increase in proportion to the higher energy requirement, equal to 300 mL/day. To compensate for additional fluid output, breastfeeding women require an additional 700 mL/day above the recommended intake values for non-lactating women.

For those who have healthy kidneys, it is somewhat difficult to drink too much water, but (especially in warm humid weather and while exercising) it is dangerous to drink too little. While overhydration is much less common than dehydration, it is also possible to drink far more water than necessary, which can result in water intoxication, a serious and potentially fatal condition. In particular, large amounts of de-ionized water are dangerous.

Micronutrients

The micronutrients are minerals, vitamins, and others.

Minerals

Dietary minerals are inorganic chemical elements required by living organisms, other than the four elements carbon, hydrogen, nitrogen, and oxygen that are present in nearly all organic molecules. The term "mineral" is archaic, since the intent is to describe simply the less common elements in the diet. Some are heavier than the four just mentioned, including several metals, which often occur as ions in the body. Some dietitians recommend that these be supplied from foods in which they occur naturally, or at least as complex compounds, or sometimes even from natural inorganic sources (such as calcium carbonate from ground oyster shells). Some minerals are absorbed much more readily in the ionic forms found in such sources. On the other hand, minerals are often artificially added to the diet as supplements; the most famous is likely iodine in iodized salt which prevents goiter.

Macrominerals

Many elements are essential in relative quantity; they are usually called "bulk minerals". Some are structural, but many play a role as electrolytes. Elements with recommended dietary allowance (RDA) greater than 150 mg/day are, in alphabetical order (with informal or folk-medicine perspectives in parentheses):

- Calcium, a common electrolyte, but also needed structurally (for muscle and digestive system health, bone strength, some forms neutralize acidity, may help clear toxins, provides signaling ions for nerve and membrane functions)
- Chlorine as chloride ions; very common electrolyte; see sodium, below
- Magnesium, required for processing ATP and related reactions (builds bone, causes strong peristalsis, increases flexibility, increases alkalinity)
- Phosphorus, required component of bones; essential for energy processing
- Potassium, a very common electrolyte (heart and nerve health)

- Sodium, a very common electrolyte; in general not found in dietary supplements, despite being needed in large quantities, because the ion is very common in food: typically as sodium chloride, or common salt. Excessive sodium consumption can deplete calcium and magnesium, leading to high blood pressure and osteoporosis.
- Sulfur, for three essential amino acids and therefore many proteins (skin, hair, nails, liver, and pancreas). Sulfur is not consumed alone, but in the form of sulfur-containing amino acids

Trace Minerals

Many elements are required in trace amounts, usually because they play a catalytic role in enzymes. Some trace mineral elements (RDA < 200 mg/day) are, in alphabetical order:

- Cobalt required for biosynthesis of vitamin B12 family of coenzymes. Animals cannot biosynthesize B12, and must obtain this cobalt-containing vitamin in their diet.
- Copper required component of many redox enzymes, including cytochrome c oxidase
- Chromium required for sugar metabolism
- Iodine required not only for the biosynthesis of thyroxine but also — it is presumed — for other important organs as breast, stomach, salivary glands, thymus, etc. For this reason iodine is needed in larger quantities than others in this list, and sometimes classified with the macrominerals
- Iron required for many enzymes, and for hemoglobin and some other proteins
- Manganese (processing of oxygen)
- Molybdenum required for xanthine oxidase and related oxidases
- Selenium required for peroxidase (antioxidant proteins)
- Zinc required for several enzymes such as carboxypeptidase, liver alcohol dehydrogenase, and carbonic anhydrase

Vitamins

As with the minerals discussed above, some vitamins are recognized as organic essential nutrients, necessary in the diet for good health. (Vitamin D is the exception: it can be synthesized in the skin, in the presence of UVB radiation.) Certain vitamin-like compounds that are recommended in the diet, such as carnitine, are thought useful for survival and health, but these are not "essential" dietary nutrients because the human body has some capacity to produce them from other compounds. Moreover, thousands of different phytochemicals have recently been discovered in food (particularly in fresh vegetables), which may have desirable properties including antioxidant activity however, experimental demonstration has been suggestive but inconclusive. Other essential nutrients that are not classified as vitamins include essential amino acids, choline, essential fatty acids and the minerals discussed in the preceding section.

Vitamin deficiencies may result in disease conditions, including goitre, scurvy, osteoporosis, impaired immune system, disorders of cell metabolism, certain forms of cancer, symptoms of premature aging, and poor psychological health (including eating disorders), among many others. Excess levels of some vitamins are also dangerous to health (notably vitamin A). Deficient or excess levels of minerals can also have serious health consequences.

Healthy Diets

Whole Plant Food Diet

Heart disease, cancer, obesity, and diabetes are commonly called "Western" diseases because these maladies were once rarely seen in developing countries. An international study in China found some regions had virtually no cancer or heart disease, while in other areas they reflected "up to a 100-fold increase" coincident with shifts from diets that were found to be entirely plant-based to heavily animal-based, respectively. In contrast, diseases of affluence like cancer and heart disease are common throughout the developed world, including the United States. Adjusted for age and exercise, large regional clusters of people in China rarely suffered from these "Western" diseases possibly because their diets are rich in vegetables, fruits, and whole grains, and have little dairy and meat products. Some studies show these to be, in high quantities, possible causes of some cancers. There are arguments for and against this controversial issue.

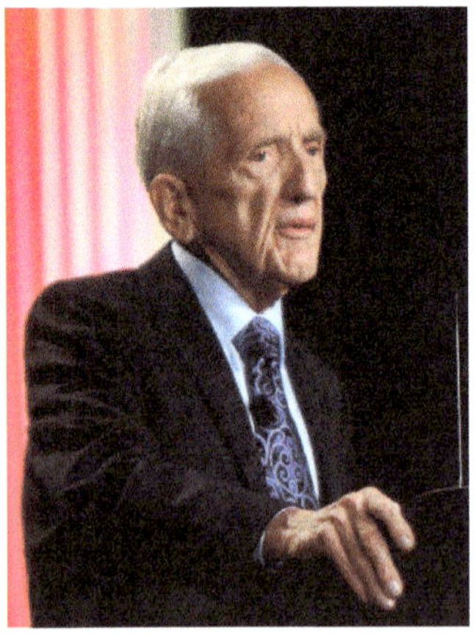

T. Colin Campbell is among the scientists who advocate a plant-based diet

The United Healthcare/Pacificare nutrition guideline recommends a whole plant food diet, and recommends using protein only as a condiment with meals. A *National Geographic* cover article from November 2005, entitled *The Secrets of Living Longer*, also recommends a whole plant food diet. The article is a lifestyle survey of three populations, Sardinians, Okinawans, and Adventists, who generally display longevity and "suffer a fraction of the diseases that commonly kill people in other parts of the developed world, and enjoy more healthy years of life." In common with all three groups is to "Eat fruits, vegetables, and whole grains."

The *National Geographic* article noted that an NIH funded study of 34,000 Seventh-day Adventists between 1976 and 1988 "...found that the Adventists' habit of consuming beans, soy milk, tomatoes, and other fruits lowered their risk of developing certain cancers. It also suggested that eating whole grain bread, drinking five glasses of water a day, and, most surprisingly, consuming four servings of nuts a week reduced their risk of heart disease."

The French "Paradox"

The French paradox is the observation that the French suffer a relatively low incidence of coronary heart disease, despite having a diet relatively rich in saturated fats. A number of explanations have been suggested:

- Saturated fat consumption does not cause heart disease.
- Reduced consumption of processed carbohydrate and other junk foods.
- Regular consumption of red wine.
- Higher consumption of artificially produced trans-fats by Americans, which has been shown to have greater lipoprotein effects per gram than saturated fat.

However, statistics collected by the World Health Organization from 1990–2000 show that the incidence of heart disease in France may have been underestimated and, in fact, may be similar to that of neighboring countries.

Phytochemicals

Phytochemicals such as polyphenols are compounds produced naturally in plants (phyto means "plant" in Greek). In general, the term is used to refer to those chemicals under research to assess whether they have biological significance. To date, there is no evidence in humans that polyphenols or other non-nutrient compounds from plants have health effects. Further, dietary supplements containing phytochemicals also have no proven health benefit.

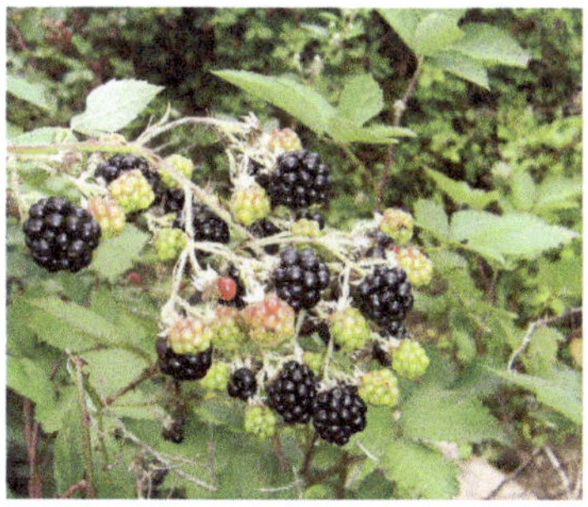

Blackberries are a source of polyphenols

While initial studies sought to reveal if antioxidant or phytochemical supplements might promote health, later large clinical trials did not detect any benefit and showed instead that excess supplementation could be harmful.

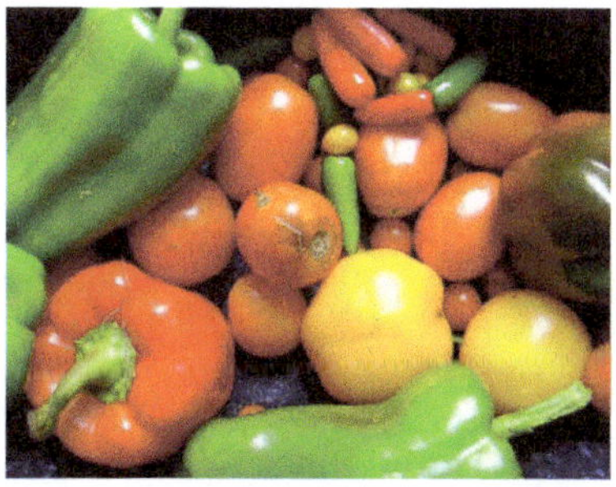

Colorful fruits and vegetables can be components of a healthy diet.

Intestinal Bacterial Flora

Animal intestines contain a large population of gut flora. In humans, the four dominant phyla are Firmicutes, Bacteroidetes, Actinobacteria, and Proteobacteria. They are essential to digestion and are also affected by food that is consumed. Bacteria in the gut perform many important functions for humans, including breaking down and aiding in the absorption of otherwise indigestible food; stimulating cell growth; repressing the growth of harmful bacteria, training the immune system to respond only to pathogens; producing vitamin B_{12}; and defending against some infectious diseases.

Animal Nutrition

Nutritional science investigates the metabolic and physiological responses of the body to diet. With advances in the fields of molecular biology, biochemistry, nutritional immunology, molecular medicine and genetics, the study of nutrition is increasingly concerned with metabolism and metabolic pathways: the sequences of biochemical steps through which substances in living things change from one form to another.

Carnivore and herbivore diets are contrasting, with basic nitrogen and carbon proportions vary for their particular foods. "The nitrogen content of plant tissues averages about 2%, while in fungi, animals, and bacteria it averages about 5% to 10%." Many herbivores rely on bacterial fermentation to create digestible nutrients from indigestible plant cellulose, while obligate carnivores must eat animal meats to obtain certain vitamins or nutrients their bodies cannot otherwise synthesize. All animals' diets must provide sufficient amounts of the basic building blocks they need, up to the point where their particular biology can synthesize the rest. Animal tissue contains chemical compounds, such as water, carbohydrates (sugar, starch, and fiber), amino acids (in proteins), fatty acids (in lipids), and nucleic acids (DNA and RNA). These compounds in turn consist of elements such as carbon, hydrogen, oxygen, nitrogen, phosphorus, calcium, iron, zinc, magnesium, manganese, and so on. All of these chemical compounds and elements occur in various forms and combinations (e.g. hormones, vitamins, phospholipids, hydroxyapatite).

Animal tissue consists of elements and compounds ingested, digested, absorbed, and circulated through the bloodstream to feed the cells of the body. Except in the unborn fetus, the digestive system is the first system involved. Digestive juices break chemical bonds in ingested molecules, and modify their conformations and energy states. Though some molecules are absorbed into the bloodstream unchanged, digestive processes release them from the matrix of foods. Unabsorbed matter, along with some waste products of metabolism, is eliminated from the body in the feces.

Studies of nutritional status must take into account the state of the body before and after experiments, as well as the chemical composition of the whole diet and of all material excreted and eliminated from the body (in urine and feces). Comparing the food to the waste can help determine the specific compounds and elements absorbed and metabolized in the body. The effects of nutrients may only be discernible over an extended period, during which all food and waste must be analyzed. The number of variables involved in such experiments is high, making nutritional studies time-consuming and expensive, which explains why the science of animal nutrition is still slowly evolving.

In particular, the consumption of whole-plant foods slows digestion and allows better absorption, and a more favorable balance of essential nutrients per Calorie, resulting in better management of cell growth, maintenance, and mitosis (cell division), as well as better regulation of appetite and blood sugar. Regularly scheduled meals (every few hours) have also proven more wholesome than infrequent or haphazard ones.

Plant Nutrition

Plant nutrition is the study of the chemical elements that are necessary for plant growth. There are several principles that apply to plant nutrition. Some elements are directly involved in plant metabolism. However, this principle does not account for the so-called beneficial elements, whose presence, while not required, has clear positive effects on plant growth.

A nutrient that is able to limit plant growth according to Liebig's law of the minimum is considered an essential plant nutrient if the plant cannot complete its full life cycle without it. There are 16 essential plant soil nutrients, besides the three major elemental nutrients carbon and oxygen that are obtained by photosynthetic plants from carbon dioxide in air, and hydrogen, which is obtained from water.

Plants uptake essential elements from the soil through their roots and from the air (consisting of mainly nitrogen and oxygen) through their leaves. Green plants obtain their carbohydrate supply from the carbon dioxide in the air by the process of photosynthesis. Carbon and oxygen are absorbed from the air, while other nutrients are absorbed from the soil. Nutrient uptake in the soil is achieved by cation exchange, wherein root hairs pump hydrogen ions (H^+) into the soil through proton pumps. These hydrogen ions displace cations attached to negatively charged soil particles so that the cations are available for uptake by the root. In the leaves, stomata open to take in carbon dioxide and expel oxygen. The carbon dioxide molecules are used as the carbon source in photosynthesis.

Although nitrogen is plentiful in the Earth's atmosphere, very few plants can use this directly. Most plants, therefore, require nitrogen compounds to be present in the soil in which they grow. This is made possible by the fact that largely inert atmospheric nitrogen is changed in a nitrogen fixation process to biologically usable forms in the soil by bacteria.

Plant nutrition is a difficult subject to understand completely, partially because of the variation between different plants and even between different species or individuals of a given clone. Elements present at low levels may cause deficiency symptoms, and toxicity is possible at levels that are too high. Furthermore, deficiency of one element may present as symptoms of toxicity from another element, and vice versa.

Environmental Nutrition

Research in the field of nutrition has greatly contributed in finding out the essential facts about how environmental depletion can lead to crucial nutrition-related health problems like contamination, spread of contagious diseases, malnutrition, etc. Moreover, environmental contamination due to discharge of agricultural as well as industrial chemicals like organocholrines, heavy metal, and radionucleotides may adversely affect the human and the ecosystem as a whole. As far as safety of the human health is concerned, then these environmental contaminants can reduce people's nutritional status and health. This could directly or indirectly cause drastic changes in their diet habits. Hence, food-based remedial as well as preventive strategies are essential to address global issues like hunger and malnutrition and to enable the susceptible people to adapt themselves to all these environmental as well as socio-economic alterations.

Advice and Guidance

U.S. Government Policies

In the US, dietitians are registered (RD) or licensed (LD) with the Commission for Dietetic Registration and the American Dietetic Association, and are only able to use the title "dietitian," as described by the business and professions codes of each respective state, when they have met specific educational and experiential prerequisites and passed a national registration or licensure examination, respectively. In California, registered dietitians must abide by the *"Business and Professions Code of Section 2585-2586.8"*.Anyone may call themselves a nutritionist, including unqualified dietitians, as this term is unregulated. Some states, such as the State of Florida, have begun to include the title "nutritionist" in state licensure requirements. Most governments provide guidance on nutrition, and some also impose mandatory disclosure/labeling requirements for processed food manufacturers and restaurants to assist consumers in complying with such guidance.

In the US, nutritional standards and recommendations are established jointly by the US Department of Agriculture and US Department of Health and Human Services. Dietary and physical activity guidelines from the USDA are presented in the concept of MyPlate, which superseded the food pyramid, which replaced the Four Food Groups. The Senate committee currently responsible for oversight of the USDA is the *Agriculture, Nutrition and Forestry Committee*. Committee hearings are often televised on C-SPAN.

The U.S. Department of Health and Human Services provides a sample week-long menu that fulfills the nutritional recommendations of the government. Canada's Food Guide is another governmental recommendation.

Government Programs

Federal and state governmental organizations have been working on nutrition literacy interventions in non-primary health care settings to address the nutrition information problem in the U.S. Some programs include:

The Family Nutrition Program (FNP) is a free nutrition education program serving low-income adults around the U.S. This program is funded by the Food Nutrition Service's (FNS) branch of the United States Department of Agriculture (USDA) usually through a local state academic institution that runs the program. The FNP has developed a series of tools to help families participating in the Food Stamp Program stretch their food dollar and form healthful eating habits including nutrition education.

Expanded Food and Nutrition Education Program (ENFEP) is a unique program that currently operates in all 50 states and in American Samoa, Guam, Micronesia, Northern Marianas, Puerto Rico, and the Virgin Islands. It is designed to assist limited-resource audiences in acquiring the knowledge, skills, attitudes, and changed behavior necessary for nutritionally sound diets, and to contribute to their personal development and the improvement of the total family diet and nutritional well-being.

An example of a state initiative to promote nutrition literacy is Smart Bodies, a public-private partnership between the state's largest university system and largest health insurer, Louisiana State Agricultural Center and Blue Cross and Blue Shield of Louisiana Foundation. Launched in 2005, this program promotes lifelong healthful eating patterns and physically active lifestyles for children and their families. It is an interactive educational program designed to help prevent childhood obesity through classroom activities that teach children healthful eating habits and physical exercise.

Education

Nutrition is taught in schools in many countries. In England and Wales, the Personal and Social Education and Food Technology curricula include nutrition, stressing the importance of a balanced diet and teaching how to read nutrition labels on packaging. In many schools, a Nutrition class will fall within the Family and Consumer Science or Health departments. In some American schools, students are required to take a certain number of FCS or Health related classes. Nutrition is offered at many schools, and, if it is not a class of its own, nutrition is included in other FCS or Health classes such as: Life Skills, Independent Living, Single Survival, Freshmen Connection, Health etc. In many Nutrition classes, students learn about the food groups, the food pyramid, Daily Recommended Allowances, calories, vitamins, minerals, malnutrition, physical activity, healthful food choices, portion sizes, and how to live a healthy life.

A 1985, US National Research Council report entitled *Nutrition Education in US Medical Schools* concluded that nutrition education in medical schools was inadequate. Only 20% of the schools surveyed taught nutrition as a separate, required course. A 2006 survey found that this number had risen to 30%.

Nutrition Literacy

At the time of this entry, we were not able to identify any specific nutrition literacy studies in the U.S. at a national level. However, the findings of the 2003 National Assessment of Adult Literacy (NAAL) provide a basis upon which to frame the nutrition literacy problem in the U.S. NAAL introduced the first ever measure of "the degree to which individuals have the capacity to obtain, process and understand basic health information and services needed to make appropriate health decisions" – an objective of Healthy People 2010 and of which nutrition literacy might be considered an important subset. On a scale of below basic, basic, intermediate and proficient, NAAL found 13 percent of adult Americans have proficient health literacy, 44% have intermediate literacy, 29 percent have basic literacy and 14 percent have below basic health literacy. The study found that health literacy increases with education and people living below the level of poverty have lower health literacy than those above it.

Another study examining the health and nutrition literacy status of residents of the lower Mississippi Delta found that 52 percent of participants had a high likelihood of limited literacy skills. While a precise comparison between the NAAL and Delta studies is difficult, primarily because of methodological differences, Zoellner et al. suggest that health literacy rates in the Mississippi

Delta region are different from the U.S. general population and that they help establish the scope of the problem of health literacy among adults in the Delta region. For example, only 12 percent of study participants identified the My Pyramid graphic two years after it had been launched by the USDA. The study also found significant relationships between nutrition literacy and income level and nutrition literacy and educational attainment further delineating priorities for the region.

These statistics point to the complexities surrounding the lack of health/nutrition literacy and reveal the degree to which they are embedded in the social structure and interconnected with other problems. Among these problems are the lack of information about food choices, a lack of understanding of nutritional information and its application to individual circumstances, limited or difficult access to healthful foods, and a range of cultural influences and socioeconomic constraints such as low levels of education and high levels of poverty that decrease opportunities for healthful eating and living.

The links between low health literacy and poor health outcomes has been widely documented and there is evidence that some interventions to improve health literacy have produced successful results in the primary care setting. More must be done to further our understanding of nutrition literacy specific interventions in non-primary care settings in order to achieve better health outcomes.

Malnutrition

Malnutrition refers to insufficient, excessive, or imbalanced consumption of nutrients by an organism. In developed countries, the diseases of malnutrition are most often associated with nutritional imbalances or excessive consumption. In developing countries, malnutrition is more likely to be caused by poor access to a range of nutritious foods or inadequate knowledge. In Mali the International Crops Research Institute for the Semi-Arid Tropics (ICRISAT) and the Aga Khan Foundation, trained women's groups to make *equinut*, a healthy and nutritional version of the traditional recipe *di-dègué* (comprising peanut paste, honey and millet or rice flour). The aim was to boost nutrition and livelihoods by producing a product that women could make and sell, and which would be accepted by the local community because of its local heritage.

Although there are more organisms in the world who are malnourished due to insufficient consumption, increasingly more organisms suffer from excessive over-nutrition; a problem caused by an over abundance of sustenance coupled with the instinctual desire (by animals in particular) to consume all that it can.

Nutritionism is the view that excessive reliance on food science and the study of nutrition can lead to poor nutrition and to ill health. It was originally credited to Gyorgy Scrinis, and was popularized by Michael Pollan. Since nutrients are invisible, policy makers rely on nutrition experts to advise on food choices. Because science has an incomplete understanding of how food affects the human body, Pollan argues, nutritionism can be blamed for many of the health problems relating to diet in the Western World today.

Insufficient

In general, *under-consumption* refers to the long-term consumption of insufficient sustenance in relation to the energy that an organism expends or expels, leading to poor health.

Excessive

In general, *over-consumption* refers to the long-term consumption of excess sustenance in relation to the energy that an organism expends or expels, leading to poor health and, in animals, obesity. It can cause excessive hair loss, brittle nails, and irregular premenstrual cycles for females.

Unbalanced

When too much of one or more nutrients is present in the diet to the exclusion of the proper amount of other nutrients, the diet is said to be unbalanced.

Illnesses Caused by Improper Nutrient Consumption

Nutrients	Deficiency	Excess
Macronutrients		
Calories	Starvation, marasmus	Obesity, diabetes mellitus, cardiovascular disease
Simple carbohydrates	Low energy levels.	Obesity, diabetes mellitus, cardiovascular disease
Complex carbohydrates	Micronutrient deficiency	Obesity, cardiovascular disease (high glycemic index foods)
Protein	Kwashiorkor	Rabbit starvation, ketoacidosis (in diabetics)
Saturated fat	Low testosterone levels, vitamin deficiencies.	Obesity, cardiovascular disease
Trans fat	None	Obesity, cardiovascular disease
Unsaturated fat	Fat-soluble vitamin deficiency	Obesity, cardiovascular disease
Micronutrients		
Vitamin A	Xerophthalmia and night blindness	Hypervitaminosis A (cirrhosis, hair loss)
Vitamin B_1	Beri-Beri	?
Vitamin B_2	Skin and corneal lesions	?
Niacin	Pellagra	Dyspepsia, cardiac arrhythmias, birth defects
Vitamin B_{12}	Pernicious anemia	?
Vitamin C	Scurvy	Diarrhea causing dehydration
Vitamin D	Rickets	Hypervitaminosis D (dehydration, vomiting, constipation)
Vitamin E	Neurological disease	Hypervitaminosis E (anticoagulant: excessive bleeding)
Vitamin K	Hemorrhage	Liver damage
Omega-3 fats	Cardiovascular Disease	Bleeding, Hemorrhages, Hemorrhagic stroke, reduced glycemic control among diabetics
Omega-6 fats	None	Cardiovascular Disease, Cancer
Cholesterol	None	Cardiovascular Disease
Macrominerals		
Calcium	Osteoporosis, tetany, carpopedal spasm, laryngospasm, cardiac arrhythmias	Fatigue, depression, confusion, nausea, vomiting, constipation, pancreatitis, increased urination, kidney stones

Magnesium	Hypertension	Weakness, nausea, vomiting, impaired breathing, and hypotension
Potassium	Hypokalemia, cardiac arrhythmias	Hyperkalemia, palpitations
Sodium	Hyponatremia	Hypernatremia, hypertension
Trace minerals		
Iron	Anemia	Cirrhosis, Hereditary hemochromatosis, heart disease
Iodine	Goiter, hypothyroidism	Iodine toxicity (goiter, hypothyroidism)

Mental Agility

Research indicates that improving the awareness of nutritious meal choices and establishing long-term habits of healthy eating have a positive effect on cognitive and spatial memory capacity, with potential to increase a student's ability to process and retain academic information.

Some organizations have begun working with teachers, policymakers, and managed foodservice contractors to mandate improved nutritional content and increased nutritional resources in school cafeterias from primary to university level institutions. Health and nutrition have been proven to have close links with overall educational success. Currently, less than 10% of American college students report that they eat the recommended five servings of fruit and vegetables daily. Better nutrition has been shown to affect both cognitive and spatial memory performance; a study showed those with higher blood sugar levels performed better on certain memory tests. In another study, those who consumed yogurt performed better on thinking tasks when compared to those that consumed caffeine-free diet soda or confections. Nutritional deficiencies have been shown to have a negative effect on learning behavior in mice as far back as 1951.

"Better learning performance is associated with diet-induced effects on learning and memory ability".

The "nutrition-learning nexus" demonstrates the correlation between diet and learning and has application in a higher education setting.

"We find that better-nourished children perform significantly better in school, partly because they enter school earlier and thus have more time to learn but mostly because of greater learning productivity per year of schooling."

91% of college students feel that they are in good health, whereas only 7% eat their recommended daily allowance of fruits and vegetables.

Nutritional education is an effective and workable model in a higher education setting.

More "engaged" learning models that encompass nutrition is an idea that is picking up steam at all levels of the learning cycle.

There is limited research available that directly links a student's Grade Point Average (G.P.A.) to their overall nutritional health. Additional substantive data is needed to prove that overall intellectual health is closely linked to a person's diet, rather than just another correlation fallacy.

Mental Disorders

Nutritional supplement treatment may be appropriate for major depression, bipolar disorder, schizophrenia, and obsessive compulsive disorder, the four most common mental disorders in developed countries. Supplements that have been studied most for mood elevation and stabilization include eicosapentaenoic acid and docosahexaenoic acid (each of which an omega-3 fatty acid contained in fish oil but not in flaxseed oil), vitamin B12, folic acid, and inositol.

Cancer

Cancer is now common in developing countries. According to a study by the International Agency for Research on Cancer, "In the developing world, cancers of the liver, stomach and esophagus were more common, often linked to consumption of carcinogenic preserved foods, such as smoked or salted food, and parasitic infections that attack organs." Lung cancer rates are rising rapidly in poorer nations because of increased use of tobacco. Developed countries "tended to have cancers linked to affluence or a 'Western lifestyle' — cancers of the colon, rectum, breast and prostate — that can be caused by obesity, lack of exercise, diet and age."

Metabolic Syndrome

Several lines of evidence indicate lifestyle-induced hyperinsulinemia and reduced insulin function (i.e., insulin resistance) as a decisive factor in many disease states. For example, hyperinsulinemia and insulin resistance are strongly linked to chronic inflammation, which in turn is strongly linked to a variety of adverse developments such as arterial microinjuries and clot formation (i.e., heart disease) and exaggerated cell division (i.e., cancer). Hyperinsulinemia and insulin resistance (the so-called metabolic syndrome) are characterized by a combination of abdominal obesity, elevated blood sugar, elevated blood pressure, elevated blood triglycerides, and reduced HDL cholesterol. The negative effect of hyperinsulinemia on prostaglandin PGE1/PGE2 balance may be significant.

The state of obesity clearly contributes to insulin resistance, which in turn can cause type 2 diabetes. Virtually all obese and most type 2 diabetic individuals have marked insulin resistance. Although the association between overweight and insulin resistance is clear, the exact (likely multifarious) causes of insulin resistance remain less clear. It is important to note that it has been demonstrated that appropriate exercise, more regular food intake, and reducing glycemic load all can reverse insulin resistance in overweight individuals (and thereby lower blood sugar levels in those with type 2 diabetes).

Obesity can unfavourably alter hormonal and metabolic status via resistance to the hormone leptin, and a vicious cycle may occur in which insulin/leptin resistance and obesity aggravate one another. The vicious cycle is putatively fuelled by continuously high insulin/leptin stimulation and fat storage, as a result of high intake of strongly insulin/leptin stimulating foods and energy. Both insulin and leptin normally function as satiety signals to the hypothalamus in the brain; however, insulin/leptin resistance may reduce this signal and therefore allow continued overfeeding despite large body fat stores. In addition, reduced leptin signalling to the brain may reduce leptin's normal effect to maintain an appropriately high metabolic rate.

There is a debate about how and to what extent different dietary factors— such as intake of processed carbohydrates, total protein, fat, and carbohydrate intake, intake of saturated and trans fatty acids, and low intake of vitamins/minerals—contribute to the development of insulin and leptin resistance. In any case, analogous to the way modern man-made pollution may possess the potential to overwhelm the environment's ability to maintain homeostasis, the recent explosive introduction of high glycemic index and processed foods into the human diet may possess the potential to overwhelm the body's ability to maintain homeostasis and health (as evidenced by the metabolic syndrome epidemic).

Hyponatremia

Excess water intake, without replenishment of sodium and potassium salts, leads to hyponatremia, which can further lead to water intoxication at more dangerous levels. A well-publicized case occurred in 2007, when Jennifer Strange died while participating in a water-drinking contest. More usually, the condition occurs in long-distance endurance events (such as marathon or triathlon competition and training) and causes gradual mental dulling, headache, drowsiness, weakness, and confusion; extreme cases may result in coma, convulsions, and death. The primary damage comes from swelling of the brain, caused by increased osmosis as blood salinity decreases. Effective fluid replacement techniques include water aid stations during running/cycling races, trainers providing water during team games, such as soccer, and devices such as Camel Baks, which can provide water for a person without making it too hard to drink the water.

Antinutrient

Antinutrients are natural or synthetic compounds that interfere with the absorption of nutrients. Nutrition studies focus on antinutrients commonly found in food sources and beverages.

Sugar Consumption in The United States

The relatively recent increased consumption of sugar has been linked to the rise of some afflictions such as diabetes, obesity, and more recently heart disease. Increased consumption of sugar has been tied to these three, among others. Obesity levels have more than doubled in the last 30 years among adults, going from 15% to 35% in the United States. Obesity and diet also happen to be high risk factors for diabetes. In the same time span that obesity doubled, diabetes numbers quadrupled in America. Increased weight, especially in the form of belly fat, and high sugar intake are also high risk factors for heart disease. Both sugar intake and fatty tissue increase the probability of elevated LDL cholesterol in the bloodstream. Elevated amounts of Low-density lipoprotein (LDL) cholesterol, is the primary factor in heart disease. In order to avoid all the dangers of sugar, moderate consumption is paramount.

Processed Foods

Since the Industrial Revolution some two hundred years ago, the food processing industry has invented many technologies that both help keep foods fresh longer and alter the fresh state of food as they appear in nature. Cooling is the primary technology used to maintain freshness, whereas many more technologies have been invented to allow foods to last longer without becoming spoiled. These latter technologies include pasteurisation, autoclavation, drying, salting, and separation of various components, all of which appearing to alter the original nutritional contents of food. Pasteurisation and autoclavation (heating techniques) have no doubt improved the safety of many common foods, preventing epidemics of bacterial infection. But some of the (new) food processing technologies have downfalls as well.

Modern separation techniques such as milling, centrifugation, and pressing have enabled concentration of particular components of food, yielding flour, oils, juices, and so on, and even separate fatty acids, amino acids, vitamins, and minerals. Inevitably, such large-scale concentration changes the nutritional content of food, saving certain nutrients while removing others. Heating techniques may also reduce food's content of many heat-labile nutrients such as certain vitamins and phytochemicals, and possibly other yet-to-be-discovered substances. Because of reduced nutritional value, processed foods are often 'enriched' or 'fortified' with some of the most critical nutrients (usually certain vitamins) that were lost during processing. Nonetheless, processed foods tend to have an inferior nutritional profile compared to whole, fresh foods, regarding content of both sugar and high GI starches, potassium/sodium, vitamins, fiber, and of intact, unoxidized (essential) fatty acids. In addition, processed foods often contain potentially harmful substances such as oxidized fats and trans fatty acids.

A dramatic example of the effect of food processing on a population's health is the history of epidemics of beri-beri in people subsisting on polished rice. Removing the outer layer of rice by polishing it removes with it the essential vitamin thiamine, causing beri-beri. Another example is the development of scurvy among infants in the late 19th century in the United States. It turned out that the vast majority of sufferers were being fed milk that had been heat-treated (as suggested by Pasteur) to control bacterial disease. Pasteurisation was effective against bacteria, but it destroyed the vitamin C.

As mentioned, lifestyle- and obesity-related diseases are becoming increasingly prevalent all around the world. There is little doubt that the increasingly widespread application of some modern food processing technologies has contributed to this development. The food processing industry is a major part of modern economy, and as such it is influential in political decisions (e.g., nutritional recommendations, agricultural subsidising). In any known profit-driven economy, health considerations are hardly a priority; effective production of cheap foods with a long shelf-life is more the trend. In general, whole, fresh foods have a relatively short shelf-life and are less profitable to produce and sell than are more processed foods. Thus, the consumer is left with the choice between more expensive, but nutritionally superior, whole, fresh foods, and cheap, usually nutritionally inferior, processed foods. Because processed foods are often cheaper, more convenient (in both purchasing, storage, and preparation), and more available, the consumption of nutritionally inferior foods has been increasing throughout the world along with many nutrition-related health complications.

Balanced Eating:

- Food Balance Wheel

Biology:

- Bioenergetics

- Digestion
- Enzyme

Dangers of Poor Nutrition

- Deficiency
    - Avitaminosis is a deficiency of vitamins.
    - Boron deficiency (medicine)
    - Chromium deficiency
    - Iron deficiency (medicine)
    - Iodine deficiency
    - Magnesium deficiency (medicine)
- Diabetes
- Eating disorders
- Illnesses related to poor nutrition
- Malnutrition
- Obesity
    - Childhood obesity
- Starvation

Food:

Food (portal)

- 5 A Day
- Canada's Food Guide
- Fast food
- Food group
- Food guide pyramid
- Food supplement
- Fruits
- Functional food
- Grains
- Junk food

- Meat
- Vegetables

Healthy Diet:

- Dieting
- Eating
- Healthy eating pyramid
- Nutritional rating systems

Nutrients:

- Carbohydrates
- Dietary minerals
    - Essential minerals
- Dietary supplements
- Evolution of dietary antioxidants
- Essential nutrients
- Fat
    - Essential fatty acids
- Macronutrients
- Micronutrients
- Nootropics
- Nutraceuticals
- Food fortification
- Phytochemicals
- Protein
    - Complete protein
    - Essential amino acids
    - Incomplete protein
    - Protein combining
    - Protein (nutrient)
- Table of food nutrients

- Vitamins
    - Megavitamin therapy
    - Vitamin C megadosage

Profession:

- Dietitian
- Nutritionist
- Food Studies

Tools:

- Nutrition scale

Organizations:

- Academy of Nutrition and Dietetics
- American Society for Nutrition
- British Dietetic Association
- Society for Nutrition Education

Related Topics

- Auxology
- Exercise
- Food preferences in older adults and seniors
- General Fitness Training
- Health (portal)
- Life extension
- Orthomolecular medicine
- Nutrition psychology
- Palatability
- Physical fitness

Diet (Nutrition)

In nutrition, diet is the sum of food consumed by a person or other organism. The word diet often implies the use of specific intake of nutrition for health or weight-management reasons (with the two often being related). Although humans are omnivores, each culture and each person holds some food preferences or some food taboos. This may be due to personal tastes or ethical reasons. Individual dietary choices may be more or less healthy.

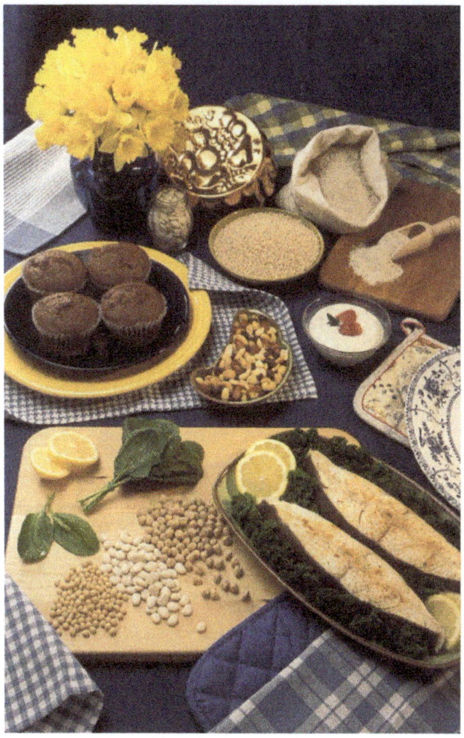

A selection of foods consumed by humans. However, the human diet can vary widely.

Complete nutrition requires ingestion and absorption of vitamins, minerals, and food energy in the form of carbohydrates, proteins, and fats. Dietary habits and choices play a significant role in the quality of life, health and longevity.

Religious and Cultural Dietary Choices

Some cultures and religions have restrictions concerning what foods are acceptable in their diet. For example, only Kosher foods are permitted by Judaism, and Halal foods by Islam. Although Buddhists are generally vegetarians, the practice varies and meat-eating may be permitted depending on the sects. In Hinduism, vegetarianism is the ideal. Jains are strictly vegetarian and consumption of roots is not permitted.

Dietary Choices

Many people choose to forgo food from animal sources to varying degrees (e.g. flexitarianism, vegetarianism, veganism, fruitarianism) for health reasons, issues surrounding morality, or to reduce their personal impact on the environment, although some of the public assumptions about which diets have lower impacts are known to be incorrect. Raw foodism is another contemporary trend. These diets may require tuning or supplementation such as vitamins to meet ordinary nutritional needs.

Weight Management

A particular diet may be chosen to seek weight loss or weight gain. Changing a subject's dietary intake, or "going on a diet", can change the energy balance and increase or decrease the amount of fat stored by the body. Some foods are specifically recommended, or even altered, for conformity to the requirements of a particular diet. These diets are often recommended in conjunction with exercise. Specific weight loss programs can be harmful to health, while others may be beneficial and can thus be coined as healthy diets. The terms "healthy diet" and "diet for weight management" are often related, as the two promote healthy weight management. Having a healthy diet is a way to prevent health problems, and will provide the body with the right balance of vitamins, minerals, and other nutrients.

Eating Disorders

An eating disorder is a mental disorder that interferes with normal food consumption. It is defined by abnormal eating habits that may involve either insufficient or excessive diet.

Health

A healthy diet may improve or maintain optimal health. In developed countries, affluence enables unconstrained caloric intake and possibly inappropriate food choices.

Health agencies recommend that people maintain a normal weight by limiting consumption of energy-dense foods and sugary drinks, eat plant-based food, limit red and processed meat, and limit alcohol.

Diet Classification Table

Food Type	Carnivorous	Ketogenic	Omnivorous	Pescetarian	Vegetarian	Vegan	Raw vegan	Islamic	Hindu	Jewish	Paleolithic	Fruitarian
Fruits and berries	No	No	Yes	Yes	Yes	Yes	Yes	Yes	Yes	Yes	Yes	Yes
Greens	No	No	Yes	Yes	Yes	Yes	Yes	Yes	Yes	Yes	Yes	Yes
Vegetables	No	No	Yes	Yes	Yes	Yes	Yes	Yes	Yes	Yes	Yes	No
Legumes	No	No	Yes	Yes	Yes	Yes	Yes	Yes	Yes	Yes	No	No
Tubers	No	No	Yes	Yes	Yes	Yes	No	Yes	Yes	Yes	Yes	No
Grains	No	No	Yes	Yes	Yes	Yes	No	Yes	Yes	Yes	No	Yes
Poultry	Yes	Yes	Yes	No	No	No	No	Yes	Maybe	Yes	Yes	No
Fish (scaled)	Yes	Yes	Yes	Yes	No	No	No	Yes	Maybe	Yes	Yes	No
Seafood (non-fish)	Yes	Yes	Yes	Yes	No	No	No	Yes	Maybe	No	Yes	No
Beef	Yes	Yes	Yes	No	No	No	No	Yes	No	Yes	Yes	No
Pork	Yes	Yes	Yes	No	No	No	No	No	No	No	Yes	No
Eggs	Yes	Yes	Yes	Yes	Maybe	No	No	Maybe	Yes	Yes	Yes	No
Dairy	No	Maybe	Yes	Yes	Maybe	No	No	Yes	Yes	Yes	No	No
Nuts	No	Maybe	Yes	Yes	Yes	Yes	Yes	Yes	Yes	Yes	Yes	Yes
Alcohol	No	Maybe	Yes	Yes	Yes	Yes	No	No	Yes	Yes	No	No

Food Science

Food science is the applied science devoted to the study of food. The Institute of Food Technologists defines food science as "the discipline in which the engineering, biological, and physical sciences are used to study the nature of foods, the causes of deterioration, the principles underlying food processing, and the improvement of foods for the consuming public". The textbook *Food Science* defines food science in simpler terms as "the application of basic sciences and engineering to study the physical, chemical, and biochemical nature of foods and the principles of food processing".

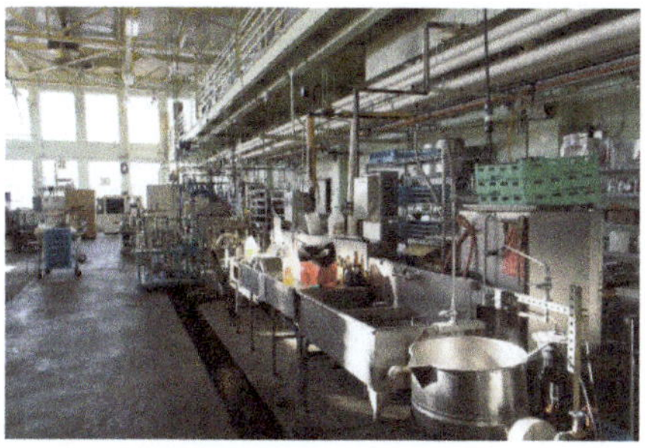

A food science laboratory

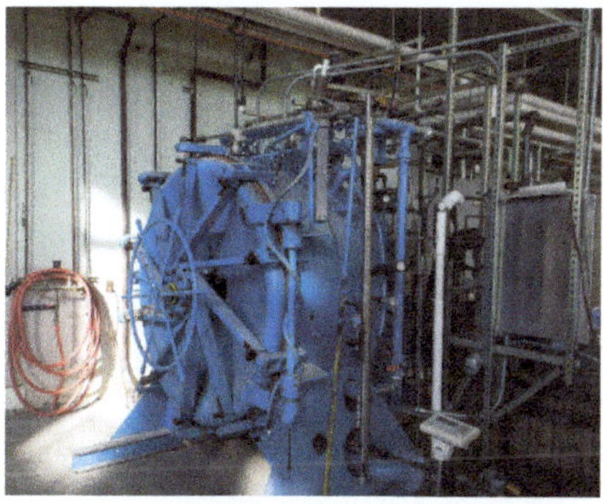

Machinery at a food science laboratory

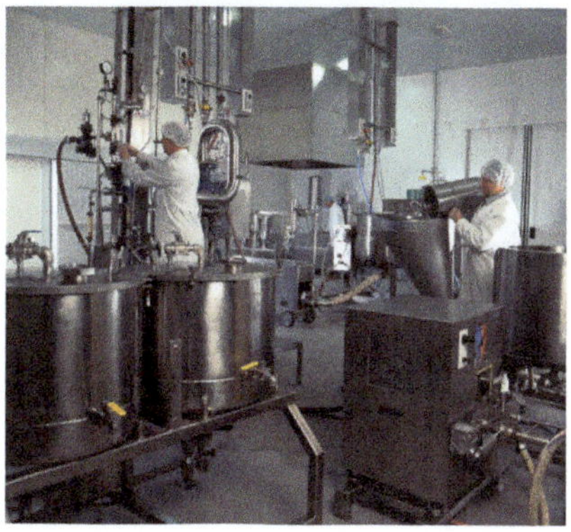

Food scientists working in Australia

Overview

Activities of food scientists include the development of new food products, design of processes to produce these foods, choice of packaging materials, shelf-life studies, sensory evaluation of products using panels or potential consumers, as well as microbiological and chemical testing. Food scientists may study more fundamental phenomena that are directly linked to the production of food products and its properties.

Food science brings together multiple scientific disciplines. It incorporates concepts from fields such as microbiology, chemical engineering, and biochemistry.

Disciplines

Some of the subdisciplines of food science are described below.

Food Chemistry

Food chemistry is the study of chemical processes and interactions of all biological and non-biological components of foods. The biological substances include such items as meat, poultry, lettuce, beer, and milk as examples. It is similar to biochemistry in its main components such as carbohydrates, lipids, and protein, but it also includes areas such as water, vitamins, minerals, enzymes, food additives, flavors, and colors. This discipline also encompasses how products change under certain food processing techniques and ways either to enhance or to prevent them from happening.

Food Physical Chemistry

Food physical chemistry is the study of both physical and chemical interactions in foods in terms of physical and chemical principles applied to food systems, as well as the application of physicochemical techniques and instrumentation for the study and analysis of foods.

Food Engineering

Food engineering is the industrial processes used to manufacture food.

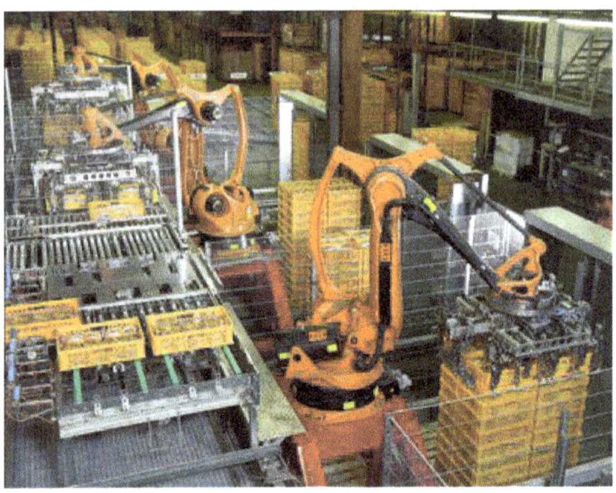

A bread factory in Germany, an example of food engineering

Food Microbiology

Food microbiology is the study of the microorganisms that inhabit, create, or contaminate food, including the study of microorganisms causing food spoilage. "Good" bacteria, however, such as probiotics, are becoming increasingly important in food science. In addition, microorganisms are essential for the production of foods such as cheese, yogurt, bread, beer, wine and, other fermented foods.

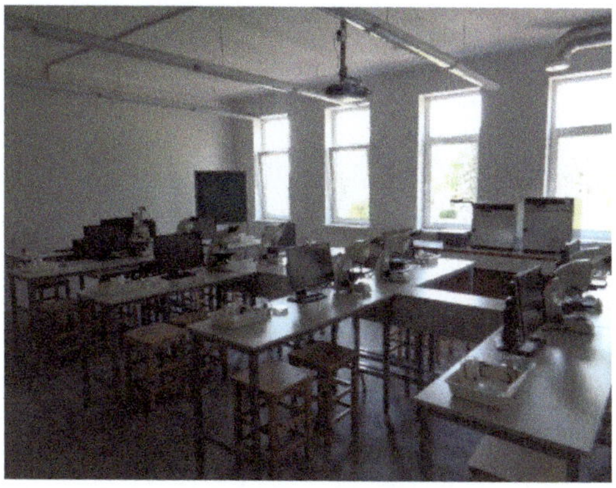

Food microbiology laboratory at the Faculty of Food Technology, Latvia University of Agriculture.

Food Packaging

Food packaging is packaging of food to preserve food after it has been processed and contain it through distribution. Its main objective is to provide physical and barrier protection for food. In most cases food packaging contains labels bearing nutritional and other information about the specific food. Food packaging is mostly done by using packaging machines.

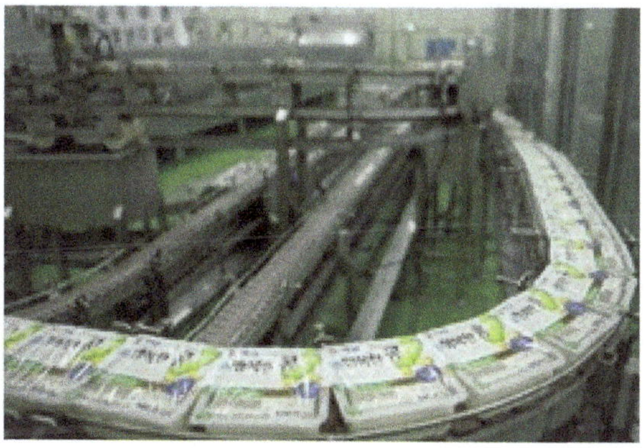

Food packaging in progress

Food Preservation

Food preservation involves the causes and prevention of quality degradation.

Food Substitution

Food substitution refers to the replacement of fat, sugar, or calories from a product while maintaining similar shape, texture, color, or taste.

Food Technology

Food technology is the technological aspects. Early scientific research into food technology concentrated on food preservation. Nicolas Appert's development in 1810 of the canning process was a decisive event. The process wasn't called canning then and Appert did not really know the principle on which his process worked, but canning has had a major impact on food preservation techniques.

Molecular Gastronomy

Molecular gastronomy is the scientific investigation of processes in cooking, social and artistic gastronomical phenomena.

New Product Development

New product development includes the invention of new food products.

Quality Control

Quality control involves the causes, prevention and communication dealing with food-borne illness.

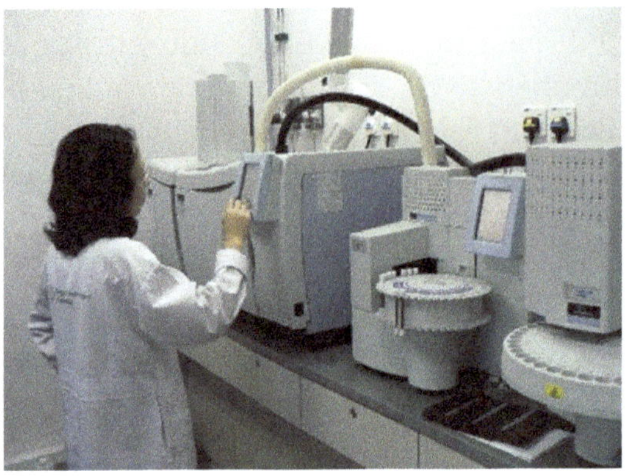

A technician performing quality control

Sensory Analysis

Sensory analysis is the study of how consumers' senses perceive food.

By Country

Australia

The Commonwealth Scientific and Industrial Research Organisation (CSIRO) is the federal government agency for scientific research in Australia. CSIRO maintains more than 50 sites across Australia and biological control research stations in France and Mexico. It has nearly 6,500 employees.

South Korea

The Korean Society of Food Science and Technology, or KoSFoST, claims to be the first society in South Korea for food science.

] programs at land-grant universities (which were state-run and largely under state mandates to allow for sex-blind admission), but then graduated and had difficulty finding jobs due to widespread sexism in the chemistry industry in the late 19th and early 20th centuries. Finding conventional career paths blocked, they found alternative employment as instructors in home economics departments and used that as a base to launch the foundation of many modern food science programs.

The main US organization regarding food science and food technology is the Institute of Food Technologists (IFT), headquartered in Chicago, Illinois, which is the US member organisation of the International Union of Food Science and Technology (IUFoST).

Popular books on some aspects of food science or kitchen science have been written by Harold McGee and Howard Hillman, among others.

References

- Whitney, Ellie; Rolfes, Sharon Rady (2013). Understanding Nutrition (13 ed.). Wadsworth, Cengage Learning. pp. 667, 670. ISBN 978-1133587521.
- Payne-Palacio, June R.; Canter, Deborah D. (2014). The Profession of Dietetics. Jones & Bartlett Learning. pp. 3, 4. ISBN 978-1-284-02608-5.
- Willett, Walter C. with Skerrett, Patrick J. (2005) [2001]. Eat, Drink, and be Healthy: The Harvard Medical School Guide To Healthy Eating. Free Press (Simon & Schuster). p. 183. ISBN 0-684-86337-5.
- Silberberg, Martin S. (2009). Chemistry: The Molecular Nature of Matter and Change (5 ed.). McGraw-Hill. p. 44. ISBN 978-0-07-304859-8.
- Nestle, Marion (2013) [2002]. Food Politics: How the Food Industry Influences Nutrition and Health. University of California Press. p. 413. ISBN 978-0-520-27596-6.
- Nelson, D. L.; Cox, M. M. (2000). Lehninger Principles of Biochemistry (3rd ed.). New York: Worth Publishing. ISBN 1-57259-153-6.
- Corbridge, D. E. C. (1995). Phosphorus: An Outline of its Chemistry, Biochemistry, and Technology (5th ed.). Amsterdam: Elsevier. ISBN 0-444-89307-5.
- Potter, Norman N.; Hotchkiss, Joseph H. (1998). Food Science. Food science texts series (5th ed.). Springer. ISBN 9780834212657.
- Fratamico PM and Bayles DO (editor). (2005). Foodborne Pathogens: Microbiology and Molecular Biology. Caister Academic Press. ISBN 978-1-904455-00-4.
- Hopkins, F. Gowland (1912). "Feeding Experiments Illustrating the Importance of Accessory Factors in Normal Dietaries" (PDF). The Journal of Physiology. 44 (5–6): 425–460. doi:10.1113/jphysiol.1912.sp001524. PMC 1512834. PMID 16993143. Retrieved March 15, 2016.
- "Joint Collection Development Policy: Human Nutrition and Food". US National Library of Medicine, National Institutes of Health. 14 October 2014. Retrieved 13 December 2014.
- Subcommittee on Vitamin Tolerance, Committee on Animal Nutrition, National Research Council (1987). "Vitamin E, in Vitamin Tolerance of Animals". National Academy of Sciences. Retrieved December 22, 2013.

2

Branches of Nutrition

Nutrition has a number of branches and some of these are nutrigenomics, sports nutrition and nutrition and pregnancy. Nutrigenomics is the study of food and its constituents on gene expression whereas the plan prescribed by a doctor to a woman before, during and after pregnancy is known as nutrition and pregnancy. The following text strategically encompasses and incorporates the major branches of nutrition.

Nutrigenomics

Nutrigenomics is a branch of nutritional genomics and is the study of the effects of foods and food constituents on gene expression. This means that nutrigenomics is research focusing on identifying and understanding molecular-level interaction between nutrients and other dietary bioactives with the genome. Nutrigenomics has also been described by the influence of genetic variation on nutrition, by correlating gene expression or SNPs with a nutrient's absorption, metabolism, elimination or biological effects. By doing so, nutrigenomics aims to develop rational means to optimise nutrition with respect to the subject's genotype.

By determining the mechanism of the effects of nutrients or the effects of a nutritional regime, nutrigenomics tries to define the causality or relationship between these specific nutrients and specific nutrient regimes (diets) on human health. Nutrigenomics has been associated with the idea of personalized nutrition based on genotype. While there is hope that nutrigenomics will ultimately enable such personalised dietary advice, it is a science still in its infancy and its contribution to public health over the next decade is thought to be major. Whilst nutrigenomics is aimed at developing an understanding of how the whole body responds to a food via systems biology, research into the effect of a single gene/single food compound relationships is known as nutrigenetics.

Definitions

Nutrigenomics has been defined as the application of high-throughput genomic tools in nutrition studies and research. It can also be seen as research to provide people with methods and tools who are looking for disease preventing and health promoting foods that match their lifestyles, cultures and genetics.

The term "high throughput tools" in nutrigenomics refers to genetic tools that enable millions of genetic screening tests to be conducted at a single time. When such high throughput screening is applied in nutrition research, it allows the examination of how nutrients affect the thousands of genes present in the human genome. Nutrigenomics involves the characterization of gene products and the physiological function and interactions of these products. This includes how nutrients impact the production and action of specific gene products and how these proteins in turn affect the response to nutrients.

Background and Preventive Health

Throughout the 20th century, nutritional science focused on finding vitamins and minerals, defining their use and preventing the deficiency diseases that they caused. As the nutrition related health problems of the developed world shifted to overnutrition, obesity and type two diabetes, the focus of modern medicine and of nutritional science changed accordingly.

To address the increasing incidence of these diet-related-diseases, the role of diet and nutrition has been and continues to be extensively studied. To prevent the development of disease, nutrition research is investigating how nutrition can optimize and maintain cellular, tissue, organ and whole body homeostasis. This requires understanding how nutrients act at the molecular level. This involves a multitude of nutrient-related interactions at the gene, protein and metabolic levels. As a result, nutrition research has shifted from epidemiology and physiology to molecular biology and genetics and nutrigenomics was born.

The emergence and development of nutrigenomics has been possible due to powerful developments in genetic research. Inter-individual differences in genetics, or genetic variability, which have an effect on metabolism and on phenotypes were recognized early in nutrition research, and such phenotypes were described. With the progress in genetics, biochemical disorders with a high nutritional relevance were linked to a genetic origin. Genetic disorders which cause pathological effects were described. Such genetic disorders include the polymorphism in the gene for the hormone Leptin which results in gross obesity. Other gene polymorphisms were described with consequences for human nutrition. The folate metabolism is a good example, where common polymorphisms (C677T and A1298C) exists for the gene that encodes the methylene-tetrahydro-folate reductase (MTHFR).

It was realized however, that there are possibly thousands of other gene polymorphisms which may result in minor deviations in nutritional biochemistry, where only marginal or additive effects would result from these deviations. The tools to study the physiological impact were not available at the time and are only now becoming available enabling the development of nutrigenomics. Such tools include those that measure the transcriptome - DNA microarray, Exon array, Tiling arrays, single nucleotide polymorphism arrays and genotyping. Tools that measure the proteome are less developed. These include methods based on gel electrophoresis, chromatography and mass spectrometry. Finally the tools that measure the metabolome are also less developed and include methods based on nuclear magnetic resonance imaging and mass spectrometry often in combination with gas and liquid chromatography.

Rationale and Aims of Nutrigenomics

In nutrigenomics, nutrients are seen as signals that tell a specific cell in the body about the diet. The nutrients are detected by a sensor system in the cell. Such a sensory system works like sensory ecology whereby the cell obtains information through the signal, the nutrient, about its environment, which is the diet. The sensory system that interprets information from nutrients about the dietary environment include transcription factors together with many additional proteins. Once the nutrient interacts with such a sensory system, it changes gene expression and metabolite production in accordance with the level of nutrient it senses. As a result, different diets should elicit different patterns of gene expression and metabolite production. Nutrigenomics seeks to describe the patterns of these effects which have been referred to as *dietary signatures*. Such dietary signatures are examined in specific cells, tissues and organisms and in this way the manner by which nutrition influences homeostasis is investigated. Genes which are affected by differing levels of nutrients need first to be identified and then their regulation is studied. Differences in this regulation as a result of differences in genes between individuals are also studied.

It is hoped that by building up knowledge in this area, nutrigenomics will promote an increased understanding of how nutrition influences metabolic pathways and homeostatic control, which will then be used to prevent the development of chronic diet related diseases such as obesity and type two diabetes. Part of the approach of nutrigenomics involves finding markers of the early phase of diet related diseases; this is the phase at which intervention with nutrition can return the patient to health. As nutrigenomics seeks to understand the effect of different genetic predispositions in the development of such diseases, once a marker has been found and measured in an individual, the extent to which they are susceptible to the development of that disease will be quantified and personalized dietary recommendation can be given for that person.

The aims of nutrigenomics also includes being able to demonstrate the effect of bioactive food compounds on health and the effect of health foods on health, which should lead to the development of functional foods that will keep people healthy according to their individual needs.

Nutrigenomics is a rapidly emerging science still in its beginning stages. It is uncertain whether the tools to study gene expression and metabolite production have been developed to the point as to enable efficient and reliable measurements. Also once such research has been achieved, it will need to be integrated together to produce results and dietary recommendations. All of these technologies are still in the process of development.

Application of Nutrigenomics

Anti-aging

Aging of cells occur because of the accumulation of excess free radicals formed due to the lack of proper nutrition to the cells and external factors like UV rays, pollution, stress, food, etc. DNA analysis is instrumental in identifying the right concoction of nutrients needed to eliminate the excess free radicals present in the cell.

The science of nutrigenomics studies the interaction between dietary components of food and genes. Scientific advances have now made it possible to apply nutrigenomics in the field of anti ageing and customize nutritional solutions in the form of supplements to meet the optimal nutrition required by the body to prevent ageing of cells by the formation of excess free radicals.

Obesity

Obesity is one of the most widely studied topics in nutrigenomics. Due to genetic variations among individuals, each person could respond to diet differently. By exploring the interaction between dietary pattern and genetic factors, nutrigenomics aim to suggest prevention measures and/ or treatment to obesity via personal nutrition.

There are studies suggesting genetic factors account for a fair proportion of inter-individual BMI.

Among different types of genetic variation between humans, SNPs are suggested to be the most important marker for the study of nutrigenomics.

Multiple studies have found association between SNPs and obesity. One of the most well known obesity associating gene is the FTO gene. Among studied individuals, it was found that those with AA genotype showed a higher BMI compared those with TT genotype when having high fat or low carbohydrate dietary intake.

The APO B SNP rs512535 is another obesity related variation. It was found that the A/G heterozygous genotype was found to have association with obesity (in terms of BMI and waist circumference). The same study also found that for individuals with habitual high fat diet (>35% of energy intaken), individuals with GG homozygotes genotype showed higher BMI compared to AA allele carriers. However, this difference is not found in low fat consuming group (<35% of energy intaken).

Besides the FTO genes and APO B, SNPs in various genes such as MC4R, SH2B1, MTCH2, SEC16B etc. have been found to be associated with obesity. Although many of these genetic variations are found in populations all over the world, there are also variations unique to certain races or populations.

Ethics

To put nutrigenomics into practice, genetic testing is required as the test results act as the reference for diagnosis. As the subject is recently commercialized by companies which sell direct to customer (DTC) genetic tests, as well as being applied by related professionals (such as dietic practitioners), there have been increased awareness in the use of this information.

These concerns include but are not limited to the lack of analytical and clinical validity of genetic tests, emotional distress of consumers, and other social concerns.

Privacy

One of the major concerns regarding genetic tests would be privacy issue. There are concerns on who has the right to have access to test results. Abuse of these tests could result in discrimination. For example, genetic information might be used by insurance companies to risk rate their clients.

Medical Claims

One of the possible ethical concerns arise would be private companies providing unverified information regarding test results. For example, there are concerns on test-providing companies making unproven medical claims, as well as selling unnecessary or over-priced supplements. Interpretations on genetic test results needs to be handled very carefully. Misinterpretation could possibly mislead patients and hence false medical claims are made. Misleading and/or inaccurate information may as well undermine customers' ability to make informed decisions.

Validity of Nutrigenomic Tests

Nutrigenomics is the study of interactions between a person's genetics and nutrition. In order to make accurate interpretations of genetic test results, sufficient genetic and nutritional knowledge is necessary for the practitioner. However, there are currently no regulations limiting who can perform these tests. As well, nutrigenomics is not currently a licensed profession. Therefore, there are concerns regarding the validity of consultation provided by private companies on genetic test results. In other words, there are concerns about how well the companies (who sell this services, and therefore have a profit motive) interpret test results.

Sports Nutrition

Sports Nutrition is the study and practice of nutrition and diet, relating to a person's athletic performance. It is concerned with the type, as well as the quantity of fluid and food taken by an athlete. In addition, it deals with the consumption of nutrients such as vitamins, minerals, supplements, which also include organic substances such as carbohydrates, proteins and fats. Nutrition is an important part of many sports training regimens, being most popular in strength sports (such as weight lifting and bodybuilding) and endurance sports (for example cycling, running, swimming, rowing).

Supplements

All athletes consider taking dietary supplements because they are looking for the "magic ingredient" to increase performance. In the extreme case of performance-enhancing supplements, athletes, particularly bodybuilders may choose to use illegal substances such as anabolic steroids, compounds which are related to the hormone testosterone, which can quickly build mass and strength, but have many adverse effects such as high blood pressure and negative gender specific effects. Blood doping, another illegal ergogenic, was discovered in the 1940s when it was used by World War II pilots.

In the 1940s early results were found regarding consumption of dietary protein for athletes involved in muscle building and resistance and strength training. Protein intake is a part of the nutrient requirements for the regular athlete and is an important component of exercise training, because it can also aid in performance and recovery. Dietary protein intake for well-trained athletes should occur before, during and after physical activity as it is advantageous in gaining muscle mass and strength. However, if too much protein and amino acid supplements are consumed (especially by the average exerciser), it can be more harmful than beneficial; health risks include: "dehydration, gout, calcium loss, liver, and renal damage [and] gastrointestinal side effects include diarrhea, bloating, and water loss" (Lawerence). A bountiful protein diet must be paired with a healthy, well-rounded meal plan and regular resistance exercise. Yet, characteristics such as the type of exercise, intensity, duration, the carbohydrate values of diet, the individual's sex and age and also the amount of background training and training environment.

Creatine may be helpful for well-trained athletes to increase exercise performance and strength in concordance with their dietary regimen. Also, the substance glutamine, found in whey protein supplements, is the most abundant free amino acid found in the human body. For well-trained and well-nourished athletes it is considered that glutamine may have a possible role in stimulated anabolic processes such muscle glycogen and protein synthesis. Other popular supplements studies done include androstenedione, chromium, and ephedra. The findings show that there are no substantial benefits from the extra intake of these supplements, yet higher health risks and costs.

High energy supplements have shown to increase the performance of physical activity. A study done at the University of Texas saw a 4.7% increase of performance in 83% of participants after drinking Red Bull Energy Drink which was more intense than the compared placebo. The energy drink most dominantly increased the epinephrine and noreprinephrine (adrenaline and its precursor) levels and beta-endorphins in the blood than before consumption. Caffeine, carbohydrates and Vitamin B are factors that may have favored performance increase with no change in perceived exertion.

Caffeine has been known since the 1900s and became popularly used since the 1970s when its power of masking fatigue became highly recognized. Similarly, the caffeine found in energy drinks shows an increased reaction performance and increased good feelings of energy, focus and alertness in quickness and reaction anaerobic power tests. In other words, consuming an energy drink with caffeine increases short time/rapid exercise performance (like short full-speed sprints and heavy power weight lifting).

Post-exercise nutrition is just as important, if not more important than pre-exercise nutrition as it pertains to recovery. Traditionally, sports drinks such as Gatorade and Powerade, are consumed during and after exercise because they effectively rehydrate the body by refueling the body with minerals and electrolytes. Gatorade was founded in the 1960s, when the University of Florida, Gainesville Gators improved their performance with "Gator Aid." A drink was made of glucose and sucrose in water and helped the football players' performance. And by the 1970s, many other sports drinks of its kind had been manufactured. However, sports drinks lack protein.

New studies in 2008 have found cow's milk, especially skim milk and chocolate milk may be effective replacements for current sports drink , as milk leads to protein the synthesis which boosts net muscle protein balance. Milk contains many electrolytes, nutrients and other elements that help to make it an effective post-exercise beverage. It is true that chocolate milk has been a proven study that is just as affective of a recovery drink as Gatorade. A recovery drink is supposed to replenish the sugar, and build muscle again so that you are ready for the next workout. Chocolate Milk includes key ingredients such as Vitamin D that helps replace fluids and electrolytes lost after the athlete has worked out.

When compared to plain water or sports drinks, research suggests that chocolate milk is more effective at replacing fluids lost as sweat and maintaining normal body fluid levels. Athletes drinking chocolate milk following exercise-induced dehydration had fluid levels about 2 percent higher (on initial body mass) than those using other post-exercise recovery beverages, allowing for prolonged performance, especially in repeated bouts of exercise or training.

Factors Influencing Nutritional Requirements

Differing conditions and objectives suggest the need for athletes to ensure that their sports nutritional approach is appropriate for their situation. Factors that may affect an athlete's nutritional needs include type of activity (aerobic vs. anaerobic), gender, weight, height, body mass index, workout or activity stage (pre-workout, intra-workout, recovery), and time of day (e.g. some nutrients are utilized by the body more effectively during sleep than while awake). Most culprits that get in the way of performance are fatigue, injury and soreness. A proper diet will reduce these disturbances in performance. The key is to get a variety of food, to get all the macronutrients, vitamins, and minerals. According to Eblere's article (2008), it is optimal to choose raw, unprocessed foods such as oranges instead of orange juice. Eating foods that are natural means the athlete is getting the most nutritional value out of the food. When foods are processed it normally means that nutritional value is reduced.

Anaerobic Exercise

During anaerobic exercise, the process of glycolysis breaks down the sugars from carbohydrates for energy without the use of oxygen. This type of exercise occurs in physical activity such as power sprints, strength resistances and quick explosive movement where the muscles are being used for power and speed, with short-time energy use. After this type of exercise, there is a need to refill glycogen storage sites in the body (the long simple sugar chains in the body that store energy), although they are not likely fully depleted.

To compensate for this glycogen reduction, athletes will often take in a large amount of carbohydrates in the period immediately following exercise. Typically, high-glycemic-index carbohydrates are preferred for their ability to rapidly raise blood glucose levels. For the purpose of protein synthesis, protein or individual amino acids are ingested as well. Branched-chain amino acids are important since they are most responsible for protein synthesis. According to Lemon et al. (1995) female endurance runners have the hardest time getting enough protein in their diet. Endurance athletes in general need more protein in their diet than the sedentary person. Research has shown that endurance athletes are recommended to have 1.2 to 1.4 g of protein per kg of body weight in order to repair damaged tissue. If the athlete consumes too few calories for the body's needs, lean tissue will be broken down for energy and repair. Protein deficiency can cause many problems such as early and extreme fatigue, particularly long recovery, and poor wound healing. Complete proteins such as meat, eggs, and soy provide the athlete with all essential amino acids for synthesising new tissues. However, vegetarian and vegan athletes frequently combine legumes with a whole grain to provide the body with a complete protein across the day's food intake. A popular example is rice and beans.

The following information on the types of carbohydrates comes from Spada's research on endurance sports nutrition (2000). He advises carbohydrates to be unprocessed and/or whole grains for optimal performance while training. This is because these carbohydrates offer the most fuel, nutritional value, and satiety. Fruits and vegetables contribute important carbohydrate foundation for an athlete's diet. They both provide vitamins and minerals that are lost through exercise and need to be replenished. Both fruits and vegetables improve healing, aid in recovery, and reduce risks of cancer, high blood pressure, and constipation. Vegetables offer a little more nutritional value than fruits for the amount of calories, therefore an athlete should strive to eat more vegetables than fruits. It is also important to look at the certain types of vegetables and fruits. Dark-colored vegetables usually have more nutritional value than pale colored ones. A general rule is the darker the color the more nutrient dense it is. Like all foods, it is very important to have a variety. To get the most nutritional value out of fruits and vegetables it is important to eat them in their natural, unprocessed form with no other nutrient (sugar) added.

Often in the continuation of this anaerobic exercise, the product from this metabolic mechanism builds up in what is called lactic acid fermentation. Lactate is produced more quickly than it is being removed and it serves to regenerate NAD^+ to the cells where it's needed. During intense exercise when oxygen is not being used, a high amount of ATP is produced and pH levels fall causing acidosis or more specifically lactic acidosis. Lactic acid build up can be treated by staying well-hydrated throughout and especially after the workout, having good cool down routine and good post-workout stretching.

Intense activity can cause significant damage to bodily tissues. In order to repair, vitamin E and other antioxidants are needed to protect muscle damage. Oxidative damage and muscle tissue breakdown happens all the time in endurance running so athletes need to eat foods high in protein in order to repair these muscle tissues. It is important for female endurance runners to consume proper nutrients in their diet that will repair, fuel, and minimize fatigue and injury. To keep a female runner's body performing at its best, ten nutrients need to be essential in diets.

Nutrition and Pregnancy

Nutrition and pregnancy refers to the nutrient intake, and dietary planning that is undertaken before, during and after pregnancy. Nutrition of the fetus begins at conception. For this reason, the nutrition of the mother is important from before conception (probably several months before) as well as throughout pregnancy and breast feeding. An ever-increasing number of studies have shown that the nutrition of the mother will have an effect on the child, up to and including the risk for cancer, cardiovascular disease, hypertension and diabetes throughout life.

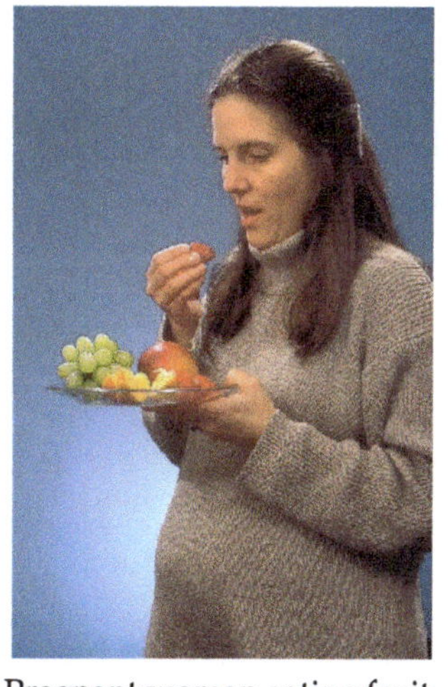

Pregnant woman eating fruit.

An inadequate or excessive amount of some nutrients may cause malformations or medical problems in the fetus, and neurological disorders and handicaps are a risk that is run by mothers who are malnourished. 23.8% of babies worldwide are estimated to be born with lower than optimal weights at birth due to lack of proper nutrition. Personal habits such as smoking, alcohol, caffeine, using certain medications and street drugs can negatively and irreversibly affect the development of the baby, which happens in the early stages of pregnancy.

Caffeine is sometimes assumed to cause harm to the unborn baby but there is not enough evidence so say if this is true. A recent review showed that more research is needed to show whether caffeine intake effects birth weight, preterm births, gestational diabetes and other outcomes.

Nutrition Before Pregnancy

Beneficial Pre-pregnancy Nutrients

As with most diets, there are chances of over-supplementing, however, as general advice, both state and medical recommendations are that mothers follow instructions listed on particular vitamin packaging as to the correct or recommended daily allowance (RDA). Daily prenatal use of iron substantially improves birth weight, potentially reducing the risk of Low birth weight.

- Folic acid supplementation is recommended prior to conception, to prevent development of spina bifida and other neural tube defects. It should be taken as at least 0.4 mg/day throughout the first trimester of pregnancy, 0.6 mg/day through the pregnancy, and 0.5 mg/day while breastfeeding in addition to eating foods rich in folic acid such as green leafy vegetables.
- Iodine levels are frequently too low in pregnant women, and iodine is necessary for normal thyroid function and mental development of the fetus, even cretinism. Pregnant women should take prenatal vitamins containing iodine.
- Vitamin D levels vary with exposure to sunlight. While it was assumed that supplementation was necessary only in areas of high latitudes, recent studies of Vitamin D levels throughout the United States and many other countries have shown a large number of women with low levels. For this reason, there is a growing movement to recommend supplementation with 1000 mg of Vitamin D daily throughout pregnancy, vitamin D is necessary to prevent rickets, a disease causing weak bones.
- A large number of pregnant women have been found to have low levels of vitamin B12, but supplementation has not yet been shown to improve pregnancy outcome or the health of the newborn, although there are suspicions.
- Polyunsaturated fatty acids, specifically docosahexaenoic acid (DHA) and eicosapentaenoic acid (EPA) are very beneficial for fetal development. Several studies have shown a small drop in preterm delivery and in low birth weight in mothers with higher intakes. The best dietary source of omega-3 fatty acids is oily fish. Some other omega-3 fatty acids not found in fish can be found in foods such as flaxseeds, walnuts, pumpkin seeds, and enriched eggs.
- Iron is needed for the healthy growth of the fetus and placenta, especially during the second and third trimesters. It is also essential before pregnancy for the production of hemoglobin.There is no evidence that a hemoglobin level of 7 grams/100 ml or higher is detrimental to pregnancy, but it must be acknowledged that maternal hemorrhage is a major source of maternal mortality worldwide, and a reserve capacity to carry oxygen is desirable. Evidence shows that giving 100 mg of elemental iron three times weekly is adequate during pregnancy.

Nutrition During Pregnancy

During the early stages of pregnancy, since the placenta is not yet formed, there is no mechanism to protect the embryo from the deficiencies which may be inherent in the mother's circulation. Thus, it is critical that an adequate amount of nutrients and energy is consumed.

Multiple micronutrient supplements taken with iron and folic acid can improve birth outcomes for women in low income countries. These supplements reduce numbers of low birth weight babies, small for gestational age babies and stillbirths in women who may not have many micronutrients in their usual diets. Undernourished women can benefit from having dietary education sessions and, balanced energy and protein supplements.

A review showed that dietary education increased the mother's protein intake and helped the baby grow more inside the womb. The balanced protein and energy supplement lowered risk of stillbirth and small babies and increased weight gain for both the mother and baby. Although more research is needed into the longer term effects on the mothers' and infants' health, the short term effects look promising.

Supplementing one's diet with foods rich in folic acid, such as oranges and dark green leafy vegetables, helps to prevent neural tube birth defects in the fetus. In addition, prenatal vitamins typically contain increased amounts of folic acid, iodine, iron, vitamin A, vitamin D, zinc, and calcium over the amounts found in standard multi-vitamins.

Zinc supplements have reduced preterm births by around 14% mainly in low income countries. No other benefits were seen. The World Health Organisation does not routinely recommend zinc supplementation for pregnant women because there is not enough good quality evidence.

For women with low calcium diets, taking calcium supplementation can reduce their risk of pre-eclampsia. It has also been suggested that calcium can reduce numbers of births that happen before the 37th week of pregnancy (preterm birth). However a more recent review looking into other benefits of calcium supplementation did not find any improvement in numbers of preterm or low birth weight babies. There is not enough good quality to research to suggest best doses and timing of calcium supplementation.

Pregnant women are advised to pay attention to the foods they eat during pregnancy, such as soft cheese and certain fish, in order to reduce the risk of exposure to substances or bacteria that may be harmful to the developing fetus. This can include food pathogens and toxic food components, alcohol, and dietary supplements such as vitamin A and potentially harmful pathogens such as listeria, toxoplasmosis, and salmonella. Dietary vitamin A is obtained in two forms which contain the preformed vitamin (retinol), that can be found in some animal products such as liver and fish liver oils, and as a vitamin A precursor in the form of carotene, which can be found in many fruits and vegetables. Intake of large amounts or, conversely, a deficiency, of retinol has been linked to birth defects and abnormalities. It is noted that a 100 g serving of liver may contain a large amount of retinol, so it is best that it is not eaten daily during pregnancy. Excessive amounts of alcohol have been proven to cause fetal alcohol syndrome. The World Health Organization recommends that alcohol should be avoided entirely during pregnancy, given the relatively unknown effects of even small amounts of alcohol during pregnancy. Although seafood contains high levels of Omega-3 fatty acids which are beneficial for both mother and the baby, but there is no consensus on consuming seafood during pregnancy. Pregnant women are advised to eat seafood in moderation.

Folic Acid

Folic acid, which is the synthetic form of the vitamin folate, is critical both in pre-and peri-conception. Deficiencies in folic acid may cause neural tube defects; women who had 0.4 mg of folic acid in their systems due to supplementing 3 months before childbirth significantly reduced the risk of NTD within the fetus. The development of every human cell is dependent on an adequate supply of folic acid. Folic acid governs the synthesis of the precursors of DNA, which is the nucleic acid that gives each cell life and character. Folic acid deficiency results in defective cellular growth and the effects are most obvious on those tissues which grow most rapidly.

Water

During pregnancy, one's mass increases by about 12 kg. Most of this added weight (6 to 9 L) is water because the plasma volume increases, 85% of the placenta is water and the fetus itself is 70-90% water. This means that hydration is an important aspect of nutrition throughout pregnancy. The European Food Safety Authority recommends an increase of 300 mL per day compared to the normal intake for non-pregnant women, taking the total adequate water intake (from food and fluids) to 2,300 mL, or approximately 1,850 mL/ day from fluids alone

Nutrition after Pregnancy

Proper nutrition is important after delivery to help the mother recover, and to provide enough food energy and nutrients for a woman to breastfeed her child. Women having serum ferritin less than 70 μg/L may need iron supplements to prevent iron deficiency anaemia during pregnancy and postpartum.

During lactation, water intake may need to be increased. Human milk is made of 88% water, and the IOM recommends that breastfeeding women increase their water intake by about 300 mL/ day to a total volume of 3000 mL/day (from food and drink); approximately 2,400 mL/day from fluids.

References

- Schaefer, Christof (2001). Drugs During Pregnancy and Lactation: Handbook of Prescription Drugs and Comparative Risk Assessment. Gulf Professional Publishing. ISBN 9780444507631.
- Shils, Maurice Edward; Shike, Moshe (2006). Modern Nutrition in Health and Disease. Lippincott Williams & Wilkins. ISBN 9780781741330.
- Briggs, Gerald G.; Freeman, Roger K.; Yaffe, Sumner J. (2011). Drugs in Pregnancy and Lactation: A Reference Guide to Fetal and Neonatal Risk. Lippincott Williams & Wilkins. ISBN 9781608317080.
- Laura Riley (2006-02-02). Stephanie Karpinske, ed. Pregnancy: The Ultimate Week-by-Week Pregnancy Guide. Meredith Books. pp. 21–22. ISBN 0-696-22221-3.
- Peña-Rosas, Juan Pablo; De-Regil, Luz Maria; Dowswell, Therese; Viteri, Fernando E. (2012). "Daily oral iron supplementation during pregnancy". The Cochrane Database of Systematic Reviews. 12: CD004736. doi:10.1002/14651858.CD004736.pub4. ISSN 1469-493X.
- Phillips, Catherine M.; Goumidi, Louisa; Bertrais, Sandrine; Field, Martyn R.; McManus, Ross; Hercberg, Serge; Lairon, Denis; Planells, Richard; Roche, Helen M. (2011-02-01). "Gene-nutrient interactions and gender may modulate the association between ApoA1 and ApoB gene polymorphisms and metabolic syndrome risk". Atherosclerosis. 214 (2): 408–414. doi:10.1016/j.atherosclerosis.2010.10.029. ISSN 1879-1484.
- Samuel, G. N.; Jordens, C. F. C.; Kerridge, I. (2010-03-01). "Direct-to-consumer personal genome testing: ethical and regulatory issues that arise from wanting to 'know' your DNA". Internal Medicine Journal. 40 (3): 220–224. doi:10.1111/j.1445-5994.2010.02190.x. ISSN 1445-5994.

3

Nutrients: A Comprehensive Study

Nutrients are constituents found in food items that are consumed by an organism to survive and to grow. Macronutrients provide an organism with the energy it requires, and also provides the necessary co-factors for metabolism. This section will provide an integrated understanding of nutrients.

Nutrients

Nutrients are components in foods that an organism uses to survive and grow. Macronutrients provide the bulk energy an organism's metabolic system needs to function while micronutrients provide the necessary cofactors for metabolism to be carried out. Both types of nutrients can be acquired from the environment. Micronutrients are used to build and repair tissues and to regulate body processes while macronutrients are converted to, and used for, energy. Methods of nutrient intake are different for plants and animals. Plants take in nutrients directly from the soil through their roots and from the atmosphere through their leaves. Animals and protists have specialized digestive systems that work to break down macronutrients for energy and utilize micronutrients for both metabolism and anabolism (constructive synthesis) in the body.

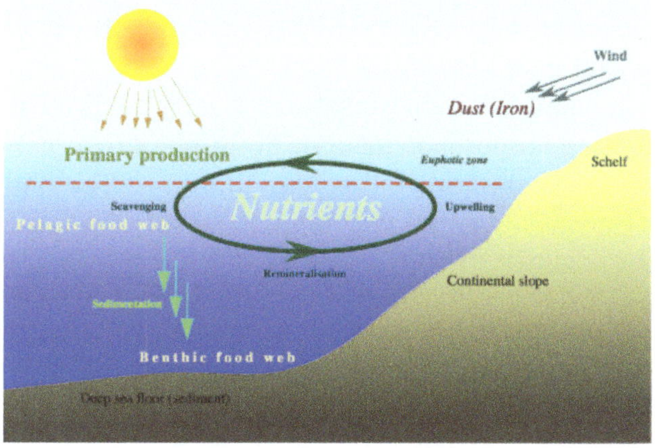

Nutrient cycle in the oceans

Organic nutrients consist of carbohydrates, fats, proteins (or their building blocks, amino acids), and vitamins. Inorganic chemical compounds such as dietary minerals, water (H2O), and oxygen may also be considered nutrients. A nutrient is considered essential if it must be obtained from an external source either because the organism cannot synthesize it or because insufficient quantities are produced. Nutrients needed in very small amounts are called micronutrients while those needed in large quantities are called macronutrients. The effects of nutrients are dose-dependent; shortages are called deficiencies.

Types of Nutrient

Macronutrients are defined in several different ways.

- The chemical elements humans consume in the largest quantities are carbon, hydrogen, nitrogen, oxygen, phosphorus, and sulphur, or CHNOPS.
- The classes of chemical compounds humans consume in the largest quantities and which provide bulk energy are carbohydrates, proteins, and fats. Water and atmospheric oxygen also must be consumed in large quantities, but are not always considered "food" or "nutrients".
- Calcium, salt (sodium and chloride), magnesium, and potassium (along with phosphorus and sulfur) are sometimes added to the list of macronutrients because they are required in large quantities compared to other vitamins and minerals. They are sometimes referred to as the macrominerals.

Substances that Provide Energy

- Carbohydrates are compounds made up of types of sugars. Carbohydrates are classified by their number of sugar units: monosaccharides (such as glucose and fructose), disaccharides (such as sucrose and lactose), oligosaccharides, and polysaccharides (such as starch, glycogen, and cellulose).
- Proteins are organic compounds that consist of amino acids joined by peptide bonds. The body cannot manufacture some of the amino acids (termed essential amino acids); the diet must supply them. Proteins, in nutrition, are broken down through digestion by proteases back into free amino acids.
- Fats consist of a glycerin molecule with three fatty acids attached. Fatty acids are unbranched hydrocarbon chains,1 connected by single bonds alone (saturated fatty acids) or by both double and single bonds (unsaturated fatty acids). Fats are needed to keep cell membranes functioning properly, to insulate body organs against shock, to keep body temperature stable, and to maintain healthy skin and hair. The body does not manufacture certain fatty acids (termed essential fatty acids) and the diet must supply them.

Although alcohol provides energy, and can thus be compared to macronutrients, it is not a substance that is essential for normal function. The acetic acid in vinegar also provides a similar amount of energy per gram, but again, it is not a nutrient because it is not essential for normal function.

Fat has an energy content of 9 kcal/g (~37.7 kJ/g); proteins and carbohydrates 4 kcal/g (~16.7 kJ/g). Ethanol (grain alcohol) has an energy content of 7 kcal/g (~29.3 kJ/g).

Substances that Support Metabolism

- Dietary minerals are generally trace elements, salts, or ions such as copper and iron. Some of these minerals are essential to human metabolism.
- Vitamins are organic compounds essential to the body. They usually act as coenzymes or

cofactors for various proteins in the body.

- Water is an essential nutrient and is the solvent in which all the chemical reactions of life take place.

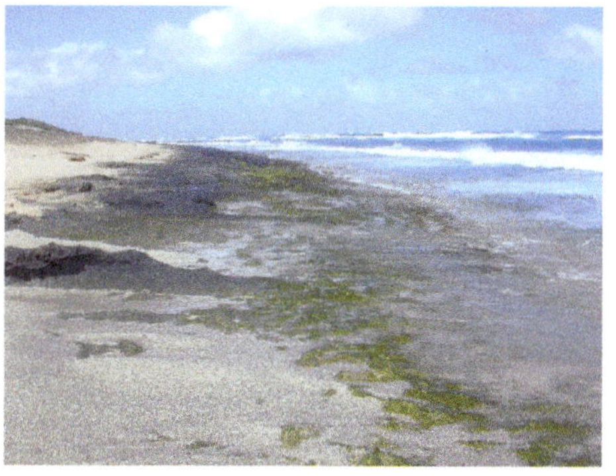

The strip of a green alga (*Enteromorpha*) along this shore indicates that there is a nearby source of nutrients (probably nitrates or ammonia from a small estuary).

Plants absorb nutrients from the soil or the atmosphere, or from water (mainly aquatic plants). An exception are the carnivorous plants, which externally digest nutrients from animals before ingesting them.

The chemical elements consumed in the greatest quantities by plants are carbon, hydrogen, and oxygen. These are present in the environment in the form of water and carbon dioxide; energy is provided by sunlight. Nitrogen, phosphorus, and sulfur are also needed in relatively large quantities. Together, the "Big Six" are the elemental macronutrients for all organisms, often represented by the acronym CHNOPS. Usually they are sourced from inorganic (e.g. carbon dioxide, water, nitrate, phosphate, sulfate) or organic (e.g. carbohydrates, lipids, proteins) compounds, although elemental diatomic molecules of nitrogen and (especially) oxygen are often used.

Other chemical elements are also necessary to carry out various life processes and build structures; see fertilizer and micronutrient for more information.

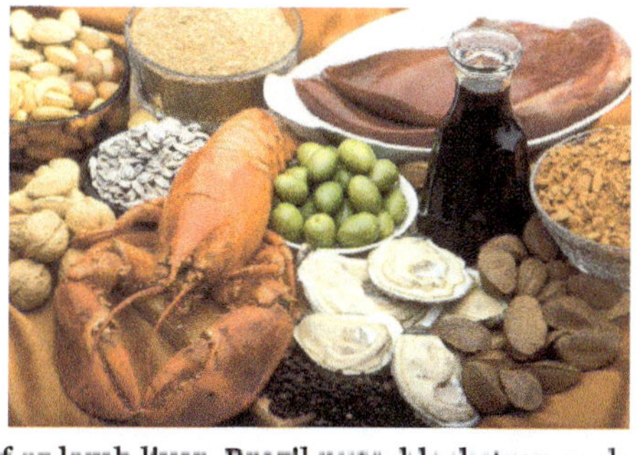

Rich sources of copper: oysters, beef or lamb liver, Brazil nuts, blackstrap molasses, cocoa, and black pepper. Good sources: lobster, nuts and sunflower seeds, green olives, and wheat bran.

Some of these are considered micronutrients in certain organisms. The mnemonic C. HOPKN'S CaFe Mg (to be used as C. Hopkins coffee mug) is used by some students to remember the list as: carbon, hydrogen, oxygen, phosphorus, potassium, nitrogen, sulfur, calcium, iron, and magnesium. Silicon, chloride, sodium, copper, zinc, and molybdenum are sometimes also included, but are in other cases considered micronutrients.

Essential and Non-essential Nutrients

Nutrients are frequently categorized as essential and nonessential.

Essential Nutrients

Essential nutrients are unable to be synthesized internally (either at all, or in sufficient quantities), and so must be consumed by an organism from its environment. Nonessential nutrients are those nutrients that can be made by the body; they may often also be absorbed from consumed food. The majority of animals ultimately derive their essential nutrients from plants, though some animals may consume mineral-based soils to supplement their diet.

For humans, these include essential fatty acids, essential amino acids, vitamins, and certain dietary minerals. Oxygen and water are also essential for human survival, but are generally not considered "food" when consumed in isolation. There are no "essential carbohydrates", animals can synthesize all the types of carbohydrates needed for growth.

Humans can derive energy from a wide variety of fats, carbohydrates, proteins, and simple chemicals such as ethanol and acetic acid.

Non-essential Nutrients

Non-essential nutrients are substances within foods can still have a significant impact on health, whether beneficial or toxic. For example, most dietary fiber is not absorbed by the human digestive tract, but is important in maintaining the bulk of a bowel movement to avoid constipation.

Interest has recently increased in phytochemicals, which include many non-essential substances which may or may not have health benefits.

Deficiencies and Toxicity

An inadequate amount of a nutrient is a deficiency. Deficiencies can be due to a number of causes including inadequacy in nutrient intake called dietary deficiency, or conditions that interfere with the utilization of a nutrient within an organism. Some of the conditions that can interfere with nutrient utilization include problems with nutrient absorption, substances that cause a greater than normal need for a nutrient, conditions that cause nutrient destruction, and conditions that cause greater nutrient excretion.

Nutrient toxicity occurs when an excess of a nutrient does harm to an organism.

Some Example of Nutrients

Carbohydrate

A carbohydrate is a biological molecule consisting of carbon (C), hydrogen (H) and oxygen (O) atoms, usually with a hydrogen–oxygen atom ratio of 2:1 (as in water); in other words, with the empirical formula $C_m(H_2O)_n$ (where *m* could be different from *n*). Some exceptions exist; for example, deoxyribose, a sugar component of DNA, has the empirical formula $C_5H_{10}O_4$. Carbohydrates are technically hydrates of carbon; structurally it is more accurate to view them as polyhydroxy aldehydes and ketones.

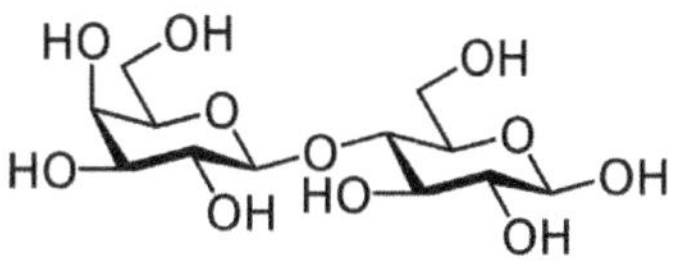

Lactose is a disaccharide found in milk. It consists of a molecule of D-galactose and a molecule of D-glucose bonded by beta-1-4 glycosidic linkage. It has a formula of $C_{12}H_{22}O_{11}$.

The term is most common in biochemistry, where it is a synonym of saccharide, a group that includes sugars, starch, and cellulose. The saccharides are divided into four chemical groups: monosaccharides, disaccharides, oligosaccharides, and polysaccharides. In general, the monosaccharides and disaccharides, which are smaller (lower molecular weight) carbohydrates, are commonly referred to as sugars. The word *saccharide* comes from the Greek word σάκχαρον (*sákkharon*), meaning "sugar." While the scientific nomenclature of carbohydrates is complex, the names of the monosaccharides and disaccharides very often end in the suffix -ose. For example, grape sugar is the monosaccharide glucose, cane sugar is the disaccharide sucrose, and milk sugar is the disaccharide lactose (see illustration).

Carbohydrates perform numerous roles in living organisms. Polysaccharides serve for the storage of energy (e.g. starch and glycogen) and as structural components (e.g. cellulose in plants and chitin in arthropods). The 5-carbon monosaccharide ribose is an important component of coenzymes (e.g. ATP, FAD and NAD) and the backbone of the genetic molecule known as RNA. The related deoxyribose is a component of DNA. Saccharides and their derivatives include many other important biomolecules that play key roles in the immune system, fertilization, preventing pathogenesis, blood clotting, and development.

In food science and in many informal contexts, the term carbohydrate often means any food that is particularly rich in the complex carbohydrate starch (such as cereals, bread and pasta) or simple carbohydrates, such as sugar (found in candy, jams, and desserts).

Often in lists of nutritional information, such as the USDA National Nutrient Database, the term "carbohydrate" (or "carbohydrate by difference") is used for everything other than water, protein, fat, ash, and ethanol. This will include chemical compounds such as acetic or lactic acid, which are not normally considered carbohydrates. It also includes "dietary fiber" which is a carbohydrate but which does not contribute much in the way of food energy (calories), even though it is often included in the calculation of total food energy just as though it were a sugar.

Structure

Formerly the name "carbohydrate" was used in chemistry for any compound with the formula $C_m(H_2O)_n$. Following this definition, some chemists considered formaldehyde (CH_2O) to be the simplest carbohydrate, while others claimed that title for glycolaldehyde. Today, the term is generally understood in the biochemistry sense, which excludes compounds with only one or two carbons and includes many biological carbohydrates which deviate from this formula. For example, while the above representative formulas would seem to capture the commonly known carbohydrates, ubiquitous and abundant carbohydrates often deviate from this. For example, carbohydrates often display chemical groups such as: *N*-acetyl (e.g. chitin), sulphate (e.g. glycosaminoglycans), carboxylic acid (e.g. sialic acid) and deoxy modifications (e.g. fucose and sialic acid).

Natural saccharides are generally built of simple carbohydrates called monosaccharides with general formula $(CH_2O)_n$ where *n* is three or more. A typical monosaccharide has the structure H–$(CHOH)_x$(C=O)–$(CHOH)_y$–H, that is, an aldehyde or ketone with many hydroxyl groups added, usually one on each carbon atom that is not part of the aldehyde or ketone functional group. Examples of monosaccharides are glucose, fructose, and glyceraldehydes. However, some biological substances commonly called "monosaccharides" do not conform to this formula (e.g. uronic acids and deoxy-sugars such as fucose) and there are many chemicals that do conform to this formula but are not considered to be monosaccharides (e.g. formaldehyde CH_2O and inositol $(CH_2O)_6$).

The open-chain form of a monosaccharide often coexists with a closed ring form where the aldehyde/ketone carbonyl group carbon (C=O) and hydroxyl group (–OH) react forming a hemiacetal with a new C–O–C bridge.

Monosaccharides can be linked together into what are called polysaccharides (or oligosaccharides) in a large variety of ways. Many carbohydrates contain one or more modified monosaccharide units that have had one or more groups replaced or removed. For example, deoxyribose, a component of DNA, is a modified version of ribose; chitin is composed of repeating units of N-acetyl glucosamine, a nitrogen-containing form of glucose.

Division

Carbohydrates are polyhydroxy aldehydes, ketones, alcohols, acids, their simple derivatives and their polymers having linkages of the acetal type. They may be classified according to their degree of polymerization and may be divided initially into three principal groups, namely sugars, oligosaccharides and polysaccharides

The major dietary carbohydrates

Class (DP*)	**Subgroup**	**Components**
Sugars (1–2)	Monosaccharides	Glucose, galactose, fructose, xylose
	Disaccharides	Sucrose, lactose, maltose, trehalose
	Polyols	Sorbitol, mannitol
Oligosaccharides (3–9)	Malto-oligosaccharides	Maltodextrins
	Other oligosaccharides	Raffinose, stachyose, fructo-oligosaccharides
Polysaccharides (>9)	Starch	Amylose, amylopectin, modified starches
	Non-starch polysaccharides	Cellulose, hemicellulose, pectins, hydrocolloids

DP * = Degree of polymerization

Monosaccharides

Monosaccharides are the simplest carbohydrates in that they cannot be hydrolyzed to smaller carbohydrates. They are aldehydes or ketones with two or more hydroxyl groups. The general chemical formula of an unmodified monosaccharide is $(C\cdot H_2O)_n$, literally a "carbon hydrate." Monosaccharides are important fuel molecules as well as building blocks for nucleic acids. The smallest monosaccharides, for which n=3, are dihydroxyacetone and D- and L-glyceraldehydes.

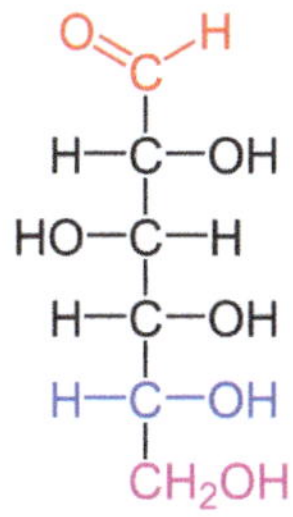

D-glucose is an aldohexose with the formula $(C{\cdot}H_2O)_6$. The red atoms highlight the aldehyde group and the blue atoms highlight the asymmetric center furthest from the aldehyde; because this -OH is on the right of the Fischer projection, this is a D sugar.

Classification of Monosaccharides

Monosaccharides are classified according to three different characteristics: the placement of its carbonyl group, the number of carbon atoms it contains, and its chiral handedness. If the carbonyl group is an aldehyde, the monosaccharide is an aldose; if the carbonyl group is a ketone, the monosaccharide is a ketose. Monosaccharides with three carbon atoms are called trioses, those with four are called tetroses, five are called pentoses, six are hexoses, and so on. These two systems of classification are often combined. For example, glucose is an aldohexose (a six-carbon aldehyde), ribose is an aldopentose (a five-carbon aldehyde), and fructose is a ketohexose (a six-carbon ketone).

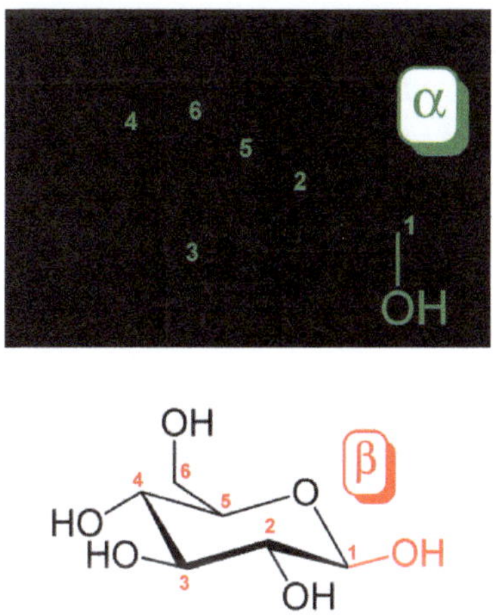

The α and β anomers of glucose. Note the position of the hydroxyl group (red or green) on the anomeric carbon relative to the CH_2OH group bound to carbon 5: they either have identical absolute configurations (R,R or S,S) (α), or opposite absolute configurations (R,S or S,R) (β).

Each carbon atom bearing a hydroxyl group (-OH), with the exception of the first and last carbons, are asymmetric, making them stereo centers with two possible configurations each (R or S). Because of this asymmetry, a number of isomers may exist for any given monosaccharide formula. Using Le Bel-van't Hoff rule, the aldohexose D-glucose, for example, has the formula $(C{\cdot}H_2O)_6$, of which four of its six carbons atoms are stereogenic, making D-glucose one of $2^4=16$ possible stereoisomers. In the case of glyceraldehydes, an aldotriose, there is one pair of possible stereoisomers, which are enantiomers and epimers. 1, 3-dihydroxyacetone, the ketose corresponding to the aldose glyceraldehydes, is a symmetric molecule with no stereo centers. The assignment of D or L is made according to the orientation of the asymmetric carbon furthest from the carbonyl group:

in a standard Fischer projection if the hydroxyl group is on the right the molecule is a D sugar, otherwise it is an L sugar. The "D-" and "L-" prefixes should not be confused with "d-" or "l-", which indicate the direction that the sugar rotates plane polarized light. This usage of "d-" and "l-" is no longer followed in carbohydrate chemistry.

Ring-straight Chain Isomerism

The aldehyde or ketone group of a straight-chain monosaccharide will react reversibly with a hydroxyl group on a different carbon atom to form a hemiacetal or hemiketal, forming a heterocyclic ring with an oxygen bridge between two carbon atoms. Rings with five and six atoms are called furanose and pyranose forms, respectively, and exist in equilibrium with the straight-chain form.

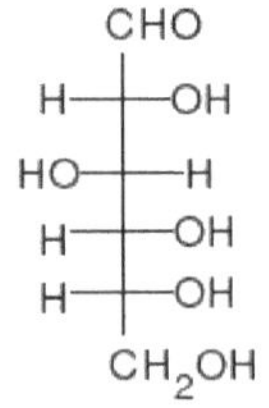

Glucose can exist in both a straight-chain and ring form.

During the conversion from straight-chain form to the cyclic form, the carbon atom containing the carbonyl oxygen, called the anomeric carbon, becomes a stereogenic center with two possible configurations: The oxygen atom may take a position either above or below the plane of the ring. The resulting possible pair of stereoisomers is called anomers. In the α anomer, the -OH substituent on the anomeric carbon rests on the opposite side (trans) of the ring from the CH_2OH side branch. The alternative form, in which the CH_2OH substituent and the anomeric hydroxyl are on the same side (cis) of the plane of the ring, is called the β anomer.

Use in Living Organisms

Monosaccharides are the major source of fuel for metabolism, being used both as an energy source (glucose being the most important in nature) and in biosynthesis. When monosaccharides are not immediately needed by many cells they are often converted to more space-efficient forms, often polysaccharides. In many animals, including humans, this storage form is glycogen, especially in liver and muscle cells. In plants, starch is used for the same purpose. The most abundant carbohydrate, cellulose, is a structural component of the cell wall of plants and many forms of algae. Ribose is a component of RNA. Deoxyribose is a component of DNA. Lyxose is a component of lyxoflavin found in the human heart. Ribulose and xylulose occur in the pentose phosphate pathway. Galactose, a component of milk sugar lactose, is found in galactolipids in plant cell membranes and in glycoproteins in many tissues. Mannose occurs in human metabolism, especially in the glycosylation of certain proteins. Fructose, or fruit sugar, is found in many plants and in humans, it is metabolized in the liver, absorbed directly into the intestines during digestion, and found in semen. Trehalose, a major sugar of insects, is rapidly hydrolyzed into two glucose molecules to support continuous flight.

Disaccharides

Two joined monosaccharides are called a disaccharide and these are the simplest polysaccharides. Examples include sucrose and lactose. They are composed of two monosaccharide units bound together by a covalent bond known as a glycosidic linkage formed via a dehydration reaction, resulting in the loss of a hydrogen atom from one monosaccharide and a hydroxyl group from the other. The formula of unmodified disaccharides is $C_{12}H_{22}O_{11}$. Although there are numerous kinds of disaccharides, a handful of disaccharides are particularly notable.

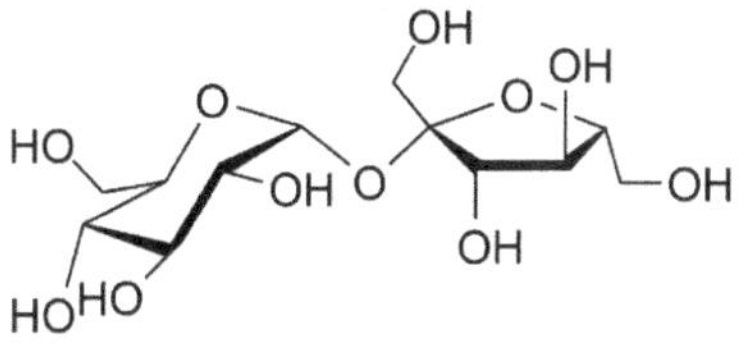

Sucrose, also known as table sugar, is a common disaccharide. It is composed of two monosaccharides: D-glucose (left) and D-fructose (right).

Sucrose, pictured to the right, is the most abundant disaccharide, and the main form in which carbohydrates are transported in plants. It is composed of one D-glucose molecule and one D-fructose molecule. The systematic name for sucrose, *O*-α-D-glucopyranosyl-(1→2)-D-fructofuranoside, indicates four things:

- Its monosaccharides: glucose and fructose
- Their ring types: glucose is a pyranose and fructose is a furanose
- How they are linked together: the oxygen on carbon number 1 (C1) of α-D-glucose is linked to the C2 of D-fructose.
- The *-oside* suffix indicates that the anomeric carbon of both monosaccharides participates in the glycosidic bond.

Lactose, a disaccharide composed of one D-galactose molecule and one D-glucose molecule, occurs naturally in mammalian milk. The systematic name for lactose is *O*-β-D-galactopyranosyl-(1→4)-D-glucopyranose. Other notable disaccharides include maltose (two D-glucoses linked α-1,4) and cellulobiose (two D-glucoses linked β-1,4). Disaccharides can be classified into two types: reducing and non-reducing disaccharides. If the functional group is present in bonding with another sugar unit, it is called a reducing disaccharide or biose.

Nutrition

Carbohydrate consumed in food yields 3.87 calories of energy per gram for simple sugars, and 3.57 to 4.12 calories per gram for complex carbohydrate in most other foods. Relatively high levels of carbohydrate are associated with processed foods or refined foods made from plants, including sweets, cookies and candy, table sugar, honey, soft drinks, breads and crackers, jams and fruit products, pastas and breakfast cereals. Lower amounts of carbohydrate are usually associated with unrefined foods, including beans, tubers, rice, and unrefined fruit. Animal-based foods generally have the lowest carbohydrate levels, although milk does contain a high proportion of lactose.

Carbohydrates are a common source of energy in living organisms; however, no carbohydrate is an essential nutrient in humans. Humans are able to obtain all of their energy requirement from protein and fats, though the potential for some negative health effects of extreme carbohydrate restriction remains, as the issue has not been studied extensively so far. However, in the case of dietary fiber – indigestible carbohydrates which are not a source of energy – inadequate intake can lead to significant increases in mortality.

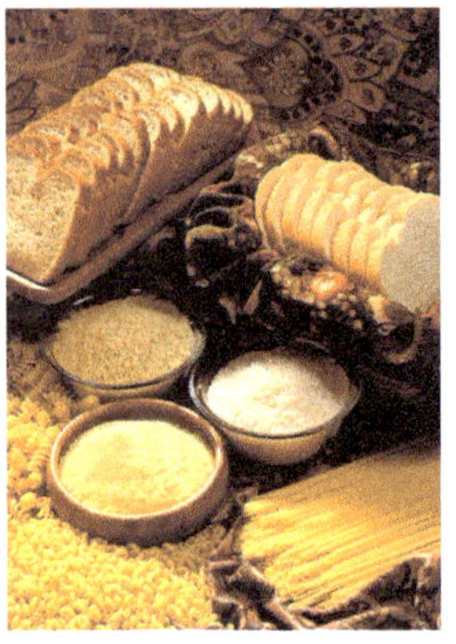

Grain products: rich sources of carbohydrates

Following a diet consisting of very low amounts of daily carbohydrate for several days will usually result in higher levels of blood ketone bodies than an isocaloric diet with similar protein content. This relatively high level of ketone bodies is commonly known as ketosis and is very often confused with the potentially fatal condition often seen in type 1 diabetics known as diabetic ketoacidosis. Somebody suffering ketoacidosis will have much higher levels of blood ketone bodies along with high blood sugar, dehydration and electrolyte imbalance.

Long-chain fatty acids cannot cross the blood–brain barrier, but the liver can break these down to produce ketones. However, the medium-chain fatty acids octanoic and heptanoic acids can cross the barrier and be used by the brain, which normally relies upon glucose for its energy. Gluconeogenesis allows humans to synthesize some glucose from specific amino acids: from the glycerol backbone in triglycerides and in some cases from fatty acids.

Organisms typically cannot metabolize all types of carbohydrate to yield energy. Glucose is a nearly universal and accessible source of energy. Many organisms also have the ability to metabolize other monosaccharides and disaccharides but glucose is often metabolized first. In *Escherichia coli*, for example, the lac operon will express enzymes for the digestion of lactose when it is present, but if both lactose and glucose are present the *lac* operon is repressed, resulting in the glucose being used first. Polysaccharides are also common sources of energy. Many organisms can easily break down starches into glucose; most organisms, however, cannot metabolize cellulose or other polysaccharides like chitin and arabinoxylans. These carbohydrate types can be metabolized by some bacteria and protists. Ruminants and termites, for example, use microorganisms to process cellulose. Even though these complex carbohydrates are not very digestible, they represent an important dietary element for humans, called dietary fiber. Fiber enhances digestion, among other benefits.

Based on the effects on risk of heart disease and obesity, the Institute of Medicine recommends that American and Canadian adults get between 45–65% of dietary energy from carbohydrates.

The Food and Agriculture Organization and World Health Organization jointly recommend that national dietary guidelines set a goal of 55–75% of total energy from carbohydrates, but only 10% directly from sugars (their term for simple carbohydrates).

Classification

Nutritionists often refer to carbohydrates as either simple or complex. However, the exact distinction between these groups can be ambiguous. The term *complex carbohydrate* was first used in the U.S. Senate Select Committee on Nutrition and Human Needs publication *Dietary Goals for the United States* (1977) where it was intended to distinguish sugars from other carbohydrates (which were perceived to be nutritionally superior). However, the report put "fruit, vegetables and whole-grains" in the complex carbohydrate column, despite the fact that these may contain sugars as well as polysaccharides. This confusion persists as today some nutritionists use the term complex carbohydrate to refer to any sort of digestible saccharide present in a whole food, where fiber, vitamins and minerals are also found (as opposed to processed carbohydrates, which provide energy but few other nutrients). The standard usage, however, is to classify carbohydrates chemically: simple if they are sugars (monosaccharides and disaccharides) and complex if they are polysaccharides (or oligosaccharides).

In any case, the simple vs. complex chemical distinction has little value for determining the nutritional quality of carbohydrates. Some simple carbohydrates (e.g. fructose) raise blood glucose slowly, while some complex carbohydrates (starches), especially if processed, raise blood sugar rapidly. The speed of digestion is determined by a variety of factors including which other nutrients are consumed with the carbohydrate, how the food is prepared, individual differences in metabolism, and the chemistry of the carbohydrate.

The USDA's *Dietary Guidelines for Americans 2010* call for moderate- to high-carbohydrate consumption from a balanced diet that includes six one-ounce servings of grain foods each day, at least half from whole grain sources and the rest from enriched.

The glycemic index (GI) and glycemic load concepts have been developed to characterize food behavior during human digestion. They rank carbohydrate-rich foods based on the rapidity and magnitude of their effect on blood glucose levels. Glycemic index is a measure of how quickly food glucose is absorbed, while glycemic load is a measure of the total absorbable glucose in foods. The insulin index is a similar, more recent classification method that ranks foods based on their effects on blood insulin levels, which are caused by glucose (or starch) and some amino acids in food.

Metabolism

Carbohydrate metabolism denotes the various biochemical processes responsible for the formation, breakdown and interconversion of carbohydrates in living organisms.

The most important carbohydrate is glucose, a simple sugar (monosaccharide) that is metabolized by nearly all known organisms. Glucose and other carbohydrates are part of a wide variety of metabolic pathways across species: plants synthesize carbohydrates from carbon dioxide and water by photosynthesis storing the absorbed energy internally, often in the form of starch or lipids. Plant components are consumed by animals and fungi, and used as fuel for cellular respiration. Oxidation of one gram of carbohydrate yields approximately 4 kcal of energy, while the oxidation of one gram of lipids yields about 9 kcal. Energy obtained from metabolism (e.g., oxidation of glucose) is usually stored temporarily within cells in the form of ATP. Organisms capable of aerobic respiration metabolize glucose and oxygen to release energy with carbon dioxide and water as byproducts.

Catabolism

Catabolism is the metabolic reaction which cells undergo to extract energy. There are two major metabolic pathways of monosaccharide catabolism: glycolysis and the citric acid cycle.

In glycolysis, oligo/polysaccharides are cleaved first to smaller monosaccharides by enzymes called glycoside hydrolases. The monosaccharide units can then enter into monosaccharide catabolism. In some cases, as with humans, not all carbohydrate types are usable as the digestive and metabolic enzymes necessary are not present.

Carbohydrate Chemistry

Carbohydrate chemistry is a large and economically important branch of organic chemistry. Some of the main organic reactions that involve carbohydrates are:

- Carbohydrate acetalisation
- Cyanohydrin reaction
- Lobry-de Bruyn-van Ekenstein transformation
- Amadori rearrangement
- Nef reaction
- Wohl degradation
- Koenigs–Knorr reaction
- Carbohydrate digestion

Fat

Fat is one of the three main macronutrients, along with carbohydrate and protein. Fats, also known as triglycerides, are esters of three fatty acid chains and the alcohol glycerol.

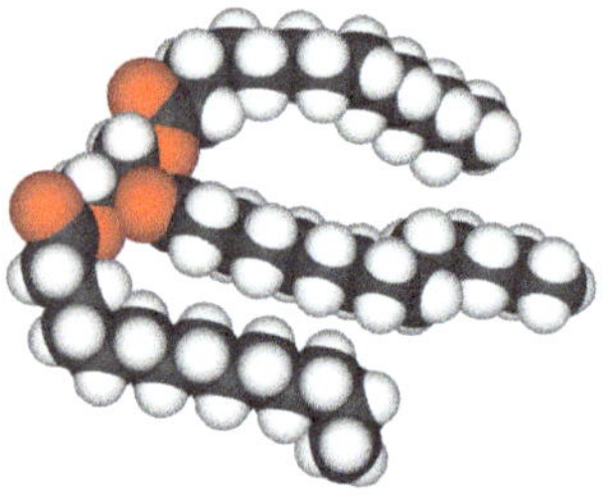

A fat, or triglyceride, molecule. Note the three fatty acid chains attached to the central glycerol portion of the molecule.

The terms “oil”, “fat”, and “lipid” are often confused. “Oil” normally refers to a fat with short or unsaturated fatty acid chains that is liquid at room temperature, while “fat” may specifically refer to fats that are solids at room temperature. “Lipid” is the general term, as a lipid is not necessarily a triglyceride. Fats, like other lipids, are generally hydrophobic, and are soluble in organic solvents and insoluble in water.

Fat is an important foodstuff for many forms of life, and fats serve both structural and metabolic functions. They are a necessary part of the diet of most heterotrophs (including humans). Some fatty acids that are set free by the digestion of fats are called essential because they cannot be synthesized in the body from simpler constituents. There are two essential fatty acids (EFAs) in human nutrition: alpha-linolenic acid (an omega-3 fatty acid) and linoleic acid (an omega-6 fatty acid). Other lipids needed by the body can be synthesized from these and other fats. Fats and other lipids are broken down in the body by enzymes called lipases produced in the pancreas.

Fats and oils are categorized according to the number and bonding of the carbon atoms in the aliphatic chain. Fats that are saturated fats have no double bonds between the carbons in the chain. Unsaturated fats have one or more double bonded carbons in the chain. The nomenclature is based on the non-acid (non-carbonyl) end of the chain. This end is called the omega end or the n-end. Thus alpha-linolenic acid is called an omega-3 fatty acid because the 3rd carbon from that end is the first double bonded carbon in the chain counting from that end. Some oils and fats have multiple double bonds and are therefore called polyunsaturated fats. Unsaturated fats can be further divided into cis fats, which are the most common in nature, and trans fats, which are rare in nature. Unsaturated fats can be altered by reaction with hydrogen effected by a catalyst. This action, called hydrogenation, tends to break all the double bonds and makes a fully saturated fat. To make vegetable shortening, then, liquid *cis*-unsaturated fats such as vegetable oils are hydrogenated to produce saturated fats, which have more desirable physical properties e.g., they melt at a desirable temperature (30–40 °C), and store well, whereas polyunsaturated oils go rancid when they react with oxygen in the air. However, trans fats are generated during hydrogenation as contaminants created by an unwanted side reaction on the catalyst during partial hydrogenation. Consumption of such trans fats has shown to increase the risk of coronary heart disease

Saturated fats can stack themselves in a closely packed arrangement, so they can solidify easily and are typically solid at room temperature. For example, animal fats tallow and lard are high in saturated fatty acid content and are solids. Olive and linseed oils on the other hand are unsaturated and liquid.

Fats serve both as energy sources for the body, and as stores for energy in excess of what the body needs immediately. Each gram of fat when burned or metabolized releases about 9 food calories (37 kJ = 8.8 kcal). Fats are broken down in the healthy body to release their constituents, glycerol and fatty acids. Glycerol itself can be converted to glucose by the liver and so become a source of energy.

Chemical Structure

There are many different kinds of fats, but each is a variation on the same chemical structure. All fats are derivatives of fatty acids and glycerol. Most fats are glycerides, particularly triglycerides (triesters of glycerol). One chain of fatty acid is bonded to each of the three -OH groups of the glycerol by the reaction of the carboxyl end of the fatty acid (-COOH) with the alcohol; I.e. three chains per molecule. Water is eliminated and the carbons are linked by an -O- bond through dehydration synthesis. This process is called esterification and fats are therefore esters. As a simple visual illustration, if the kinks and angles of these chains were straightened out, the molecule would have the shape of a capital letter E. The fatty acids would each be a horizontal line; the glycerol "backbone" would be the vertical line that joins the horizontal lines. Fats therefore have "ester" bonds.

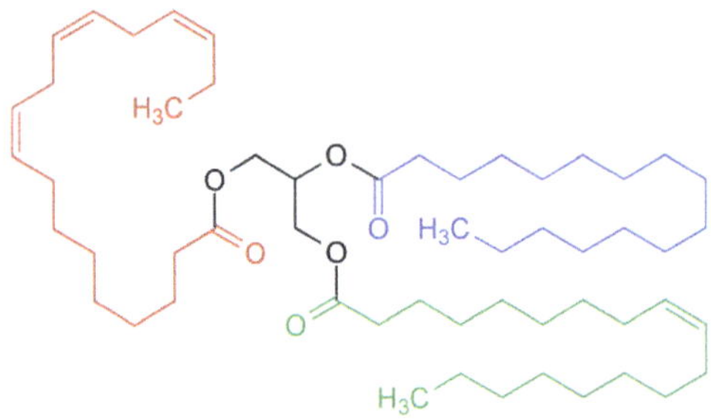

Example of a natural triglyceride with three different fatty acids. One fatty acids is saturated (blue highlighted), another contains one double bond within the carbon chain (green highlighted). The third fatty acid (a polyunsaturated fatty acid, highlighted in red) contains three double bonds within the carbon chain. All carbon-carbon double bonds shown are *cis* isomers.

The properties of any specific fat molecule depend on the particular fatty acids that constitute it. Fatty acids form a family of compounds are composed of increasing numbers of carbon atoms linked into a zig-zag chain (hydrogen atoms to the side). The more carbon atoms there are in any fatty acid, the longer its chain will be. Long chains are more susceptible to intermolecular forces of attraction (in this case, van der Waals forces), and so the longer ones melt at a higher temperature (melting point).

Examples of fatty acids.		
***trans* Unsaturated (Example shown: Elaidic acid)**	***cis* Unsaturated (Example shown: Oleic acid)**	**Saturated (Example shown: Stearic acid)**
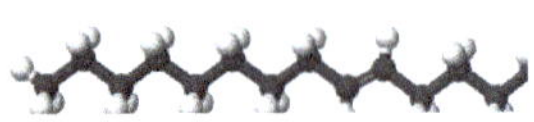	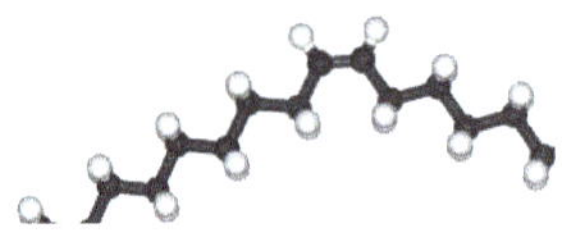	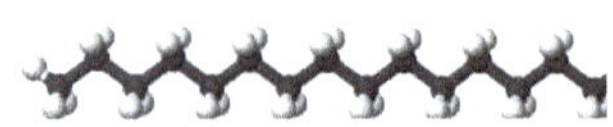
Elaidic acid is the principal *trans* unsaturated fatty acid often found in partially hydrogenated vegetable oils.	Oleic acid is a *cis* unsaturated fatty acid making up 55–80% of olive oil.	Stearic acid is a saturated fatty acid found in animal fats and is the intended product in full hydrogenation. Stearic acid is neither *cis* nor *trans* because it has no carbon-carbon double bonds.

Fatty acid chains may also differ by length, often categorized as short to very long.

- Short-chain fatty acids (SCFA) are fatty acids with aliphatic tails of fewer than six carbons (i.e. butyric acid).
- Medium-chain fatty acids (MCFA) are fatty acids with aliphatic tails of 6–12 carbons, which can form medium-chain triglycerides.
- Long-chain fatty acids (LCFA) are fatty acids with aliphatic tails 13 to 21 carbons.

- Very long chain fatty acids (VLCFA) are fatty acids with aliphatic tails longer than 22 carbons

Any of these aliphatic fatty acid chains may be glycerated and the resultant fats may have tails of different lengths from very short triformin to very long, e.g., cerotic acid, or *hexacosanoic acid*, a 26-carbon long-chain saturated fatty acid. Long chain fats are exemplified by tallow (lard) whose chains are 17 carbons long. Most fats found in food, whether vegetable or animal, are made up of medium to long-chain fatty acids, usually of equal or nearly equal length. Many cell types can use either glucose or fatty acids for this energy. In particular, heart and skeletal muscle prefer fatty acids. Despite long-standing assertions to the contrary, fatty acids can also be used as a source of fuel for brain cells.

Importance for Living Organisms

Fats are also sources of essential fatty acids, an important dietary requirement. They provide energy as noted above. Vitamins A, D, E, and K are fat-soluble, meaning they can only be digested, absorbed, and transported in conjunction with fats.

Fats play a vital role in maintaining healthy skin and hair, insulating body organs against shock, maintaining body temperature, and promoting healthy cell function.

Fat also serves as a useful buffer against a host of diseases. When a particular substance, whether chemical or biotic, reaches unsafe levels in the bloodstream, the body can effectively dilute—or at least maintain equilibrium of—the offending substances by storing it in new fat tissue. This helps to protect vital organs, until such time as the offending substances can be metabolized or removed from the body by such means as excretion, urination, accidental or intentional bloodletting, sebum excretion, and hair growth.

Adipose Tissue

In animals, adipose, or fatty tissue is the body's means of storing metabolic energy over extended periods of time. Adipocytes (fat cells) store fat derived from the diet and from liver metabolism. Under energy stress these cells may degrade their stored fat to supply fatty acids and also glycerol to the circulation. These metabolic activities are regulated by several hormones (e.g., insulin, glucagon and epinephrine).

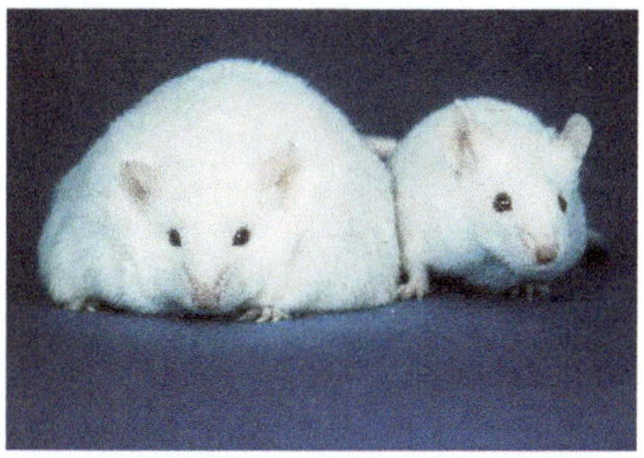

The obese mouse on the left has large stores of adipose tissue. For comparison, a mouse with a normal amount of adipose tissue is shown on the right.

The location of the tissue determines its metabolic profile: visceral fat is located within the abdominal wall (i.e., beneath the wall of abdominal muscle) whereas "subcutaneous fat" is located beneath the skin (and includes fat that is located in the abdominal area beneath the skin but *above* the abdominal muscle wall). Visceral fat was recently discovered to be a significant producer of signaling chemicals (i.e., hormones), among which several are involved in inflammatory tissue responses. One of these is resistin which has been linked to obesity, insulin resistance, and Type 2 diabetes. This latter result is currently controversial, and there have been reputable studies supporting all sides on the issue.

Protein (Nutrient)

Proteins are essential nutrients for the human body. They are one of the building blocks of body tissue, and can also serve as a fuel source. As a fuel, proteins provide as much energy density as carbohydrates: 4 kcal (17 kJ) per gram; in contrast, lipids provide 9 kcal (37 kJ) per gram. The most important aspect and defining characteristic of protein from a nutritional standpoint is its amino acid composition.

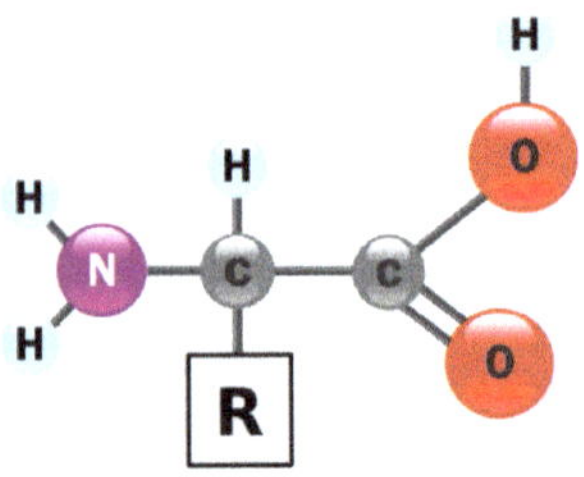

Amino acids are the building blocks of protein.

Proteins are polymer chains made of amino acids linked together by peptide bonds. During human digestion, proteins are broken down in the stomach to smaller polypeptide chains via hydrochloric acid and protease actions. This is crucial for the synthesis of the essential amino acids that cannot be biosynthesized by the body.

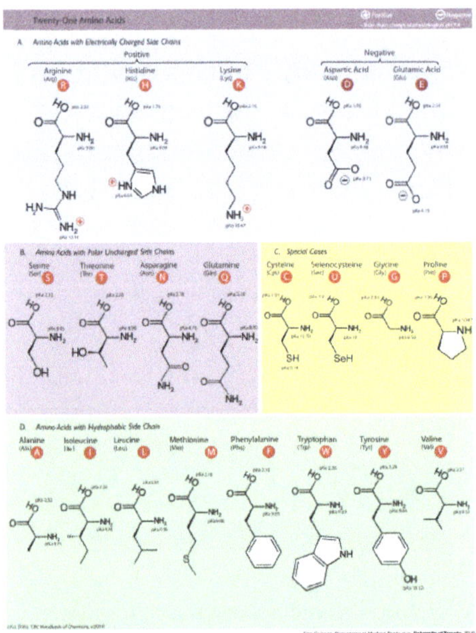

Amino acids are necessary nutrients. Present in every cell, they are also precursors to nucleic acids, co-enzymes, hormones, immune response, repair and other molecules essential for life.

There are nine essential amino acids which humans must obtain from their diet in order to prevent protein-energy malnutrition. They are phenylalanine, valine, threonine, tryptophan, methionine, leucine, isoleucine, lysine, and histidine. There are five dispensable amino acids which humans are able to synthesize in the body. These five are alanine, aspartic acid, asparagine, glutamic acid and serine. There are six conditionally essential amino acids whose synthesis can be limited under special pathophysiological conditions, such as prematurity in the infant or individuals in severe catabolic distress. These six are arginine, cysteine, glycine, glutamine, proline and tyrosine.

Humans need the essential amino acids in certain ratios. Some protein sources contain amino acids in a more or less 'complete' sense. This has given rise to various ranking systems for protein sources, as described in the article.

Sources of protein include grains, legumes and nuts, as well as animal sources such as meats, dairy products, fish and eggs. Vegetarians and vegans can get enough essential amino acids by eating a variety of plant proteins. It is commonly believed that athletes should consume a higher-than-normal protein intake to maintain optimal physical performance.

Protein Functions in Body

Protein is a nutrient needed by the human body for growth and maintenance. Aside from water, proteins are the most abundant kind of molecules in the body. Protein can be found in all cells of the body and is the major structural component of all cells in the body, especially muscle. This also includes body organs, hair and skin. Proteins are also used in membranes, such as glycoproteins. When broken down into amino acids, they are used as precursors to nucleic acid, co-enzymes, hormones, immune response, cellular repair, and other molecules essential for life. Additionally, protein is needed to form blood cells.

Protein Function in Exercise

Proteins are believed to increase performance in terms of athletics. Amino acids, the building blocks of proteins, are used for building muscle tissue and repairing damaged tissues. Protein is only used as anaerobic fuel when carbohydrates are low, or as aerobic fuel when lipid resources are also low.

Sources

Protein can be found in a wide range of food. The best combination of protein sources depends on the region of the world, access, cost, amino acid types and nutrition balance, as well as acquired tastes. Some foods are high in certain amino acids, but their digestibility and the anti-nutritional factors present in these foods make them of limited value in human nutrition. Therefore, one must consider digestibility and secondary nutrition profile such as calories, cholesterol, vitamins and essential mineral density of the protein source. On a worldwide basis, plant protein foods contribute over 60 percent of the per capita supply of protein, on average. In North America, animal-derived foods contribute about 70 percent of protein sources.

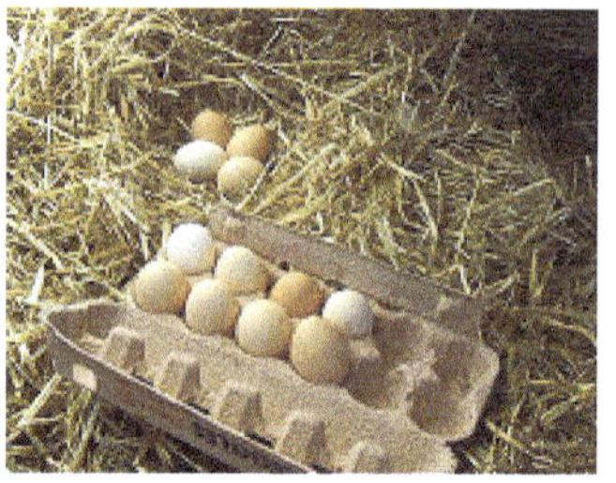

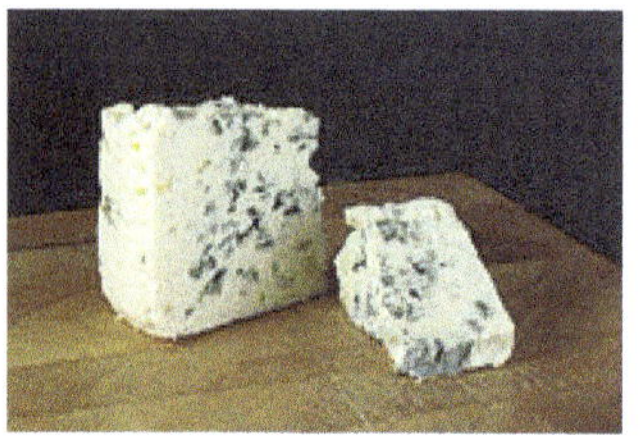

Animal sources of protein.

Meat, products from milk, eggs, soy, and fish are sources of complete protein.

Whole grains and cereals are another source of proteins. However, these tend to be limiting in the amino acid lysine or threonine, which are available in other vegetarian sources and meats. Examples of food staples and cereal sources of protein, each with a concentration greater than 7 percent, are (in no particular order) buckwheat, oats, rye, millet, maize (corn), rice, wheat, bulgar, sorghum, amaranth, and quinoa.

Vegetarian sources of proteins include legumes, nuts, seeds and fruits. Legumes, some of which are called pulses in certain parts of the world, have higher concentrations of amino acids and are more complete sources of protein than whole grains and cereals. Examples of vegetarian foods with protein concentrations greater than 7 percent include soybeans, lentils, kidney beans, white beans, mung beans, chickpeas, cowpeas, lima beans, pigeon peas, lupines, wing beans, almonds, Brazil nuts, cashews, pecans, walnuts, cotton seeds, pumpkin seeds, hemp seeds, sesame seeds, and sunflower seeds.

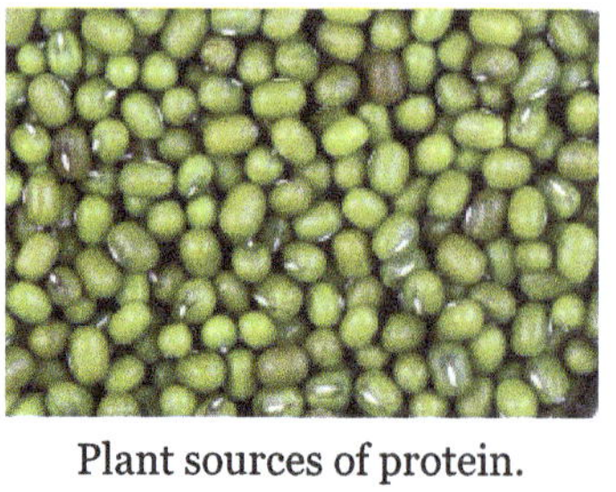

Plant sources of protein.

Food staples that are poor sources of protein include roots and tubers such as yams, cassava and sweet potato. Plantains, another major staple, are also a poor source of essential amino acids. Fruits, while rich in other essential nutrients, are another poor source of amino acids. The protein content in roots, tubers and fruits is between 0 and 2 percent. Food staples with low protein content must be complemented with foods with complete, quality protein content for a healthy life, particularly in children for proper development.

A good source of protein is often a combination of various foods, because different foods are rich in different amino acids. A good source of dietary protein meets two requirements:

- The requirement for the nutritionally indispensable amino acids (histidine, isoleucine, leucine, lysine, methionine, phenylalanine, threonine, tryptophan, and valine) under all conditions and for conditionally indispensable amino acids (cystine, tyrosine, taurine, glycine, arginine, glutamine, proline) under specific physiological and pathological conditions
- The requirement for nonspecific nitrogen for the synthesis of the nutritionally dispensable amino acids (aspartic acid, asparagine, glutamic acid, alanine, serine) and other physiologically important nitrogen-containing compounds such as nucleic acids, creatine, and porphyrins.

Healthy people eating a balanced diet rarely need protein supplements. Except for a few amino acids, most are readily available in human diet. The limiting amino acids are lysine, threonine, tryptophan and sulfur-containing amino acids.

The table below presents the most important food groups as protein sources, from a worldwide perspective. It also lists their respective performance as source of the commonly limiting amino acids, in milligrams of limiting amino acid per gram of total protein in the food source. The table reiterates the need for a balanced mix of foods to ensure adequate amino acid source.

Food source	**Lysine**	**Threonine**	**Tryptophan**	**Sulfur-containing amino acids**
Legumes	64	38	12	25
Cereals and whole grains	31	32	12	37
Nuts and seeds	45	36	17	46
Fruits	45	29	11	27
Animal	85	44	12	38
Protein source with highest density of respective amino acid.				
Protein source with lowest density of respective amino acid.				

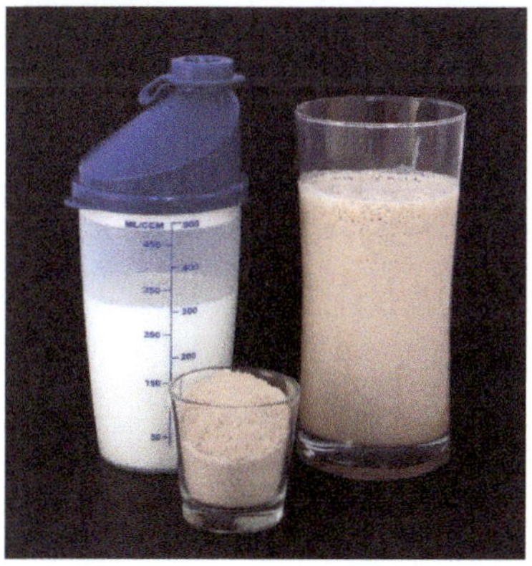

Protein milkshakes, made from protein powder (center) and milk (left), are a common bodybuilding supplement.

Protein powders – such as casein, whey, egg, rice and soy – are processed and manufactured sources of protein. These protein powders may provide an additional source of protein for bodybuilders. The type of protein is important in terms of its influence on protein metabolic response and possibly on the muscle's exercise performance. The different physical and/or chemical properties within the various types of protein may affect the rate of protein digestion. As a result, the amino acid availability and the accumulation of tissue protein is altered because of the various protein metabolic responses.

Protein Quality

The most important aspect and defining characteristic of protein from a nutritional standpoint is its amino acid composition. There are multiple systems which rate proteins by their usefulness to an organism based on their relative percentage of amino acids and, in some systems, the digestibility of the protein source. They include biological value, net protein utilization, and PDCAAS (Protein Digestibility Corrected Amino Acids Score). Also see complete protein, nitrogen balance and protein combining. The PDCAAS was developed by the FDA as an improvement over the Protein efficiency ratio (PER) method. The PDCAAS rating is a fairly recent evaluation method; it was adopted by the US Food and Drug Administration (FDA) and the Food and Agricultural Organization of the United Nations/World Health Organization (FAO/WHO) in 1993 as "the preferred 'best'" method to determine protein quality. These organizations have suggested that other methods for evaluating the quality of protein are inferior.

Digestion

Most proteins are decomposed to single amino acids by digestion in the gastro-intestinal tract.

Digestion typically begins in the stomach when pepsinogen is converted to pepsin by the action of hydrochloric acid, and continued by trypsin and chymotrypsin in the small intestine. Before the absorption in the small intestine, most proteins are already reduced to single amino acid or peptides of several amino acids. Most peptides longer than four amino acids are not absorbed. Absorption into the intestinal absorptive cells is not the end. There, most of the peptides are broken into single amino acids.

Absorption of the amino acids and their derivatives into which dietary protein is degraded is done by the gastrointestinal tract. The absorption rates of individual amino acids are highly dependent on the protein source; for example, the digestibilities of many amino acids in humans, the difference between soy and milk proteins and between individual milk proteins, beta-lactoglobulin and casein. For milk proteins, about 50% of the ingested protein is absorbed between the stomach and the jejunum and 90% is absorbed by the time the digested food reaches the ileum. Biological value (BV) is a measure of the proportion of absorbed protein from a food which becomes incorporated into the proteins of the organism's body.

Newborn

Newborns of mammals are exceptional in protein digestion and assimilation in that they can absorb intact proteins at the small intestine. This enables passive immunity from milk.

Dietary Requirements

An education campaign launched by the United States Department of Agriculture about 100 years ago, on cottage cheese as a lower-cost protein substitute for meat.

Considerable debate has taken place regarding issues surrounding protein intake requirements. The amount of protein required in a person's diet is determined in large part by overall energy intake, the body's need for nitrogen and essential amino acids, body weight and composition, rate of growth in the individual, physical activity level, individual's energy and carbohydrate intake, as well as the presence of illness or injury. Physical activity and exertion as well as enhanced muscular mass increase the need for protein. Requirements are also greater during childhood for growth and development, during pregnancy or when breast-feeding in order to nourish a baby, or when the body needs to recover from malnutrition or trauma or after an operation.

If not enough energy is taken in through diet, as in the process of starvation, the body will use protein from the muscle mass to meet its energy needs, leading to muscle wasting over time. If the individual does not consume adequate protein in nutrition, then muscle will also waste as more vital cellular processes (e.g. respiration enzymes, blood cells) recycle muscle protein for their own requirements.

According to US & Canadian Dietary Reference Intake guidelines, women aged 19–70 need to consume 46 grams of protein per day, while men aged 19–70 need to consume 56 grams of protein per day to avoid a deficiency. The generally accepted daily protein dietary allowance, measured as intake per kilogram of body weight, is 0.8 g/kg. However, this recommendation is based on structural requirements, but disregards use of protein for energy metabolism. This requirement is for a normal sedentary person.

Active People

Several studies have concluded that active people and athletes may require elevated protein intake (compared to 0.8 g/kg) due to increase in muscle mass and sweat losses, as well as need for body repair and energy source. Suggested amounts vary between 1.6 g/kg and 1.8 g/kg, while a proposed *maximum* daily protein intake would be approximately 25% of energy requirements i.e. approximately 2 to 2.5 g/kg. However, many questions still remain to be resolved.

In addition, some have suggested that athletes using restricted-calorie diets for weight loss should further increase their protein consumption, possibly to 1.8–2.0 g/kg, in order to avoid loss of lean muscle mass.

Aerobic Exercise Protein Needs

Endurance athletes differ from strength-building athletes in that endurance athletes do not build muscle mass from training. Research suggests that individuals performing endurance activity require more protein intake than sedentary individuals so that muscles broken down during endurance workouts can be repaired. Although the protein requirement for athletes still remains controversial, research does show that endurance athletes can benefit from increasing protein intake because the type of exercise endurance athletes participate in still alters the protein metabolism pathway. The overall protein requirement increases because of amino acid oxidation in endurance-trained athletes. Endurance athletes who exercise over a long period (2–5 hours per training session) use protein as a source of 5–10% of their total energy expended. Therefore, a slight increase in protein intake may be beneficial to endurance athletes by replacing the protein lost in energy expenditure and protein lost in repairing muscles. Some scientists suggest that endurance athletes may increase daily protein intake to a maximum of 1.2–1.4 g per kg body weight.

Anaerobic Exercise Protein Needs

Research also indicates that individuals performing strength-training activity require more protein than sedentary individuals. Strength-training athletes may increase their daily protein intake to a maximum of 1.4–1.8 g per kg body weight to enhance muscle protein synthesis, or to make up for the loss of amino acid oxidation during exercise. Many athletes maintain a high-protein diet as part of their training, and so protein deficiency is less likely among this group than among non-athletes. In fact, some athletes who specialize in anaerobic sports (e.g., weightlifting) assume a very high level of protein intake is necessary, and may over-consume. Research indicates that many athletes consume more protein than they need even without the use of protein supplements.

Special Populations

Phenylketonuria

Individuals with phenylketonuria (PKU) must keep their intake of phenylalanine extremely low to prevent a mental disability and other metabolic complications.

Maple Syrup Urine Disease

Maple syrup urine disease is associated with genetic anomalies in the metabolism of branched-chain amino acids (BCAAs). They have high blood levels of BCAAs and must severely restrict their intake of BCAAs in order to prevent mental retardation and death.

Excess Consumption

Research indicates that a high protein diet is carcinogenic, and that the cancer risk is somewhat decreased if it's non-animal protein. When a high dietary protein intake is consumed, there is an increase in urea excretion, which suggests that amino acid oxidation is increased.High levels of protein intake increase the activity of branched-chain ketoacid dehydrogenase. As a result, oxidation is facilitated, and the amino group of the amino acid is excreted to the liver. This process suggests that excess protein consumption results in protein oxidation and that the protein is excreted. The body is unable to store excess protein. Protein is digested into amino acids, which enter the bloodstream. Excess amino acids are converted to other usable molecules by the liver in a process called deamination. Deamination converts nitrogen from the amino acid into ammonia, which is converted by the liver into urea in the urea cycle. Excretion of urea is performed by the kidneys. These organs can normally cope with any extra workload, but, if kidney disease occurs, a decrease in protein will often be prescribed. When there is excess protein intake, amino acids can be converted to glucose or ketones, in addition to being oxidized for fuel. When food protein intake is periodically high or low, the body tries to keep protein levels at an equilibrium by using the "labile protein reserve", which serves as a short-term protein store to be used for emergencies or daily variations in protein intake. However, that reserve is not utilized as longer-term storage for future needs.

Many researchers have also found that excessive intake of protein increases calcium excretion in urine. It has been thought that this occurs to maintain the pH imbalance from the oxidation of sulfur amino acids. Also, it is inconclusive whether bone resorption contributes to bone loss and osteoporosis. However, it is also found that a regular intake of calcium would be able to stabilize this loss.

Another issue arising from over-consumption of protein is a higher risk of kidney stone formation from calcium in the renal circulatory system. It has been found that high animal protein intake in healthy individuals increases the probability of forming kidney stones by 250 percent.

An epidemiological study from 2006 has found no relationship between total protein intake and blood pressure; it did, however, find an inverse relationship between vegetable protein intake and blood pressure.

Saying they eat too much protein, the *2015–2020 Dietary Guidelines for Americans* asked men and teenage boys to increase their consumption of vegetables or other underconsumed foods.

Testing in Foods

The classic assays for protein concentration in food are the Kjeldahl method and the Dumas method. These tests determine the total nitrogen in a sample. The only major component of most food which contains nitrogen is protein (fat, carbohydrate and dietary fibre do not contain nitrogen). If the amount of nitrogen is multiplied by a factor depending on the kinds of protein expected in the food the total protein can be determined. This value is known as the "crude protein" content. On food labels the protein is given by the nitrogen multiplied by 6.25, because the average nitrogen content of proteins is about 16%. The Kjeldahl test is typically used because it is the method the AOAC International has adopted and is therefore used by many food standards agencies around the world, though the Dumas method is also approved by some standards organizations.

Accidental contamination and intentional adulteration of protein meals with non-protein nitrogen sources that inflate crude protein content measurements have been known to occur in the food industry for decades. To ensure food quality, purchasers of protein meals routinely conduct quality control tests designed to detect the most common non-protein nitrogen contaminants, such as urea and ammonium nitrate.

In at least one segment of the food industry, the dairy industry, some countries (at least the U.S., Australia, France and Hungary), have adopted "true protein" measurement, as opposed to crude protein measurement, as the standard for payment and testing: "True protein is a measure of only the proteins in milk, whereas crude protein is a measure of all sources of nitrogen and includes nonprotein nitrogen, such as urea, which has no food value to humans. ... Current milk-testing equipment measures peptide bonds, a direct measure of true protein." Measuring peptide bonds in grains has also been put into practice in several countries including Canada, the UK, Australia, Russia and Argentina where near-infrared reflectance (NIR) technology, a type of infrared spectroscopy is used. The Food and Agriculture Organization of the United Nations (FAO) recommends that only amino acid analysis be used to determine protein in, *inter alia*, foods used as the sole source of nourishment, such as infant formula, but also provides: "When data on amino acids analyses are not available, determination of protein based on total N content by Kjeldahl (AOAC, 2000) or similar method ... is considered acceptable."

The limitations of the Kjeldahl method were at the heart of the Chinese protein export contamination in 2007 and the 2008 China milk scandal in which the industrial chemical melamine was added to the milk or glutens to increase the measured "protein".

Protein Deficiency

Protein deficiency and malnutrition can lead to variety of ailments including mental retardation and kwashiorkor. Symptoms of kwashiorkor include apathy, diarrhea, inactivity, failure to grow, flaky skin, fatty liver, and edema of the belly and legs. This edema is explained by the action of lipoxygenase on arachidonic acid to form leukotrienes and the normal functioning of proteins in fluid balance and lipoprotein transport.

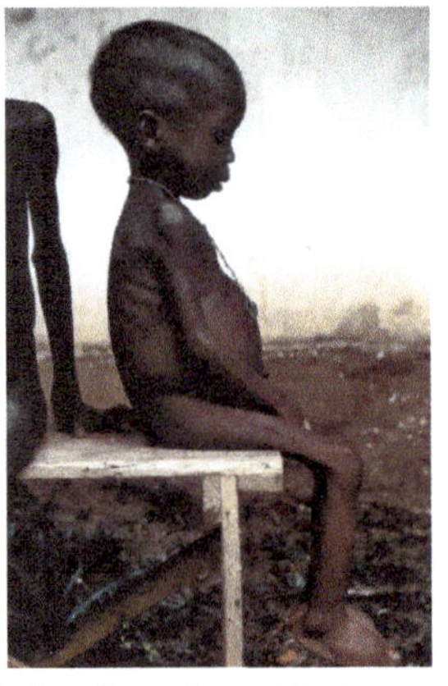

A child in Nigeria during the Biafra War suffering from kwashiorkor – one of the three protein energy malnutrition ailments afflicting over 10 million children in developing countries.

PEM is fairly common worldwide in both children and adults and accounts for 6 million deaths annually. In the industrialized world, PEM is predominantly seen in hospitals, is associated with disease, or is often found in the elderly.

Mineral (Nutrient)

A mineral is a chemical element required as an essential nutrient by organisms, other than carbon, hydrogen, nitrogen, oxygen and sulfur present in common organic molecules. These elements are classed as *minerals* in the four groups of essential nutrients; the others are vitamins, essential fatty acids, and essential amino acids.

Major chemical elements in order of abundance in the human body include calcium, phosphorus, potassium, sodium, chlorine, and magnesium. Important trace elements, necessary for mammalian life, include iron, cobalt, copper, zinc, manganese, molybdenum, iodine, and selenium. Because inorganic mineral content of foods do not form volatile combustion products, nutrition analysis methods involving combustion may report the total mineral content of food as "crude ash".

Over twenty minerals are necessary for mammals, and several more for various other types of life. The total number of chemical elements that are absolutely needed is not known for any organism. Ultratrace elements of some minerals such as boron and chromium are known to clearly have a role but the exact biochemical nature is unknown, and others such as arsenic, bromine, and silicon are suspected to have a role in health, but with weaker evidence.

Most chemical elements that are ingested by organisms are in the form of simple compounds. Larger chemical compounds of elements need to be broken down for absorption. Plants absorb dissolved elements in soils, which are subsequently picked up by the herbivores that eat them, and the elements move up the food chain. Larger organisms may also consume soil (geophagia) and visit salt licks to obtain limiting minerals they are unable to acquire through other components of their diet.

Bacteria play an essential role in the weathering of primary elements that results in the release of nutrients for their own nutrition and for the nutrition of others in the ecological food chain. One element, cobalt, is available for use by animals only after having been processed into complex molecules (e.g., vitamin B12) by bacteria. Scientists are only recently starting to appreciate the magnitude and role that microorganisms have in the global cycling and formation of biominerals.

Essential Chemical Elements for Humans

At least twenty chemical elements are known to be *required* to support human biochemical processes by serving structural and functional roles as well as electrolytes. However, as many as twenty-nine elements in total (including the common hydrogen, carbon, nitrogen and oxygen) are suggested to be used by mammals, as a result of studies of biochemical, special uptake, and metabolic handling studies. However, many of these additional elements have no well-defined biochemical function known at present. Most of the known and suggested mineral nutrients are of relatively low atomic weight, and are reasonably common on land, or at least, common in the ocean (iodine, sodium):

Nutritional elements in the periodic table																		
H																		He
Li	Be												B	C	N	O	F	Ne
Na	Mg												Al	Si	P	S	Cl	Ar
K	Ca	Sc		Ti	V	Cr	Mn	Fe	Co	Ni	Cu	Zn	Ga	Ge	As	Se	Br	Kr
Rb	Sr	Y		Zr	Nb	Mo	Tc	Ru	Rh	Pd	Ag	Cd	In	Sn	Sb	Te	I	Xe
Cs	Ba	La	*	Hf	Ta	W	Re	Os	Ir	Pt	Au	Hg	Tl	Pb	Bi	Po	At	Rn
Fr	Ra	Ac	**	Rf	Db	Sg	Bh	Hs	Mt	Ds	Rg	Cn	Uut	Fl	Uup	Lv	Uus	Uuo
			*	Ce	Pr	Nd	Pm	Sm	Eu	Gd	Tb	Dy	Ho	Er	Tm	Yb	Lu	
			**	Th	Pa	U	Np	Pu	Am	Cm	Bk	Cf	Es	Fm	Md	No	Lr	

The four organic basic elements
Quantity elements
Essential trace elements
Suggested function from deprivation effects or active metabolic handling, but no clearly-identified biochemical function in humans
Limited circumstantial evidence for trace benefits or biological action in mammals

The following play important roles in biological processes:

DV = Daily Value (formerly Recommended Daily Allowance); UL = Tolerable Upper Intake Level

(figures shown are for adults age 31-50, male or female neither pregnant nor lactating)

Dietary element	DV	UL	Amount	Category	High nutrient density dietary sources	Insufficiency	Excess
Potassium	3500	NE	Quantity	A systemic electrolyte and is essential in coregulating ATP with sodium	Sweetpotato, tomato, potato, beans, lentils, dairy products, seafood, banana, prune, carrot, orange	hypo kalemia	hyper kalemia
Chlorine	3400	3600	Quantity	Needed for production of hydrochloric acid in the stomach and in cellular pump functions	Table salt (sodium chloride) is the main dietary source.	hypo chloremia	hyper chloremia
Sodium	2400	2300	Quantity	A systemic electrolyte and is essential in coregulating ATP with potassium	Table salt (sodium chloride, the main source), sea vegetables, milk, and spinach.	hypo natremia	hypernatremia
Calcium	1000	2500	Quantity	Needed for muscle, heart and digestive system health, builds bone, supports synthesis and function of blood cells	Dairy products, eggs, canned fish with bones (salmon, sardines), green leafy vegetables, nuts, seeds, tofu, thyme, oregano, dill, cinnamon.	hypo calcaemia	hypercalcaemia
Phosphorus	1000	4000	Quantity	A component of bones, cells, in energy processing, in DNA and ATP (as phosphate) and many other functions	Red meat, dairy foods, fish, poultry, bread, rice, oats. In biological contexts, usually seen as phosphate	hypophos phatemia	hyper phosphatemia
Magnesium	400	350	Quantity	Required for processing ATP and for bones	Spinach, legumes, nuts, seeds, whole grains, peanut butter, avocado	hypomagnesemia, magnesium deficiency	hyper magnesemia

Dietary element	DV	UL	Amount	Category	High nutrient density dietary sources	Insufficiency	Excess
Iron	18	45	Trace	Required for many proteins and enzymes, notably hemoglobin to prevent anemia	Meat, seafood, nuts, beans, dark chocolate	iron deficiency	iron overload disorder
Zinc	15	40	Trace	Pervasive and required for several enzymes such as carboxypeptidase, liver alcohol dehydrogenase, and carbonic anhydrase	Oysters*, red meat, poultry, nuts, whole grains, dairy products	zinc deficiency	zinc toxicity
Manganese	2	350	Trace	A cofactor in enzyme functions	Grains, legumes, seeds, nuts, leafy vegetables, tea, coffee	manganese deficiency	manganism
Copper	2	11	Trace	Required component of many redox enzymes, including cytochrome c oxidase	Liver, seafood, oysters, nuts, seeds; some: whole grains, legumes	copper deficiency	copper toxicity
Iodine	0.150	1.1	Trace	Required for synthesis of thyroid hormones, thyroxine and triiodothyronine and to prevent goiter: • Iodine in biology	Seaweed (kelp or kombu)*, grains, eggs, iodized salt	iodine deficiency	iodism Hyper thyroidism
Chromium	0.120	NE	Trace	Involved in glucose and lipid metabolism, although its mechanisms of action in the body and the amounts needed for optimal health are not well defined	Broccoli, grape juice (especially red), meat, whole grain products	Chromium deficiency	Chromium toxicity
Molybdenum	0.075	2	Trace	The oxidases xanthine oxidase, aldehyde oxidase, and sulfite oxidase	Legumes, whole grains, nuts	molybdenum deficiency	molybdenum toxicity
Selenium	0.070	0.4	Trace	Essential to activity of antioxidant enzymes like glutathione peroxidase	Brazil nuts, seafoods, organ meats, meats, grains, dairy products, eggs	selenium deficiency	selenosis

Dietary element	DV	UL	Amount	Category	High nutrient density dietary sources	Insufficiency	Excess
Cobalt	none	NE	Trace	Required in the synthesis of vitamin B_{12}, but because bacteria are required to synthesize the vitamin, it is usually considered part of vitamin B_{12}			Cobalt poisoning

* One serving exceeds UL (tolerable upper intake level).

Blood Concentrations of Minerals

Minerals are present in a healthy human being's blood at certain mass and molar concentrations. The figure below presents the concentrations of each of the chemical elements discussed in this article, from center-right to the right. Depending on the concentrations, some are in upper part of the picture, while others are in the lower part. The figure includes the relative values of other constituents of blood such as hormones. In the figure, minerals are color highlighted in purple.

Dietary Nutrition

Dietitians may recommend that minerals are best supplied by ingesting specific foods rich with the chemical element(s) of interest. The elements may be naturally present in the food (e.g., calcium in dairy milk) or added to the food (e.g., orange juice fortified with calcium; iodized salt, salt fortified with iodine). Dietary supplements can be formulated to contain several different chemical elements (as compounds), a combination of vitamins and/or other chemical compounds, or a single element (as a compound or mixture of compounds), such as calcium (as calcium carbonate, calcium citrate, etc.) or magnesium (as magnesium oxide, etc.), chromium (usually as chromium(III) picolinate), or iron (as iron bis-glycinate).

The dietary focus on chemical elements derives from an interest in supporting the biochemical reactions of metabolism with the required elemental components. Appropriate intake levels of certain chemical elements have been demonstrated to be required to maintain optimal health. Diet can meet all the body's chemical element requirements, although supplements can be used when some requirements (e.g., calcium, which is found mainly in dairy products) are not adequately met by the diet, or when chronic or acute deficiencies arise from pathology, injury, etc. Research has supported that altering inorganic mineral compounds (carbonates, oxides, etc.) by reacting them with organic ligands (amino acids, organic acids, etc.) improves the bioavailability of the supplemented mineral.

Typical Maximum Nutrient Losses due to cooking					
Vitamin & Minerals	**Freeze**	**Dry**	**Cook**	**Cook+Drain**	**Reheat**
Vitamin A	5%	50%	25%	35%	10%
Vit A- Retinol Activity Equivalent	5%	50%	25%	35%	10%

Typical Maximum Nutrient Losses due to cooking					
Vitamin & Minerals	**Freeze**	**Dry**	**Cook**	**Cook+Drain**	**Reheat**
Vit A- Alpha Carotene	5%	50%	25%	35%	10%
Vit A- Beta Carotene	5%	50%	25%	35%	10%
Vit A- Beta Cryptoxanthin	5%	50%	25%	35%	10%
Vit A- Lycopene	5%	50%	25%	35%	10%
Vit A- Lutein+Zeaxanthin	5%	50%	25%	35%	10%
Vitamin C	30%	80%	50%	75%	50%
Thiamin	5%	30%	55%	70%	40%
Riboflavin	0%	10%	25%	45%	5%
Niacin	0%	10%	40%	55%	5%
Vitamin B6	0%	10%	50%	65%	45%
Folate	5%	50%	70%	75%	30%
Food Folate	5%	50%	70%	75%	30%
Folic Acid	5%	50%	70%	75%	30%
Vitamin B12	0%	0%	45%	50%	45%
Calcium	5%	0%	20%	25%	0%
Iron	0%	0%	35%	40%	0%
Magnesium	0%	0%	25%	40%	0%
Phosphorus	0%	0%	25%	35%	0%
Potassium	10%	0%	30%	70%	0%
Sodium	0%	0%	25%	55%	0%
Zinc	0%	0%	25%	25%	0%
Copper	10%	0%	40%	45%	0%

Elements Considered Possibly Essential but Not Confirmed

Many ultratrace elements have been suggested as essential, but such claims have usually not been confirmed. Definitive evidence for efficacy comes from the characterization of a biomolecule containing the element with an identifiable and testable function. One problem with identifying efficacy is that some elements are innocuous at low concentrations and are pervasive (examples: silicon and nickel in solid and dust), so proof of efficacy is lacking because deficiencies are difficult to reproduce.

Element	Description	Excess
Bromine	Possibly important to basement membrane architecture and tissue development.	bromism
Arsenic	Essential in rat, hamster, goat and chicken models, but no biochemical mechanism known in humans.	arsenic poisoning
Nickel	Nickel is an essential component of several enzymes, including urease and hydrogenase. Although not required by humans, some are thought to be required by gut bacteria, such as urease required by some varieties of Bifidobacterium. In humans, nickel may be a cofactor or structural component of certain metalloenzymes involved in hydrolysis, redox rections, and gene expression. Nickel deficiency depressed growth in goats, pigs, and sheep, and diminished circulating thyroid hormone concentration in rats.	Nickel toxicity

Fluorine	Fluorine (as fluoride) is not generally considered an essential element because humans do not require it for growth or to sustain life. However, if one considers the prevention of dental cavities an important criterion in determining essentiality, then fluoride might well be considered an essential trace element. However, recent research indicates that the primary action of fluoride occurs topically (at the surface).	Fluoride poisoning
Boron	Boron is an essential plant nutrient, required primarily for maintaining the integrity of cell walls. Boron has been shown to be essential to complete the life cycle in representatives of all phylogenetic kingdoms, including the model species danio rerio (zebrafish) and Xenopus laevis (African clawed frog). In animals, supplemental boron has been shown to reduce calcium excretion and activate vitamin D.	Nontoxic
Lithium	It is not known whether lithium has a physiological role in any species, but nutritional studies in mammals have indicated its importance to health, leading to a suggestion that it be classed as an essential trace element.	Lithium toxicity
Strontium	Strontium has been found to be involved in the utilization of calcium in the body. It has promoting action on calcium uptake into bone at moderate dietary strontium levels, but a rachitogenic (rickets-producing) action at higher dietary levels.	Rachitogenic (causing Rickets)
Other	Silicon and vanadium have established, albeit specialized, biochemical roles as structural or functional cofactors in other organisms, and are possibly, even probably, used by mammals (including humans). By contrast, tungsten and cadmium have specialized biochemical uses in certain lower organisms, but these elements appear not to be utilized by humans. Other elements considered to be possibly essential include aluminium, germanium, lead, rubidium, and tin.	Multiple

Mineral Ecology

Recent studies have shown a tight linkage between living organisms and chemical elements on this planet. This led to the redefinition of minerals as "an element or compound, amorphous or crystalline, formed through 'biogeochemical' processes. The addition of `bio' reflects a greater appreciation, although an incomplete understanding, of the processes of mineral formation by living forms." Biologists and geologists have only recently started to appreciate the magnitude of mineral biogeoengineering. Bacteria have contributed to the formation of minerals for billions of years and critically define the biogeochemical mineral cycles on this planet. Microorganisms can precipitate metals from solution contributing to the formation of ore deposits in addition to their ability to catalyze mineral dissolution, to respire, precipitate, and form minerals.

Most minerals are inorganic in nature. Mineral nutrients refers to the smaller class of minerals that are metabolized for growth, development, and vitality of living organisms. Mineral nutrients are recycled by bacteria that are freely suspended in the vast water columns of the worlds oceans. They absorb dissolved organic matter containing mineral nutrients as they scavenge through the dying individuals that fall out of large phytoplankton blooms. Flagellates are effective bacteriovores and are also commonly found in the marine water column. The flagellates are preyed upon by zooplankton while the phytoplankton concentrates on the larger particulate matter that is suspended in the water column as they are consumed by larger zooplankton, with fish as the top predator. Mineral nutrients cycle through this marine food chain, from bacteria and phytoplankton to flagellates and zooplankton who are then eaten by fish. The bacteria are important in this chain because only they have the physiological ability to absorb the dissolved mineral nutrients from the sea. These recycling principals from marine environments apply to many soil and freshwater ecosystems as well.

Micronutrient

Micronutrients are nutrients required by organisms throughout life in small quantities to orchestrate a range of physiological functions. For people, they include dietary trace minerals in amounts generally less than 100 milligrams per day, as opposed to macrominerals, which are required in larger quantities. The microminerals or trace elements include at least iron, cobalt, chromium, copper, iodine, manganese, selenium, zinc and molybdenum. Micronutrients also include vitamins, which are organic compounds required as nutrients in trace amounts.

Public Health Initiatives for Humans

At the 1990 World Summit for Children, the gathered nations identified deficiencies in two microminerals and one micronutrient – iodine, iron, and vitamin A – as being particularly common and posing public health risks in developing countries. The Summit set goals for elimination of these deficiencies. The Ottawa-based Micronutrient Initiative was formed in response to this challenge with the mission to undertake research and fund and implement micronutrient programming.

As programming around these micronutrients grew, new research in the 1990s led to the implementation of folate and zinc supplementation programmes as well.

Priority programs include supplementation with vitamin A for children 6–59 months, zinc supplementation as a treatment for diarrhoeal disease, iron and folate supplementation for women of child-bearing age, salt iodization, staple food fortification, multiple micronutrient powders, biofortification of crops and behaviour-centred nutrition education.

Salt Iodization

Salt iodization is the recommended strategy for ensuring adequate human iodine intake. To iodize salt, potassium iodate is added to salt after it is refined and dried and before it is packed. Although large-scale iodization is most efficient, given the proliferation of small scale salt producers in developing countries, technology for small-scale iodization has also been developed. International organizations work with national governments to identify and support small salt producers in adopting iodization activity.

In 1990, less than 20 percent of households in developing countries were consuming iodized salt. By 1994, international partnerships had formed in a global campaign for Universal Salt Iodization. By 2008, it was estimated that 72 per cent of households in developing countries were consuming iodized salt and the number of countries in which iodine deficiency disorders were a public health concern reduced by more than half from 110 to 47 countries.

Vitamin A supplementation

In 1997, national vitamin A supplementation programming received a boost when experts met to discuss rapid scale-up of supplementation activity and the Micronutrient Initiative, with support from the Government of Canada, began to ensure vitamin A supply to UNICEF.

In areas with vitamin A deficiency, it is recommended that children aged 6–59 months receive two doses annually. In many countries, vitamin A supplementation is combined with immunization and campaign-style health events.

Global vitamin A supplementation efforts have targeted 103 priority countries. In 1999, 16 per cent of children in these countries received two annual doses of vitamin A. By 2007, the rate increased to 62 per cent.

The Micronutrient Initiative, with funding from the Government of Canada, supplies 75 per cent of the vitamin A required for supplementation in developing countries.

Double-fortified Salt

Double-fortified salt (DFS) is a public health tool for delivering nutritional iron. DFS is fortified with both iodine and iron. It was developed by Venkatesh Mannar, Executive Director of the Micronutrient Initiative and University of Toronto Professor Levente Diosady, who discovered a process for coating iron particles with a vegetable fat to prevent the negative interaction of iodine and iron.

In India, Tata Salt Plus, priced at an economical rate of Rs 20 per kg, is an iodine plus iron fortified salt, developed by the National Institute of Nutrition, Hyderabad through double fortification technology. This technology was offered to Tata Chemicals under a long-term MoU after due studies on bio-availability across the population strata conducted and published by NIN.

It was first used in public programming in 2004. In September 2010 DFS was produced in the Indian State of Tamil Nadu and distributed through a state school feeding program. DFS has also been used to combat Iron Deficiency Anemia (IDA) in the Indian state of Bihar. In September 2010, Venkatesh Mannar was named a Laureat of the California-based Tech Awards for his work in developing Double-Fortified Salt.

Micro-enriched Fertilization

The returns of applying micronutrient-enriched fertilizers could be huge for human health, social and economic development. Research has shown that enriching fertilizers with micronutrients had not only an impact on plant deficiencies but also on humans and animals, through the food chain. A 1994 report by the World Bank estimated that micronutrient malnutrition costs developing economies at least 5 percent of gross domestic product. The Asian Development Bank has summarized the benefits of eliminating micronutrient deficiencies as follows:

Along with a growing understanding of the extent and impact of micronutrient malnutrition, several interventions have demonstrated the feasibility and benefits of correction and prevention. Distributing inexpensive capsules, diversifying to include more micronutrient-rich foods, or fortifying commonly consumed foods can make an enormous difference. Correcting iodine, vitamin A, and iron deficiencies can improve the population-wide intelligence quotient by 10-15 points, reduce maternal deaths by one fourth, decrease infant and child mortality by 40 percent, and increase people's work capacity by almost half. The elimination of these deficiencies will reduce health care and education costs, improve work capacity and productivity, and accelerate equitable economic growth and national development. Improved nutrition is essential to sustained economic growth.

Micronutrient deficiency elimination is as cost effective as the best public health interventions and fortification is the most cost-effective strategy.

Addressing Zinc Deficiencies through Zinc Fertilization

Experiments show that soil and foliar application of zinc fertilizer can effectively reduce the phytate zinc ratio in grain. People who eat bread prepared from zinc enriched wheat show a significant increase in serum zinc, suggesting that the zinc fertilizer strategy is a promising approach to address zinc deficiencies in humans.

Where zinc deficiency is a limiting factor, zinc fertilization can increase crop yields. Balanced crop nutrition supplying all essential nutrients, including zinc, is a cost effective management strategy. Even with zinc-efficient varieties, zinc fertilizers are needed when the available zinc in the topsoil becomes depleted.

Micronutrients for Plants

There are about seven nutrients essential to plant growth and health that are only needed in very small quantities. Though these are present in only small quantities, they are all necessary:

- Boron is believed to be involved in carbohydrate transport in plants; it also assists in metabolic regulation. Boron deficiency will often result in bud dieback.
- Chlorine is necessary for osmosis and ionic balance; it also plays a role in photosynthesis.
- Copper is a component of some enzymes. Symptoms of copper deficiency include browning of leaf tips and chlorosis.
- Iron is essential for chlorophyll synthesis, which is why an iron deficiency results in chlorosis.
- Manganese activates some important enzymes involved in chlorophyll formation. Manganese deficient plants will develop chlorosis between the veins of its leaves. The availability of manganese is partially dependent on soil pH.
- Molybdenum is essential to plant health. Molybdenum is used by plants to reduce nitrates into usable forms. Some plants use it for nitrogen fixation, thus it may need to be added to some soils before seeding legumes.
- Zinc participates in chlorophyll formation, and also activates many enzymes. Symptoms of zinc deficiency include chlorosis and stunted growth.

Micronutrient Deficiencies in Crops

Micronutrient deficiencies are widespread. 51% of world cereal soils are deficient in zinc and 30% of cultivated soils globally are deficient in iron. Steady growth of crop yields during recent decades (in particular through the Green Revolution) compounded the problem by progressively depleting soil micronutrient pools.

In general, farmers only apply micronutrients when crops show deficiency symptoms, while micronutrient deficiencies decrease yields before symptoms appear. Some common farming practices (such as liming acid soils) contribute to widespread occurrence of micronutrient deficiencies in crops by decreasing the availability of the micronutrients present in the soil. Also, extensive use of glyphosate is increasingly suspected to impair micronutrient uptake by crops, especially with regard to manganese, iron and zinc.

References

- Mark Kern (12 May 2005). CRC desk reference on sports nutrition. CRC Press. pp. 117–. ISBN 978-0-8493-2273-0. Retrieved 12 October 2010.
- David Sadava; H. Craig Heller; David M. Hillis; May Berenbaum (2009). Life: The Science of Biology. Macmillan. pp. 767–. ISBN 978-1-4292-1962-4. Retrieved 12 October 2010.
- John Griffith Vaughan; Catherine Geissler; Barbara Nicholson; Elisabeth Dowle; Elizabeth Rice (2009). The new Oxford book of food plants. Oxford University Press US. pp. 212–. ISBN 978-0-19-954946-7. Retrieved 13 October 2010.
- Campbell, Neil A.; Brad Williamson; Robin J. Heyden (2006). Biology: Exploring Life. Boston, Massachusetts: Pearson Prentice Hall. ISBN 0-13-250882-6.
- Food and Nutrition Board (2002/2005). Dietary Reference Intakes for Energy, Carbohydrate, Fiber, Fat, Fatty Acids, Cholesterol, Protein and Amino Acids. Washington, D.C.: The National Academies Press. Page 769. ISBN 0-309-08537-3.
- Steinke, Waggle; et al. (1992). New protein foods in human health: nutrition, prevention and therapy. CRC Press. pp. 91–100. ISBN 978-0-8493-6904-9.
- Amino acid content of foods and biological data on proteins (FAO nutritional studies number 24). Food and Agriculture Organization. 1985. ISBN 92-5-001102-4.
- Smith, Jack L.; Gropper, Sareen Annora Stepnick; Groff, James L. (2009). Advanced nutrition and human metabolism. Belmont, CA: Wadsworth Cengage Learning. ISBN 0-495-11657-2.
- Jeffery Schwartz; Bryant, Carol A.; DeWalt, Kathleen Musante; Anita Courtney (2003). The cultural feast: an introduction to food and society. Belmont, California: Thomson/Wadsworth. pp. 282, 283. ISBN 0-534-52582-2.
- Nelson, David L.; Michael M. Cox (2000-02-15). Lehninger Principles of Biochemistry, Third Edition (3 Har/Com ed.). W. H. Freeman. p. 1200. ISBN 1-57259-931-6.
- Corbridge, D. E. C. (1995-02-01). Phosphorus: An Outline of Its Chemistry, Biochemistry, and Technology (5th ed.). Amsterdam: Elsevier Science Pub Co. p. 1220. ISBN 0-444-89307-5.
- Schlenker, Eleanor; Gilbert, Joyce Ann (28 August 2014). Williams' Essentials of Nutrition and Diet Therapy. Elsevier Health Sciences. pp. 162–3. ISBN 978-0-323-29401-0.
- Jameson, J. Larry; De Groot, Leslie J. (25 February 2015). Endocrinology: Adult and Pediatric. Elsevier Health Sciences. p. 1510. ISBN 978-0-323-32195-2.
- Kim, Myoung Jin; Anderson, John; Mallory, Caroline (1 February 2014). Human Nutrition. Jones & Bartlett Publishers. p. 241. ISBN 978-1-4496-4742-1.
- Gropper, Sareen S.; Smith, Jack L. (1 June 2012). Advanced Nutrition and Human Metabolism. Cengage Learning. pp. 527–8. ISBN 1-133-10405-3. Retrieved 10 July 2016.
- Lippard, Stephen J.; Jeremy M. Berg (1994). Principles of Bioinorganic Chemistry. Mill Valley, CA: University Science Books. p. 411. ISBN 0-935702-72-5.
- Berdanier, Carolyn D.; Dwyer, Johanna T.; Heber, David (19 April 2016). Handbook of Nutrition and Food,

Third Edition. CRC Press. pp. 211–26. ISBN 978-1-4665-0572-8.

- Sigel, Astrid; Sigel, Helmut; Sigel, Roland K. O. (27 January 2014). Interrelations between Essential Metal Ions and Human Diseases. Springer Science & Business Media. p. 349. ISBN 978-94-007-7500-8. Retrieved 4 July 2016.
- Erdman, John W., Jr.; MacDonald, Ian A.; Zeisel, Steven H. (30 May 2012). Present Knowledge in Nutrition. John Wiley & Sons. p. 1324. ISBN 978-0-470-96310-4. Retrieved 4 July 2016.

4

Food Industry: An Overview

The food industry has progressed over the years; only hunter- gatherers and the farmers who survive on what they grow are considered to be separate from this industry. Some of the topics covered in this chapter are food fortification, food grading, food processing, food packaging, food coloring and food technology. This following content is an overview of the subject matter incorporating all the major aspects of the food industry.

Food Industry

The food industry is a complex, global collective of diverse businesses that supply most of the food consumed by the world population. Only subsistence farmers, those who survive on what they grow, and hunter-gatherers can be considered outside of the scope of the modern food industry.

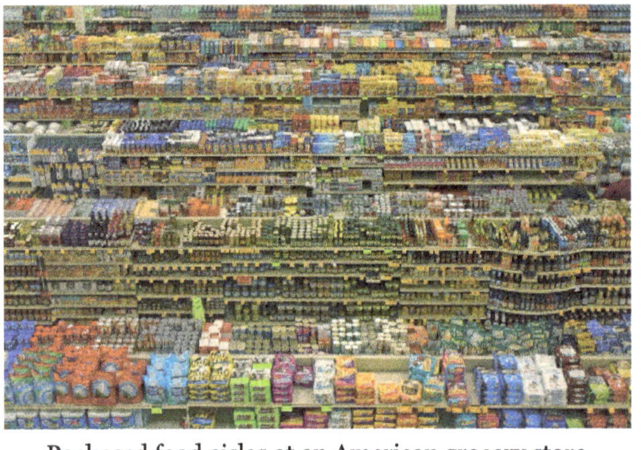

Packaged food aisles at an American grocery store

The food industry includes:

- Agriculture: raising of crops and livestock, and seafood
- Manufacturing: agrichemicals, agricultural construction, farm machinery and supplies, seed, etc.
- Food processing: preparation of fresh products for market, and manufacture of prepared food products
- Marketing: promotion of generic products (e.g., milk board), new products, advertising, marketing campaigns, packaging, public relations, etc.
- Wholesale and distribution: logistics, transportation, warehousing
- Foodservice (which includes Catering)

- Grocery, farmers' markets, public markets and other retailing
- Regulation: local, regional, national, and international rules and regulations for food production and sale, including food quality, food safety, marketing/advertising, and industry lobbying activities
- Education: academic, consultancy, vocational
- Research and development: food technology
- Financial services: credit, insurance

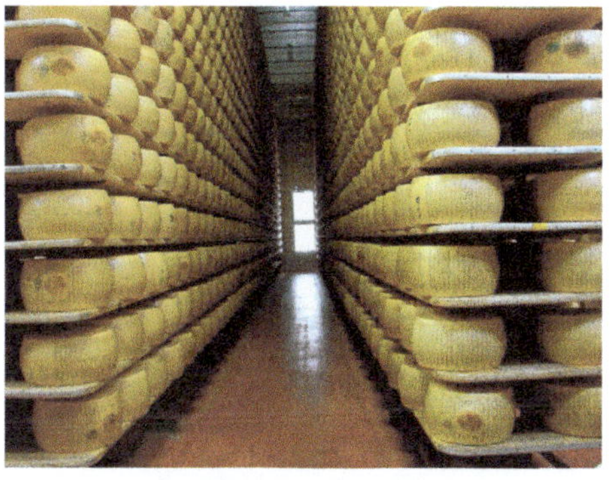

Parmigiano reggiano Cheese in a modern factory

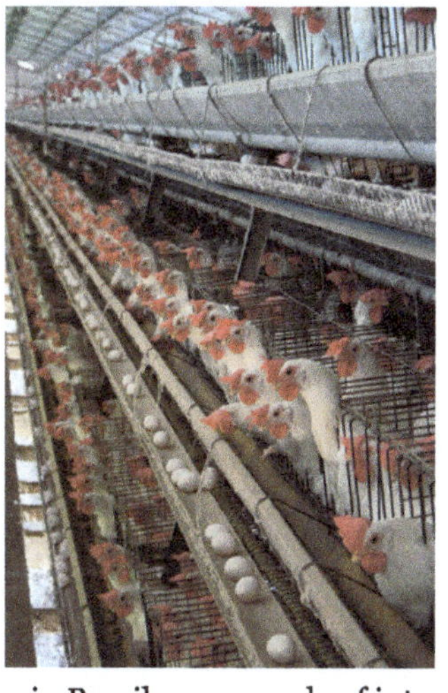

Hens in a battery cage in Brazil, an example of intensive animal farming

Definitions

It is challenging to find an inclusive way to cover all aspects of food production and sale. The Food Standards Agency, a government body in India, describes it thusly:

> "...the whole food industry – from farming and food production, packaging and distribution, to retail and catering."

The Economic Research Service of the USDA uses the term *food system* to describe the same thing:

> "The U.S. food system is a complex network of farmers and the industries that link to them.

Those links include makers of farm equipment and chemicals as well as firms that provide services to agribusinesses, such as providers of transportation and financial services. The system also includes the food marketing industries that link farms to consumers, and which include food and fiber processors, wholesalers, retailers, and foodservice establishments."

Agriculture and Agronomy

Agriculture is the process of producing food, feeding products, fiber and other desired products by the cultivation of certain plants and the raising of domesticated animals (livestock). The practice of agriculture is also known as "farming". Scientists, inventors, and others devoted to improving farming methods and implements are also said to be engaged in agriculture. 1 in 3 people worldwide are employed in agriculture, yet it only contributes 3% to global GDP.

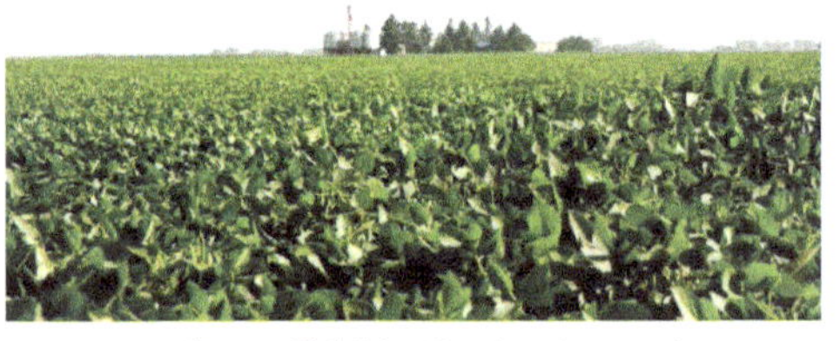

A soybean field in Junin, Argentina

Agronomy is the science and technology of producing and using plants for food, fuel, fibre, and land reclamation. Agronomy encompasses work in the areas of plant genetics, plant physiology, meteorology, and soil science. Agronomy is the application of a combination of sciences. Agronomists today are involved with many issues including producing food, creating healthier food, managing environmental impact of agriculture, and extracting energy from plants.

Food Processing

Food processing includes the methods and techniques used to transform raw ingredients into food for human consumption. Food processing takes clean, harvested or slaughtered and butchered components and uses them to produce marketable food products. There are several different ways in which food can be produced.

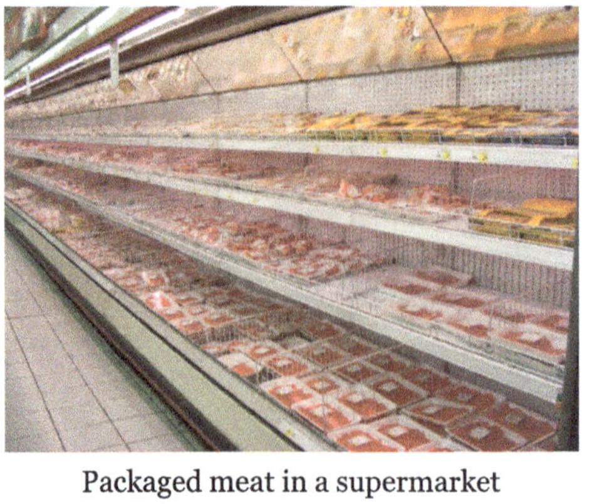

Packaged meat in a supermarket

One off production: This method is used when customers make an order for something to be made to their own specifications, for example a wedding cake. The making of one-off products could take days depending on how intricate the design is.

Batch production: This method is used when the size of the market for a product is not clear, and where there is a range within a product line. A certain number of the same goods will be produced to make up a batch or run, for example a bakery may bake a limited number of cupcakes. This method involves estimating consumer demand.

Mass production: This method is used when there is a mass market for a large number of identical products, for example chocolate bars, ready meals and canned food. The product passes from one stage of production to another along a production line.

Just-in-time (JIT) (production): This method of production is mainly used in restaurants. All components of the product are available in-house and the customer chooses what they want in the product. It is then prepared in a kitchen, or in front of the buyer as in sandwich delicatessens, pizzerias, and sushi bars.

Wholesale and Distribution

A vast global cargo network connects the numerous parts of the industry. These include suppliers, manufacturers, warehousers, retailers and the end consumers. Wholesale markets for fresh food products have tended to decline in importance in urbanizing countries, including Latin America and some Asian countries as a result of the growth of supermarkets, which procure directly from farmers or through preferred suppliers, rather than going through markets.

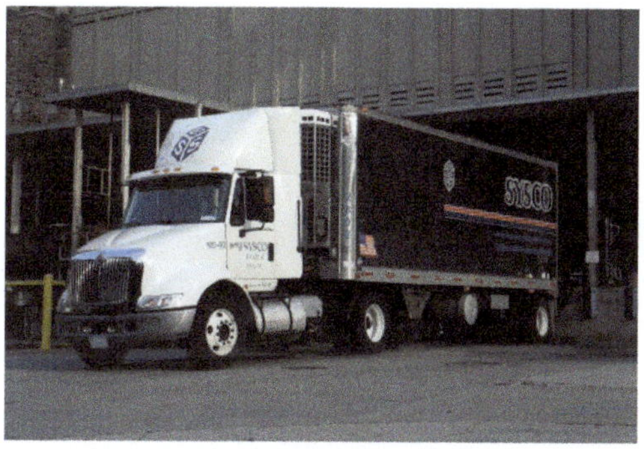

A foodservice truck at a loading dock. Trucks commonly distribute food products to commercial businesses and organizations.

The constant and uninterrupted flow of product from distribution centers to store locations is a critical link in food industry operations. Distribution centers run more efficiently, throughput can be increased, costs can be lowered, and manpower better utilized if the proper steps are taken when setting up a material handling system in a warehouse.

Retail

With worldwide urbanization, food buying is increasingly removed from food production. During the 20th century, the supermarket became the defining retail element of the food industry. There, tens of thousands of products are gathered in one location, in continuous, year-round supply.

Food preparation is another area where the change in recent decades has been dramatic. Today, two food industry sectors are in apparent competition for the retail food dollar. The grocery industry sells fresh and largely raw products for consumers to use as ingredients in home cooking. The food service industry by contrast offers prepared food, either as finished products, or as partially prepared components for final "assembly". Restaurants, cafes, bakeries and mobile food trucks provide opportunities for consumers to purchase food.

Food Industry Technologies

Modern food production is defined by sophisticated technologies. These include many areas. Agricultural machinery, originally led by the tractor, has practically eliminated human labor in many areas of production. Biotechnology is driving much change, in areas as diverse as agrochemicals, plant breeding and food processing. Many other types of technology are also involved, to the point where it is hard to find an area that does not have a direct impact on the food industry. As in other fields, computer technology is also a central force, with computer networks and specialized software providing the support infrastructure to allow global movement of the myriad components involved.

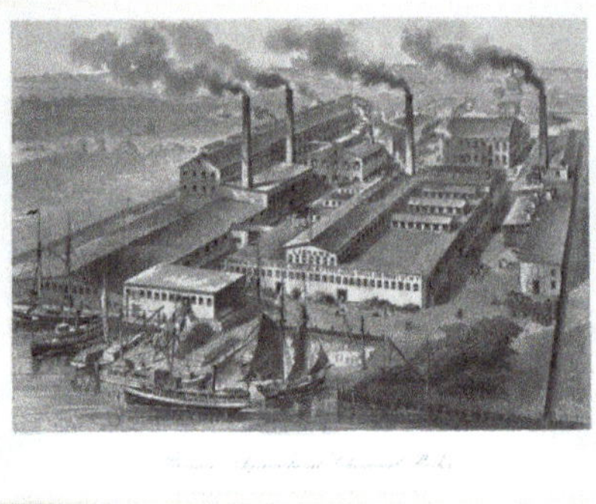

The Passaic Agricultural Chemical Works, an agrochemical company, in Newark, New Jersey, 1876

Marketing

As consumers grow increasingly removed from food production, the role of product creation, advertising, and publicity become the primary vehicles for information about food. With processed food as the dominant category, marketers have almost infinite possibilities in product creation.

Labor and Education

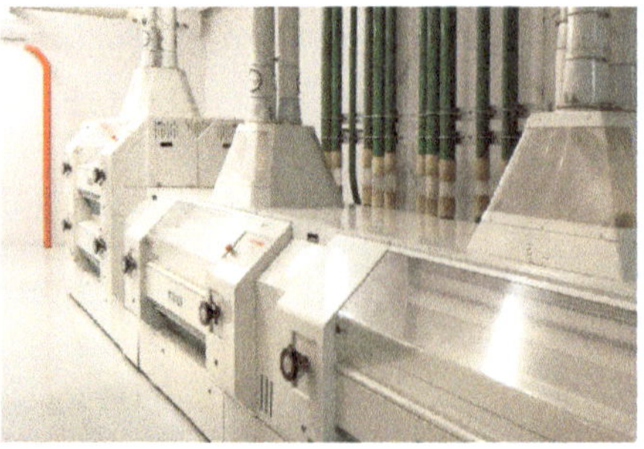

Some equipment at Tartu Mill, the largest grain milling company in the Baltic states. Modern food processing factories are often highly automated and need few workers.

Until the last 100 years, agriculture was labor intensive. Farming was a common occupation and millions of people were involved in food production. Farmers, largely trained from generation to generation, carried on the family business. That situation has changed dramatically today. In America in 1870, 70-80 percent of the US population was employed in agriculture. As of 2008, less than 2 percent of the population is directly employed in agriculture., and about 80% of the population lives in cities. The food industry as a complex whole requires an incredibly wide range of skills. Several hundred occupation types exist within the food industry.

Food Fortification

Food fortification or enrichment is the process of adding micronutrients (essential trace elements and vitamins) to food. It may be a purely commercial choice to provide extra nutrients in a food, while other times it is a public health policy which aims to reduce the number of people with dietary deficiencies within a population.

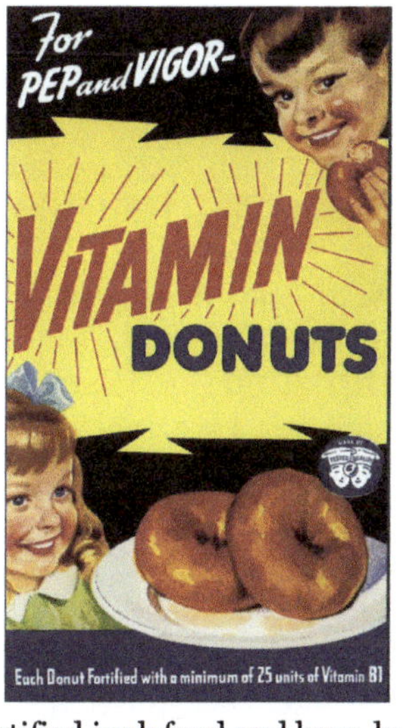

Manufacturers once proposed selling fortified junk food and beer, but USFDA policies of the time forbade it

Diets that lack variety can be deficient in certain nutrients. Sometimes the staple foods of a region can lack particular nutrients, due to the soil of the region or because of the inherent inadequacy of the normal diet. Addition of micronutrients to staples and condiments can prevent large-scale deficiency diseases in these cases.

While it is true that both fortification and enrichment refer to the addition of nutrients to food, the true definitions do slightly vary. As defined by the World Health Organization (WHO) and the Food and Agricultural Organization of the United Nations (FAO), fortification refers to "the practice of deliberately increasing the content of an essential micronutrient, ie. vitamins and minerals (including trace elements) in a food irrespective of whether the nutrients were originally in the food before processing or not, so as to improve the nutritional quality of the food supply and to provide a public health benefit with minimal risk to health," whereas enrichment is defined as "synonymous with fortification and refers to the addition of micronutrients to a food which are lost during processing."

Food fortification was identified as the second strategy of four by the WHO and FAO to begin decreasing the incidence of nutrient deficiencies at the global level.

As outlined by the FAO, the most common fortified foods are:

- Cereals and cereal based products
- Milk and Milk products
- Fats and oils
- Accessory food items
- Tea and other beverages
- Infant formulas

Types

The four main methods of food fortification (named as to indicate the procedure that is used in order to fortify the food):

1. Biofortification (i.e. breeding crops to increase their nutritional value, which can include both conventional selective breeding, and modern genetic modification)
2. Synthetic biology (i.e. addition of probiotic bacteria to foods)
3. Commercial and industrial fortification (i.e. flour, rice, oils (common cooking foods))
4. Home fortification (e.g. vitamin D drops)

Rationale

The WHO and FAO, among many other nationally recognized organizations, have recognized that there are over 2 billion people worldwide who suffer from a variety of micronutrient deficiencies. In 1992, 159 countries pledged at the FAO/WHO International Conference on Nutrition to make efforts to help combat these issues of micronutrient deficiencies, highlighting the importance of decreasing the number of those with iodine, vitamin A, and iron deficiencies. A significant statistic that led to these efforts was the discovery that approximately 1 in 3 people worldwide were at risk for either an iodine, vitamin A, or iron deficiency. Although it is recognized that food fortification alone will not combat this deficiency, it is a step towards reducing the prevalence of these deficiencies and their associated health conditions.

In Canada, The Food and Drug Regulations have outlined specific criterion which justifies food fortification:

1. To replace nutrients which were lost during manufacturing of the product (i.e. the manufacturing of flour)
2. To act as a public health intervention

3. To ensure the nutritional equivalence of substitute foods (i.e. to make butter and margarine similar in content, soy milk and cow's milk, etc.)
4. To ensure the appropriate vitamin and mineral nutrient composition of foods for special dietary purposes (i.e., gluten-free products, low sodium, or any other products specifically designed for special dietary requirements from an individual).

There are also several advantages to approaching nutrient deficiencies among populations via food fortification as opposed to other methods. These may include, but are not limited to: treating a population without specific dietary interventions therefore not requiring a change in dietary patterns, continuous delivery of the nutrient, does not require individual compliance, and potential to maintain nutrient stores more efficiently if consumed on a regular basis.

Criticism

Several organizations such as the WHO, FAO, Health Canada, and the Nestlé Research Center acknowledge that there are limitations to food fortification. Within the discussion of nutrient deficiencies the topic of nutrient toxicities can also be immediately questioned. Fortification of nutrients in foods may deliver toxic amounts of nutrients to an individual and also cause its associated side effects. As seen with the case of excessive fluoride intakes below, the result can be irreversible staining to the teeth. Although this may be a minor toxic effect to health, there are several that are more severe.

The WHO states that limitations to food fortification may include: human rights issues indicating that consumers have the right to choose if they want fortified products or not, the potential for insufficient demand of the fortified product, increased production costs leading to increased retail costs, the potential that the fortified products will still not be a solution to nutrient deficiencies amongst low income populations who may not be able to afford the new product, and children who may not be able to consume adequate amounts thereof.

Food safety worries led to legislation in Denmark in 2004 restricting foods fortified with extra vitamins or minerals. Products banned include: Rice Crispies, Shreddies, Horlicks, Ovaltine and Marmite.

Limited Absorption

One factor that limits the benefits of food fortification is that isolated nutrients added back into a processed food that has had many of its nutrients removed, does not always result in the added nutrients being as bioavailable as they would be in the original, whole food. An example is skim milk that has had the fat removed, and then had vitamin A and vitamin D added back. Vitamins A and D are both fat-soluble and non-water-soluble, so a person consuming skim milk in the absence of fats may not be able to absorb as much of these vitamins as one would be able to absorb from drinking whole milk. On the other hand, the nutrient added as a fortificant may have a higher bioavailability than from foods, which is the case with folic acid used to increase folate intakes.

Phytochemicals such as polyphenols, phytic acid in cereal grains and tannin in tea can also impact nutrient absorption, limiting the bioavailability of intrinsic and additional nutrients, and reducing the effectiveness of fortification programs.

Excess Intake of Micronutrients

Ecological studies have shown that increased B vitamin fortification is correlated with the prevalence of obesity and diabetes. Daily consumption of iron per capita in the United States has dramatically surged since World War II and nearly doubled over the past century due to increases in iron fortification and increased consumption of meat. Existing evidence suggests that excess iron intake may play a role in the development of obesity, cardiovascular disease, diabetes and cancer.

Fortification of foods with folic acid has been mandated in many countries solely to improve the folate status of pregnant women to prevent neural tube defects—a relatively rare birth defect which affected 0.5% of US births before fortification began. However, when fortification is introduced, several hundred thousand people are exposed to an increased intake of folic acid for each neural tube defect pregnancy that is prevented. In humans, increased folic acid intake leads to elevated blood concentrations of naturally occurring folates and of unmetabolized folic acid. High blood concentrations of folic acid may decrease natural killer cell cytotoxicity, and high folate status may reduce the response to drugs used to treat malaria, rheumatoid arthritis, psoriasis, and cancer. A combination of high folate levels and low vitamin B-12 status may be associated with an increased risk of cognitive impairment and anemia in the elderly and, in pregnant women, with an increased risk of insulin resistance and obesity in their children. Folate has a dual effect on cancer, protecting against cancer initiation but facilitating progression and growth of preneoplastic cells and subclinical cancers. Furthermore, intake of folic acid from fortification have turned out to be significantly greater than originally modeled in pre mandate predictions. Therefore, a high folic acid intake due to fortification may be harmful for more people than the policy is designed to help.

Different Forms of Micronutrients

There is a concern that micronutrients are legally defined in such a way that does not distinguish between different forms, and that fortified foods often have nutrients in a balance that would not occur naturally. For example, in the U.S., food is fortified with folic acid, which is one of the many naturally-occurring forms of folate, and which only contributes a minor amount to the folates occurring in natural foods. In many cases, such as with folate, it is an open question of whether or not there are any benefits or risks to consuming folic acid in this form.

In many cases, the micronutrients added to foods in fortification are synthetic.

In some cases, certain forms of micronutrients can be actively toxic in a sufficiently high dose, even if other forms are safe at the same or much higher doses. There are examples of such toxicity in both synthetic and naturally-occurring forms of vitamins. Retinol, the active form of Vitamin A, is toxic in a much lower dose than other forms, such as beta carotene. Menadione, a phased-out synthetic form of Vitamin K, is also known to be toxic.

Food Supplements

There are several main groups of food supplements like:

- Vitamins and co-vitamins
- Essential minerals

- Essential fatty acids
- Essential amino acids
- Phytonutrients
- Enzymes

Examples of Fortification In Foods

Many foods and beverages worldwide have been fortified, whether a voluntary action by the product developers or by law. Although some may view these additions as strategic marketing schemes to sell their product, there is a lot of work that must go into a product before simply fortifying it. In order to fortify a product, it must first be proven that the addition of this vitamin or mineral is beneficial to health, safe, and an effective method of delivery. The addition must also abide by all food and labeling regulations and support nutritional rationale. From a food developer's point of view, they also need to consider the costs associated with this new product and whether or not there will be a market to support the change.

Examples of foods and beverages that have been fortified and shown to have positive health effects:

Iodized Salt

"Iodine deficiency disorder (IDD) is the single greatest cause of preventable mental retardation. Severe deficiencies cause cretinism, stillbirth and miscarriage. But even mild deficiency can significantly affect the learning ability of populations........ Today over 1 billion people in the world suffer from iodine deficiency, and 38 million babies born every year are not protected from brain damage due to IDD."—Kul Gautam, Deputy Executive Director, UNICEF, October 2007

Iodised salt has been used in the United States since before World War II. It was discovered in 1821 that goiters could be treated by the use of iodized salts. However, it was not until 1916 that the use of iodized salts could be tested in a research trial as a preventative measure against goiters. By 1924, it became readily available in the US.

Currently in Canada and the US, the RDA for iodine is as low as 90 μg/day for children (4–8 years) and as high as 290 μg/day for breast-feeding mothers.

Diseases that are associated with an iodine deficiency include: mental retardation, hypothyroidism, and goiter. There is also a risk of various other growth and developmental abnormalities.

Folic Acid

Folic acid (also known as folate) functions in reducing blood homocysteine levels, forming red blood cells, proper growth and division of cells, and preventing neural tube defects (NTDs).

In many industrialized countries, the addition of folic acid to flour has prevented a significant number of NTDs in infants. Two common types of NTDs, spina bifida and anencephaly, affect approximately 2500-3000 infants born in the US annually. Research trials have shown the ability to reduce the incidence of NTDs by supplementing pregnant mothers with folic acid by 72%.

The RDA for folic acid ranges from as low as 150 μg/day for children aged 1–3 years old, to 400 μg/day for males and females over the age of 19, and 600 μg/day during pregnancy.

Diseases associated with folic acid deficiency include: megaloblastic or macrocytic anemia, cardiovascular disease, certain types of cancer, and NTDs in infants.

Niacin

Niacin has been added to bread in the USA since 1938 (when voluntary addition started), a programme which substantially reduced the incidence of pellagra. As early as 1755, pellagra was recognized by doctors as being a niacin deficiency disease. Although not officially receiving its name of pellagra until 1771. Pellagra was seen amongst poor families who used corn as their main dietary staple. Although corn itself does contain niacin, it is not a bioavailable form unless it undergoes Nixtamalization (treatment with alkali, traditional in Native American cultures) and therefore was not contributing to the overall intake of niacin.

The RDA for niacin is 2 mg NE(niacin equivalents)/day (AI) for infants aged 0–6 months, 16 mg NE/day for males, and 14 mg NE/day for females who are over the age of 19.

Diseases associated with niacin deficiency include: Pellagra which consisted of signs and symptoms called the 3D's-"Dermatitis, dementia, and diarrhea. Others may include vascular or gastrointestinal diseases.

Common diseases which present a high frequency of niacin deficiency: alcoholism, anorexia nervosa, HIV infection, gastrectomy, malabsorptive disorders, certain cancers and their associated treatments.

Vitamin D

Since Vitamin D is a fat-soluble vitamin, it cannot be added to a wide variety of foods. Foods that it is commonly added to are margarine, vegetable oils and dairy products. During the late 1800s, after the discovery of curing conditions of scurvy and beriberi had occurred, researchers were aiming to see if the disease, later known as rickets, could also be cured by food. Their results showed that sunlight exposure and cod liver oil were the cure. It was not until the 1930s that vitamin D was actually linked to curing rickets. This discovery led to the fortification of common foods such as milk, margarine, and breakfast cereals. This took the astonishing statistics of approximately 80–90% of children showing varying degrees of bone deformations due to vitamin D deficiency to being a very rare condition.

The current RDA for infants aged 0–6 months is 10 μg (400 International Units (IU))/day and for adults over 19 years of age it is 15 μg (600 IU)/day.

Diseases associated with a vitamin D deficiency include rickets, osteoporosis, and certain types of cancer (breast, prostate, colon and ovaries). It has also been associated with increased risks for fractures, heart disease, type 2 diabetes, autoimmune and infectious diseases, asthma and other wheezing disorders, myocardial infarction, hypertension, congestive heart failure, and peripheral vascular disease.

Fluoride

Although fluoride is not considered an essential mineral, it is seen as possibly useful in prevention of tooth decay and maintaining adequate dental health. In the mid-1900s it was discovered that towns with a high level of fluoride in their water supply was causing the residents' teeth to have both brown spotting and a strange resistance to dental caries. This led to the fortification of water supplies with fluoride with safe amounts to retain the properties of resistance to dental caries but avoid the staining cause by fluorosis (a condition caused by excessive fluoride intake). The tolerable upper intake level (UL) set for fluoride ranges from 0.7 mg/day for infants aged 0–6 months and 10 mg/day for adults over the age of 19.

Conditions commonly associated with fluoride deficiency are dental caries and osteoporosis.

Others

Some other examples of fortified foods:

- Calcium is frequently added to fruit juices, carbonated beverages and rice.
- White rice is frequently enriched to replace some of the lost nutrients during milling or adding extras in.
- "Golden rice" is a variety of rice which has been genetically modified to produce beta carotene.
- Amylase rich flour is utilized for food making to increase dietary consumption.

Fortification for Body Building

Despite having some scientific basis, but with controversial ethics, is the science of using foods and food supplements to achieve a defined health goal. A common example of this use of food supplements is the extent to which body builders will use amino acid mixtures, vitamins and phytochemicals to enhance natural hormone production, increase muscle and reduce fat. The literature is not concrete on an appropriate method for use of fortification for body builders and therefore may not be recommended due to safety concerns.

Fortification for Medical Treatment

There is interest in the use of food supplements in established medical conditions. This nutritional supplementation using foods as medicine (nutraceuticals) has been effectively used in treating disorders affecting the immune system up to and including cancers. This goes beyond the definition of "food supplement", but should be included for the sake of completeness.

Food Grading

Food grading involves the inspection, assessment and sorting of various foods regarding quality, freshness, legal conformity and market value. Food grading often occurs by hand, in which foods are assessed and sorted. Machinery is also used to grade foods, and may involve sorting products by size, shape and quality. For example, machinery can be used to remove spoiled food from fresh product.

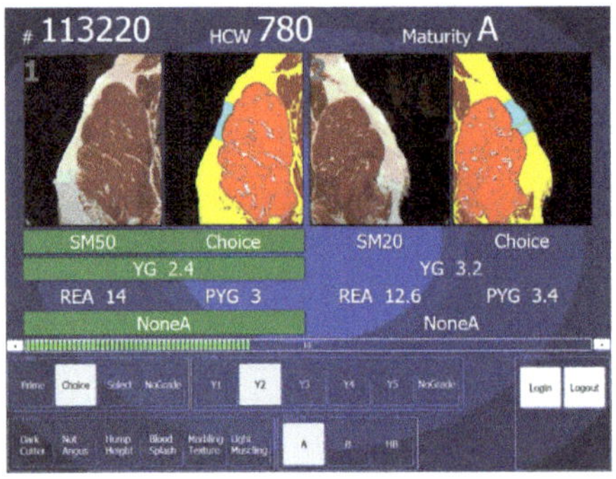

A screenshot from the electronic grading system showing USDA Choice, Yield Grade 2 beef. The left is the natural color view of the cut; the right is the instrument enhanced view that details the amount of marbling, size, and fat thickness.

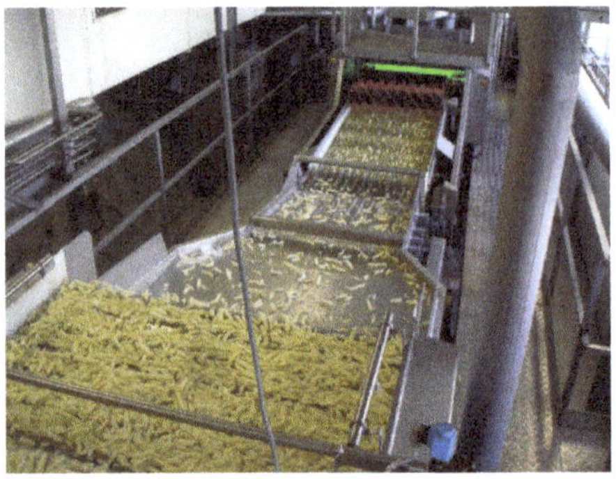

Optical sorting achieves non-destructive, 100 percent inspection in-line at full production volumes

By Food Type

Beef

Beef grading in the United States is performed by the United States Department of Agriculture's (USDA) Agricultural and Marketing Service. There are eight beef quality grades, with U.S. Prime being the highest grade and U.S. Canner being the lowest grade. Beef grading is a complex and detailed process, requiring graders to think and calculate quickly with great accuracy. Using technology to complement and supplement the onsite human graders generates an efficient and more precise process.

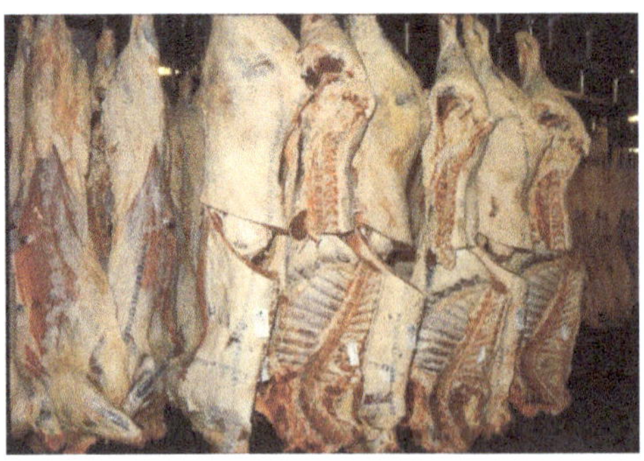

Inspected beef carcasses tagged by the USDA

Beer

In beer grading, the letter "X" is used on some beers, and was traditionally a mark of beer strength, with the more Xs the greater the strength. Some sources suggest that the origin of the mark was in the breweries of medieval monasteries Another plausible explanation is contained in a treatise entitled "The Art of Brewing" published in London in 1829. It says; *"The duties on ale and beer, which were first imposed in 1643... at a certain period, in distinguishing between small beer and strong, all ale or beer, sold at or above ten shillings per barrel, was reckoned to be* strong *and was, therefore, subjected to a higher duty. The cask which contained this strong beer was then first marked with an X signifying ten; and hence the present quack-like denominations of XX (double X) and XXX (treble X) on the casks and accounts of the strong-ale brewers".*

In mid-19th century England, the use of "X" and other letters had evolved into a standardised grading system for the strength of beer. Today, it is used as a trade mark by a number of brewers in the United Kingdom, the Commonwealth and the United States.

European Bitterness Units scale, often abbreviated as EBU, is a scale for measuring the perceived bitterness of beer, with lower values being generally "less bitter" and higher values "more bitter". The scale and method are defined by the European Brewery Convention, and the numerical value should be the same as of the International Bitterness Units scale (IBU), defined in co-operation with the American Society of Brewing Chemists. However, the exact process of determining EBU and IBU values differs slightly, which may in theory result with slightly smaller values for EBU than IBU.

The International Bittering Units scale, or simply IBU scale, provides a measure of the bitterness of beer, which is provided by the hops used during brewing. Bittering units are measured through the use of a spectrophotometer and solvent extraction.

Butter

Coconut Milk

Several grades of coconut milk exist: from thick at 20-22% fat to thin at 5-7% fat level.

Coffee

Coffee growers, traders, and roasters grade beans based on size, color, and a variety of other characteristics. Coffees of exceptional quality are traded as "specialty coffees" and fetch a higher price in the international market.

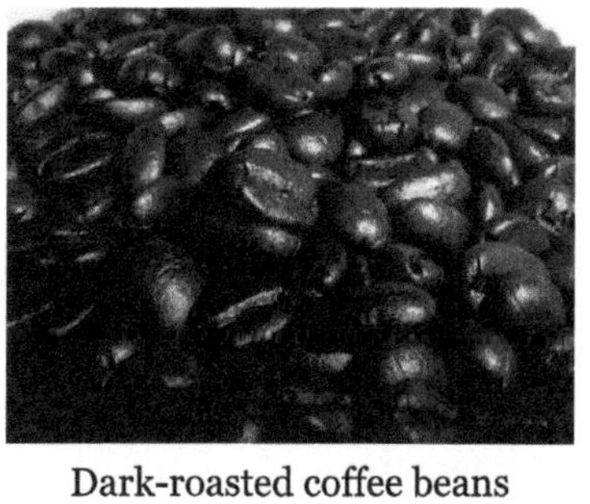

Dark-roasted coffee beans

After the roast, Coffee grading involves assessment of roasted coffee seed colorization and then labeling as light, medium light, medium, medium dark, dark, or very dark. A more accurate method of discerning the degree of roast involves measuring the reflected light from roasted seeds illuminated with a light source in the near infrared spectrum. This elaborate light meter uses a process known as spectroscopy to return a number that consistently indicates the roasted coffee's relative degree of roast or flavor development.

Eggs

In the United States, egg grading is performed by the USDA, and is based upon the interior quality of the egg, the appearance and condition of the egg shell. Eggs of any quality grade may differ in weight (size). Egg grading is performed by candling, which involves observing the interior of eggs by placing them in front of a bright light.

Guar Gum

Guar gum grading involves analysis for coloration, viscosity, moisture, granulation, protein content and insolubles ash.

Honey

Honey grading in the United States is performed voluntarily based upon USDA standards (USDA does offer inspection and grading "as on-line (in-plant) or lot inspection...upon application, on a fee-for-service basis.") . Honey is graded based upon a number of factors, including water content, flavor and aroma, absence of defects and clarity. Honey is also classified by color though it is not a factor in the grading scale. U.S. honey grade scales are Grade A, Grade B, Grade C and Grade substandard.

Lobster

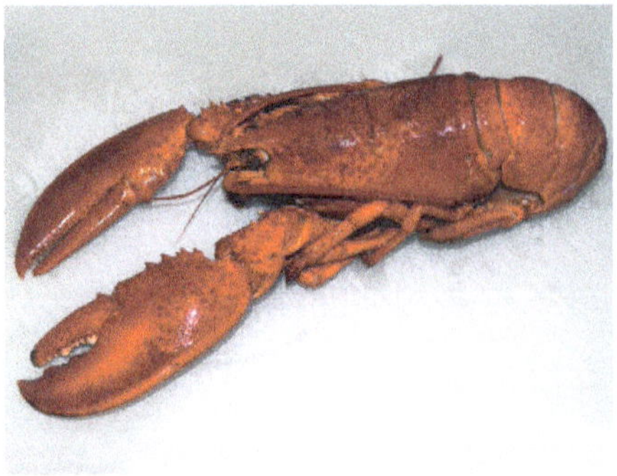

A lobster

In the U.S., lobster grading involves denoting lobsters as new-shell, hard-shell or old-shell, and because lobsters which have recently shed their shells are the most delicate, there is an inverse relationship between the price of American lobster and its flavour. New-shell lobsters have paper-thin shells and a worse meat-to-shell ratio, but the meat is very sweet. However, the lobsters are so delicate that even transport to Boston almost kills them, making the market for new-shell lobsters strictly local to the fishing towns where they are offloaded. Hard-shell lobsters with firm shells, but with less sweet meat, can survive shipping to Boston, New York and even Los Angeles, so they command a higher price than new-shell lobsters. Meanwhile, old-shell lobsters, which have not shed since the previous season and have a coarser flavour, can be air-shipped anywhere in the world and arrive alive, making them the most expensive. One seafood guide notes that an eight-dollar lobster dinner at a restaurant overlooking fishing piers in Maine is consistently delicious, while “the eighty-dollar lobster in a three-star Paris restaurant is apt to be as much about presentation as flavor”.

Maple Syrup

In Canada, the grading of maple syrup involves classification by the Canadian Food Inspection Agency (CFIA) of maple syrups into one of three grades, each with several colour classes: Canada No. 1, including Extra Light, Light, and Medium; No. 2 Amber; and finally No. 3 Dark or any other ungraded category. Producers in Quebec and Ontario may follow either federal or provincial grading guidelines, which differ slightly.

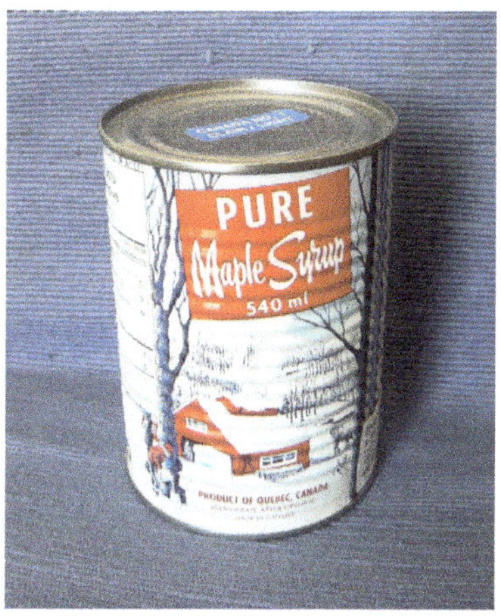

Maple syrup from Quebec, graded as No. 1, Light (enlarge image to read the label atop the can)

The United States uses different grading standards. Maple syrup is divided into two major grades: Grade A and Grade B. Grade A is further divided into three subgrades: Light Amber (sometimes known as Fancy), Medium Amber, and Dark Amber. The Vermont Agency of Agriculture Food and Markets uses a similar grading system of color, and is roughly equivalent, especially for lighter syrups, but using letters: “AA”, “A”, etc. The Vermont grading system differs from the US system in maintaining a slightly higher standard of product density (measured on the Baumé scale). New Hampshire maintains a similar standard, but not a separate state grading scale. The Vermont-graded product has 0.9 percent more sugar and less water in its composition than US-graded. One grade of syrup not for table use, called commercial or Grade C, is also produced under the Vermont system. Vermont inspectors enforce strict syrup grading regulations, and can fine producers up to US$1000 for labelling syrup incorrectly.

Milk

In the United States, there are two grades of milk, with Grade A primarily used for direct sales and consumption in stores, and Grade B used for indirect consumption, such as in cheese making or other processing.

The differences between the two grades are defined in the Wisconsin administrative code for Agriculture, Trade, and Consumer Protection, chapter 60. Grade B generally refers to milk that is cooled in milk cans, which are immersed in a bath of cold flowing water that typically is drawn up from an underground water well rather than using mechanical refrigeration.

Oranges

The USDA has established the following grades for Florida oranges, which primarily apply to oranges sold as fresh fruit: US Fancy, US No. 1 Bright, US No. 1, US No. 1 Golden, US No. 1 Bronze, US No. 1 Russet, US No. 2 Bright, US No. 2, US No. 2 Russet, and US No. 3. The general characteristics graded are color (both hue and uniformity), firmness, maturity, varietal characteristics, texture, and shape. Fancy, the highest grade, requires the highest grade of color and an absence of blemishes, while the terms Bright, Golden, Bronze, and Russet concern solely discoloration.

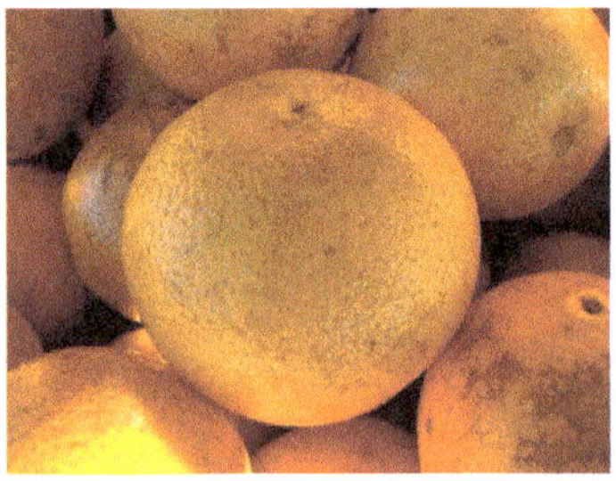

Florida navel oranges

Peas

Pea grading involves sorting peas by size, in which smallest peas are graded as the highest quality for their tenderness. Brines may be used, in which peas are floated in them, from which their density can be determined.

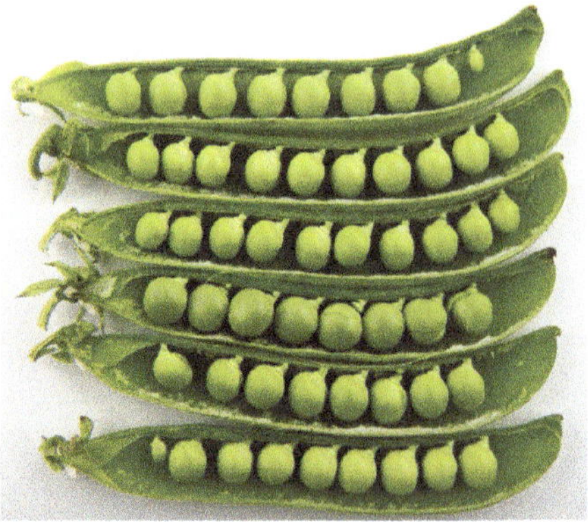

Peas

Potatoes

In the U.S., potato grading for Idaho potatoes is performed in which No. 1 potatoes are the highest quality and No. 2 are rated as lower in quality due to their appearance (e.g. blemishes or bruises, pointy ends). Density assessment can be performed by floating them in brines. High density potatoes are desirable in the production of dehydrated mashed potatoes, potato crisps and french fries.

Rice

The main criteria used by many countries and millers in rice grading are degree of milling, appearance (color), damaged (broken) and percentage of chalky kernels. In the United States rice is marketed according to three main properties size, color and condition (kernels damage), these properties are directly related to quality, milling percentage and other processing conditions. All properties are considered important in grading. For instance, chalky kernels are not desirable because they give lower milling yields after processing and easily break during handling.

Spices

Cinnamon

In Sri Lanka, cinnamon grading is performed by dividing cinnamon quills into four groups, which are then further divided into specific grades.

Vanilla

Several vanilla fruit grading systems are in use. Each country which produces vanilla has its own grading system, and individual vendors, in turn, sometimes use their own criteria for describing the quality of the fruits they offer for sale.

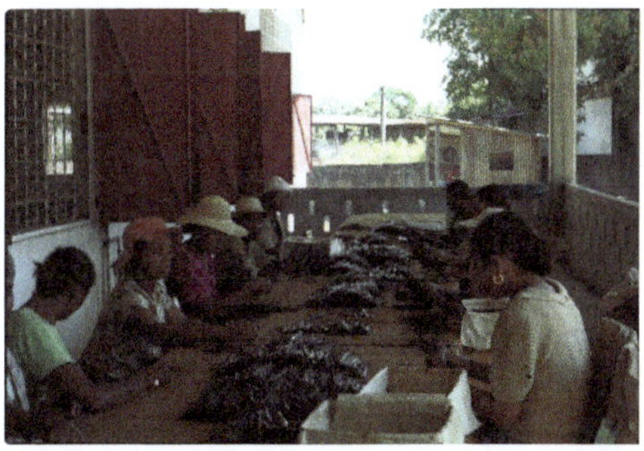

People grading vanilla beans in Sambava, Madagascar

Tea

In the western black tea industry, tea leaf grading is the process of evaluating products based on the quality and condition of the tea leaves themselves. The highest grades are referred to as "orange pekoe", and the lowest as "fannings" or "dust". This grading system is based upon the size of processed and dried black tea leaves. Despite a purported Chinese origin, these grading terms are typically used for teas from Sri Lanka, India and countries other than China; they are not generally known within Chinese-speaking countries.

Black Tea

Black tea grading is usually based upon one of four scales of quality. Whole-leaf teas are the highest quality, followed by broken leaves, fannings, and dusts. Whole-leaf teas are produced with little or no alteration to the tea leaf. This results in a finished product with a coarser texture than that of bagged teas. Whole-leaf teas are widely considered the most valuable, especially if they contain leaf tips. Broken leaves are commonly sold as medium-grade loose teas. Smaller broken varieties may be included in tea bags.

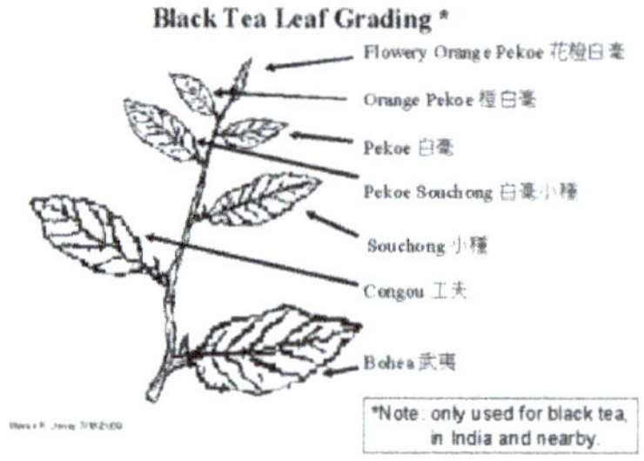

A black tea leaf grading diagram

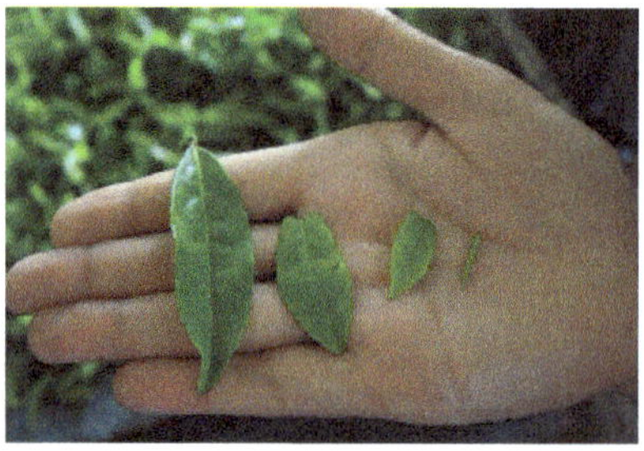

Fresh tea leaves of different sizes

Rooibos

Rooibos grades are largely related to the proportion of "needle" or leaf to stem content in the mix. A higher leaf content will result in a darker liquor, richer flavour and less "dusty" aftertaste. The high-grade rooibos is exported and does not reach local markets, with major consumers being in the EU, particularly Germany, where it is used in creating flavoured blends for loose-leaf tea markets. In development within South Africa are a small number of specialty tea companies producing similar blends.

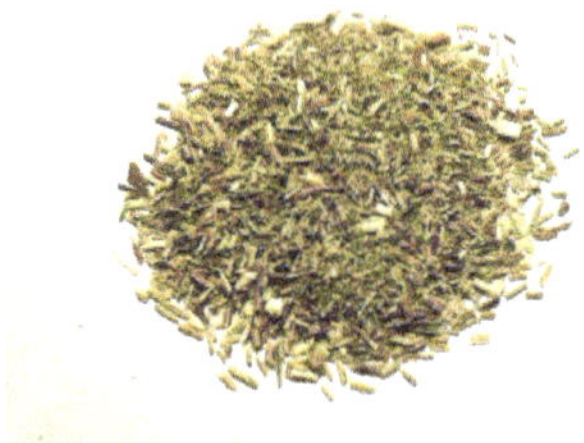

Organic green rooibos tea leaves

Food Additives and Preservatives

Carrageenan

There are two basic grades of carrageenan, refined carrageenan (RC) and semi-refined carrageenan (SRC). In the United States, RC and SRC are both labeled as carrageenan. In the European Union, RC is designated by the E number E-407, and SRC is E-407a. RC has a 2% maximum for acid-insoluble material and is produced through an alcohol precipitation process or potassium chloride gel press process. SRC contains a much higher level of cellulosic content and is produced in a less complex process. Indonesia, the Philippines, and Chile are three main sources of raw material and extracted carrageenan.

Lye

Lye is used to cure foods such as lutefisk, olives (making them less bitter), canned mandarin oranges, hominy, lye rolls, century eggs, and pretzels. It is also used as a tenderizer in the crust of baked Cantonese moon cakes, and in lye-water "zongzi" (glutinous rice dumplings wrapped in bamboo leaves), chewy southern Chinese noodles popular in Hong Kong and southern China, and Japanese ramen noodles. In the United States, food-grade lye must meet the requirements outlined in the Food Chemicals Codex (FCC), as prescribed by the U.S. Food and Drug Administration (FDA). Lower or more caustic grades of lye are commonly used as drain de-cloggers and oven cleaners. As a result, such grades should not be used for food preparation, as they would be too poisonous for human consumption.

Sodium Bisulfate

Sodium bisulfate is used as a food additive to leaven cake mixes (make them rise) as well as being used in meat and poultry processing and most recently in browning prevention of fresh-cut produce. The food-grade product meets the requirements set out in the Food Chemicals Codex. It is denoted by E number E514ii in the EU and is approved for use in Australia and New Zealand where it is listed as additive 514. Food-grade sodium bisulfate is used in a variety of food products, including beverages, dressings, sauces, and fillings. It has many synonyms (bisulfate of soda, sodium bisulfate, sodium acid sulfate, monosodium hydrogen sulfate, monosodium salt, sodium hydrogen sulfate, sodium hydrosulfate, sodium pyrosulfate, sulfuric acid, sulfuric acid sodium salt (1:1)).

By Country

- In India, AGMARK is a certification mark employed on agricultural products, assuring that they conform to a set of standards approved by the Directorate of Marketing and Inspection, an agency of the Government of India.

Food Processing

Food processing is the transformation of raw ingredients, by physical or chemical means into food, or of food into other forms. Food processing combines raw food ingredients to produce marketable food products that can be easily prepared and served by the consumer. Food processing typically involves activities such as mincing and macerating, liquefaction, emulsification, and cooking (such as boiling, broiling, frying, or grilling); pickling, pasteurization, and many other kinds of preservation; and canning or other packaging. (Primary-processing such as dicing or slicing, freezing or drying when leading to secondary products are also included.)

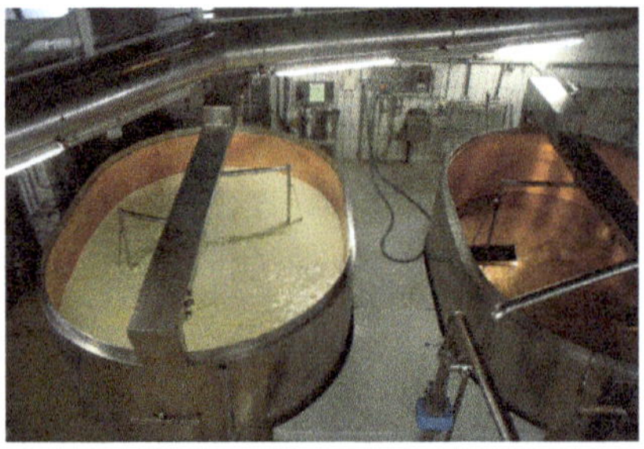

Industrial cheese production

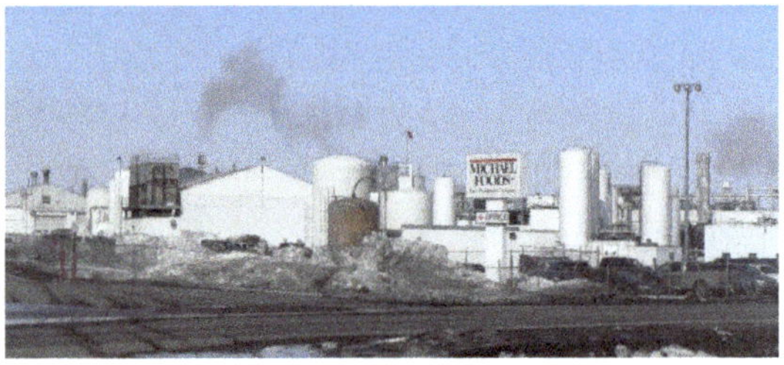

Michael Foods egg-processing plant in Wakefield, Nebraska

History

Food processing dates back to the prehistoric ages when crude processing incorporated fermenting, sun drying, preserving with salt, and various types of cooking (such as roasting, smoking, steaming, and oven baking), Such basic food processing involved chemical enzymatic changes to the basic structure of food in its natural form, as well served to build a barrier against surface microbial activity that caused rapid decay. Salt-preservation was especially common for foods that constituted warrior and sailors' diets until the introduction of canning methods. Evidence for the existence of these methods can be found in the writings of the ancient Greek, Chaldean, Egyptian and Roman civilizations as well as archaeological evidence from Europe, North and South America and Asia. These tried and tested processing techniques remained essentially the same until the advent of the industrial revolution. Examples of ready-meals also date back to before the preindustrial revolution, and include dishes such as Cornish pasty and Haggis. Both during ancient times and today in modern society these are considered processed foods.

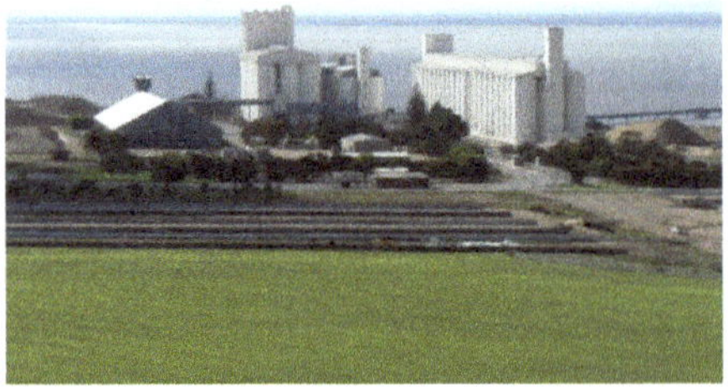

Grain silos in Ardrossan, Scotland

Modern food processing technology developed in the 19th and 20th centuries was developed in a large part to serve military needs. In 1809 Nicolas Appert invented a hermetic bottling technique that would preserve food for French troops which ultimately contributed to the development of tinning, and subsequently canning by Peter Durand in 1810. Although initially expensive and somewhat hazardous due to the lead used in cans, canned goods would later become a staple around the world. Pasteurization, discovered by Louis Pasteur in 1864, improved the quality of preserved foods and introduced the wine, beer, and milk preservation.

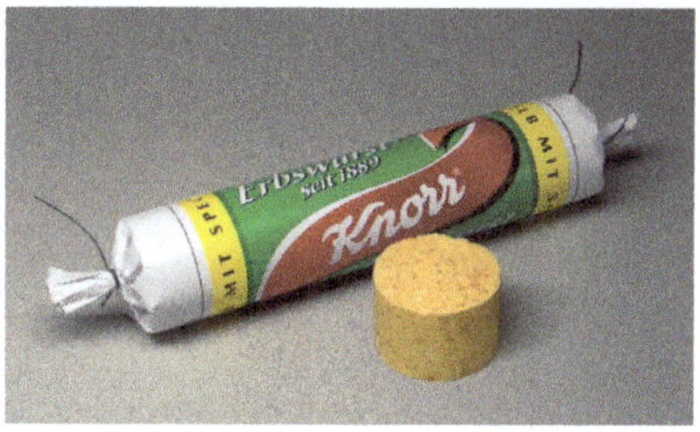

A form of pre-made split-pea soup that has become traditional

In the 20th century, World War II, the space race and the rising consumer society in developed countries (including the United States) contributed to the growth of food processing with such advances as spray drying, juice concentrates, freeze drying and the introduction of artificial sweeteners, colouring agents, and such preservatives as sodium benzoate. In the late 20th century, products such as dried instant soups, reconstituted fruits and juices, and self cooking meals such as MRE food ration were developed.

In western Europe and North America, the second half of the 20th century witnessed a rise in the pursuit of convenience. Food processing companies marketed their products especially towards middle-class working wives and mothers. Frozen foods (often credited to Clarence Birdseye) found their success in sales of juice concentrates and "TV dinners". Processors utilised the perceived value of time to appeal to the postwar population, and this same appeal contributes to the success of convenience foods today.

Benefits and Drawbacks

Benefits

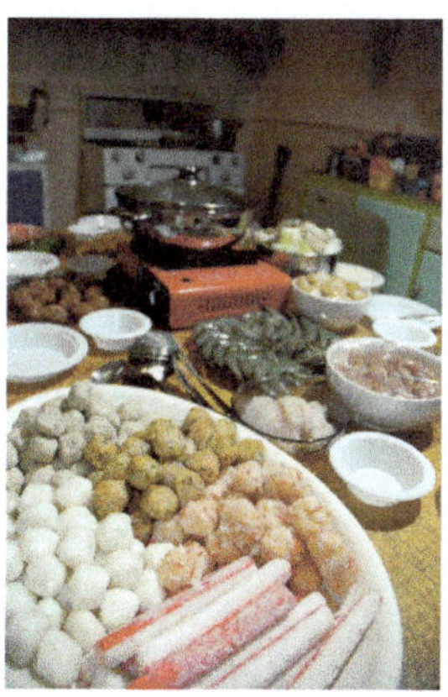
Processed seafood - fish, squid, prawn balls and simulated crab sticks (surimi)

Benefits of food processing include toxin removal, preservation, easing marketing and distribution tasks, and increasing food consistency. In addition, it increases yearly availability of many foods, enables transportation of delicate perishable foods across long distances and makes many kinds of foods safe to eat by de-activating spoilage and pathogenic micro-organisms. Modern supermarkets would not exist without modern food processing techniques, and long voyages would not be possible.

Processed foods are usually less susceptible to early spoilage than fresh foods and are better suited for long distance transportation from the source to the consumer. When they were first introduced, some processed foods helped to alleviate food shortages and improved the overall nutrition of populations as it made many new foods available to the masses.

Processing can also reduce the incidence of food borne disease. Fresh materials, such as fresh produce and raw meats, are more likely to harbour pathogenic micro-organisms (e.g. Salmonella) capable of causing serious illnesses.

The extremely varied modern diet is only truly possible on a wide scale because of food processing. Transportation of more exotic foods, as well as the elimination of much hard labour gives the modern eater easy access to a wide variety of food unimaginable to their ancestors.

The act of processing can often improve the taste of food significantly.

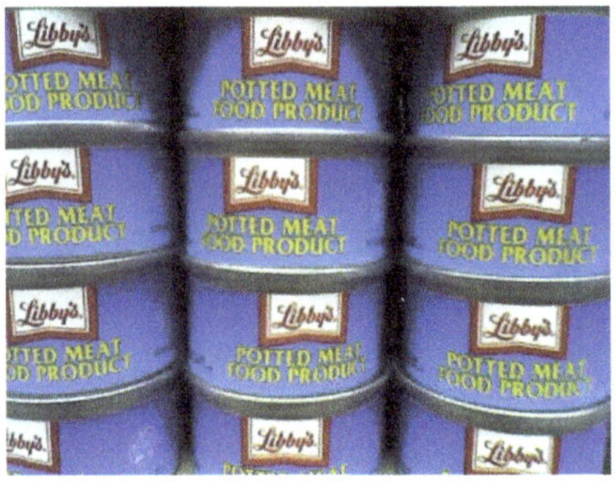

Libby's brand 'Potted Meat Food Product'

Mass production of food is much cheaper overall than individual production of meals from raw ingredients. Therefore, a large profit potential exists for the manufacturers and suppliers of processed food products. Individuals may see a benefit in convenience, but rarely see any direct financial cost benefit in using processed food as compared to home preparation.

Processed food freed people from the large amount of time involved in preparing and cooking "natural" unprocessed foods. The increase in free time allows people much more choice in life style than previously allowed. In many families the adults are working away from home and therefore there is little time for the preparation of food based on fresh ingredients. The food industry offers products that fulfill many different needs: e.g. fully prepared ready meals that can be heated up in the microwave oven within a few minutes.

Modern food processing also improves the quality of life for people with allergies, diabetics, and other people who cannot consume some common food elements. Food processing can also add extra nutrients such as vitamins.

Drawbacks

Any processing of food can affect its nutritional density. The amount of nutrients lost depends on the food and processing method. For example, heat destroys vitamin C. Therefore, canned fruits possess less vitamin C than their fresh alternatives. The USDA conducted a study in 2004, creating a nutrient retention table for several foods.

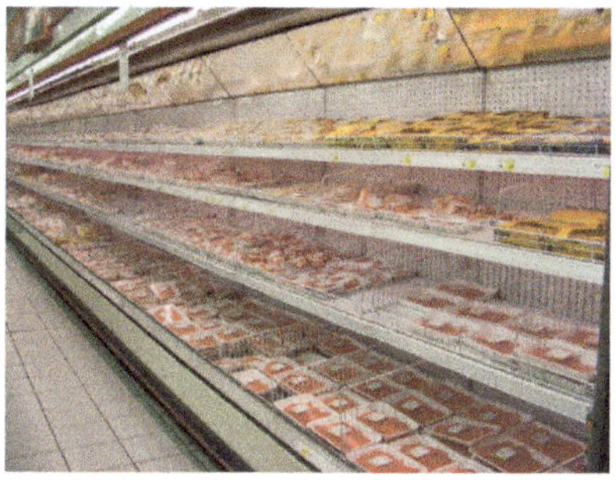

Meat packages in a Roman supermarket

New research highlighting the importance to human health of a rich microbial environment in the intestine indicates that abundant food processing (not fermentation of foods) endangers that environment.

Using food additives represents another safety concern. The health risks of any given additive vary greatly from person to person; for example using sugar as an additive endangers diabetics. In the European Union, only European Food Safety Authority (EFSA) approved food additives (e.g., sweeteners, preservatives, stabilizers) are permitted at specified levels for use in food products. Approved additives receive an E number (E for Europe), simplifying communication about food additives included in the ingredients' list for all the different languages spoken in the EU. As effects of chemical additives are learnt, changes to laws and regulatory practices are made to make such processed foods more safe.

Food processing is typically a mechanical process that utilizes large mixing, grinding, chopping and emulsifying equipment in the production process. These processes inherently introduce a number of contamination risks. As a mixing bowl or grinder is used over time the food contact parts will tend to fail and fracture. This type of failure will introduce into the product stream small to large metal contaminants. Further processing of these metal fragments will result in downstream equipment failure and the risk of ingestion by the consumer. Food manufacturers utilize industrial metal detectors to detect and reject automatically any metal fragment. Large food processors will utilize many metal detectors within the processing stream to reduce both damage to processing machinery as well as risk to consumer health.

Typical Maximum Nutrient Losses due to cooking					
Vitamin & Minerals	**Freeze**	**Dry**	**Cook**	**Cook+Drain**	**Reheat**
Vitamin A	5%	50%	25%	35%	10%
Vit A- Retinol Activity Equivalent	5%	50%	25%	35%	10%
Vit A- Alpha Carotene	5%	50%	25%	35%	10%
Vit A- Beta Carotene	5%	50%	25%	35%	10%
Vit A- Beta Cryptoxanthin	5%	50%	25%	35%	10%
Vit A- Lycopene	5%	50%	25%	35%	10%
Vit A- Lutein+Zeaxanthin	5%	50%	25%	35%	10%
Vitamin C	30%	80%	50%	75%	50%

Thiamin	5%	30%	55%	70%	40%
Riboflavin	0%	10%	25%	45%	5%
Niacin	0%	10%	40%	55%	5%
Vitamin B6	0%	10%	50%	65%	45%
Folate	5%	50%	70%	75%	30%
Food Folate	5%	50%	70%	75%	30%
Folic Acid	5%	50%	70%	75%	30%
Vitamin B12	0%	0%	45%	50%	45%
Calcium	5%	0%	20%	25%	0%
Iron	0%	0%	35%	40%	0%
Magnesium	0%	0%	25%	40%	0%
Phosphorus	0%	0%	25%	35%	0%
Potassium	10%	0%	30%	70%	0%
Sodium	0%	0%	25%	55%	0%
Zinc	0%	0%	25%	25%	0%
Copper	10%	0%	40%	45%	0%

Performance Parameters for Food Processing

When designing processes for the food industry the following performance parameters may be taken into account:

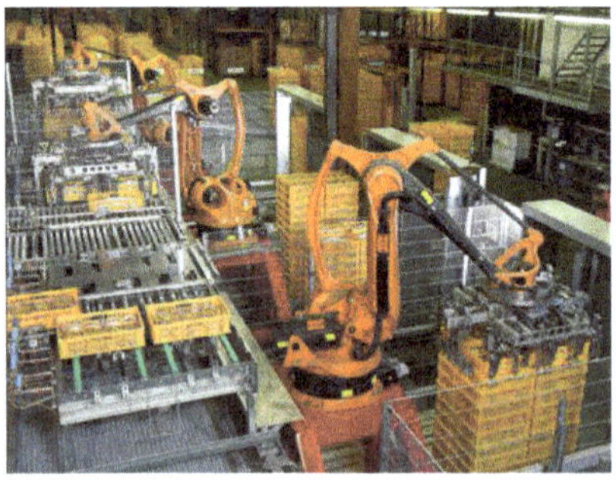

Factory automation - robotics palettizing bread

- Hygiene, e.g. measured by number of micro-organisms per mL of finished product
- Energy efficiency measured e.g. by "ton of steam per ton of sugar produced"
- Minimization of waste, measured e.g. by "percentage of peeling loss during the peeling of potatoes"
- Labour used, measured e.g. by "number of working hours per ton of finished product"
- Minimization of cleaning stops measured e.g. by "number of hours between cleaning stops"

De-agglomerating Batter Mixes in Food Processing

Problems often occur during preparation of batter mixes because flour and other powdered ingredients tend to form lumps or agglomerates as they are being mixed during production. A conventional mixer/agitator cannot break down these agglomerates, resulting in a lumpy batter. If lumpy batter is used to enrobe products, it causes an unsatisfactory appearance with misshapen or oversize products that do not fit properly into packaging. This can force production to a standstill. Furthermore, batter mix is generally recirculated from an enrobing system back to a holding vessel; lumps then have a tendency to build up, reducing the flow of material and raising potential sanitation issues.

Using a high shear in-line mixer in place of a conventional agitator or mixer can quickly solve problems of agglomeration with dry ingredients. A single pass through a self-pumping, in-line mixer adds high shear to batter, which de-agglomerates the mix, resulting in a homogeneous, smooth batter. With a consistent, smooth batter, finished product appearance is improved; the effectiveness and hygiene of the recirculation system is increased; and a better yield of raw materials is achieved. By increasing overall product quality, the amount of raw materials needed is decreased, thereby lowering manufacturing costs and increasing shelf life. Increased shelf life is achieved by creating and maintaining an emulsion, often by adding a food stabilizer.

High shear in-line mixers process food to be made faster and cheaper while increasing consistency of the finished food. Powder and liquid mixing systems are capable of rapidly incorporating large quantities of powders at high concentrations – agglomerate free and fully hydrated. Advances in technology have made processing equipment easy to clean, leading to a much safer processed food.

Trends in Modern Food Processing

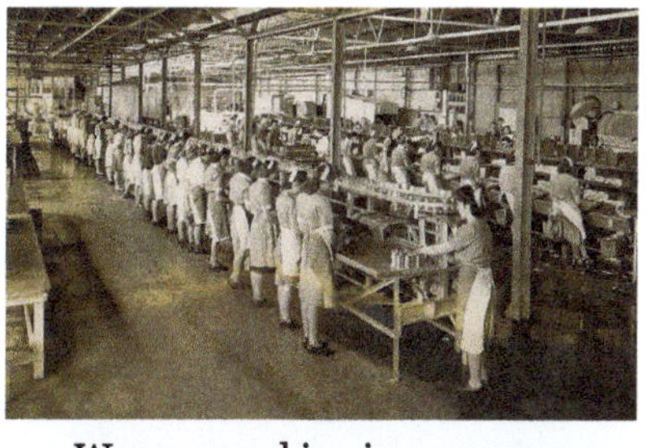

Women working in a cannery

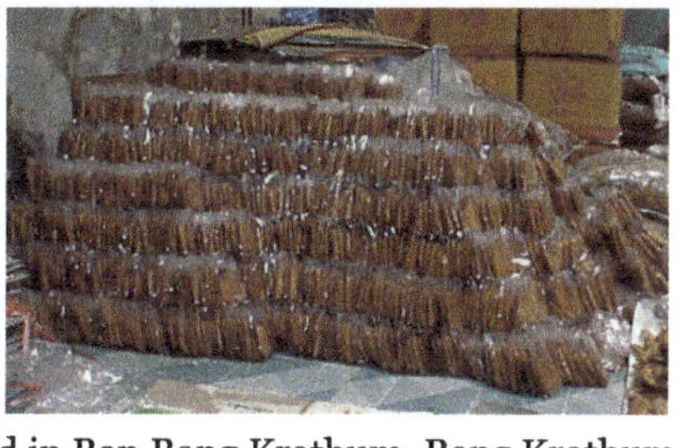

Dried bananas packaged in Ban Bang Krathum, Bang Krathum, Phitsanulok, Thailand

Health

- Reduction of fat content in final product by using baking instead of deep-frying in the production of potato chips, another processed food.
- Maintaining the natural taste of the product by using less artificial sweetener than was used before.

Hygiene

The rigorous application of industry and government endorsed standards to minimise possible risk and hazards. The international standard adopted is HACCP.

Efficiency

- Rising energy costs lead to increasing usage of energy-saving technologies, e.g. frequency converters on electrical drives, heat insulation of factory buildings and heated vessels, energy recovery systems, keeping a single fish frozen all the way from China to Switzerland.
- Factory automation systems (often Distributed control systems) reduce personnel costs and may lead to more stable production results.

Fermentation in Food Processing

Fermentation in food processing is the process of converting carbohydrates to alcohol or organic acids using microorganisms—yeasts or bacteria—under anaerobic conditions. Fermentation usually implies that the action of microorganisms is desired. The science of fermentation is known as zymology or zymurgy.

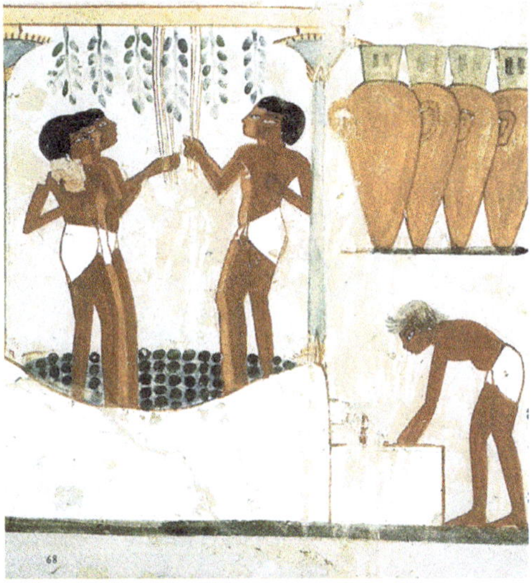

Grapes being trodden to extract the juice and made into wine in storage jars. Tomb of Nakht, 18th dynasty, Thebes, Ancient Egypt

The term fermentation sometimes refers specifically to the chemical conversion of sugars into ethanol, producing alcoholic drinks such as wine, beer, and cider. However, similar processes take place in the leavening of bread (CO_2 produced by yeast activity), and in the preservation of sour foods with the production of lactic acid, such as in sauerkraut and yogurt.

Apart from alcohol, widely consumed fermented foods include vinegar, olives, yogurt, bread, and cheese. In various parts of the world, more localised foods prepared by fermentation may also be based on beans, dough, grain, vegetables, fruit, honey, dairy products, fish, meat, or tea.

History and Prehistory

Natural fermentation precedes human history. Since ancient times, humans have exploited the fermentation process. The earliest evidence of an alcoholic drink, made from fruit, rice, and honey, dates from 7000 to 6600 BC, in the Neolithic Chinese village of Jiahu, and winemaking dates from 6000 BC, in Georgia, in the Caucasus area. Seven-thousand-year-old jars containing the remains of wine, now on display at the University of Pennsylvania, were excavated in the Zagros Mountains in Iran. There is strong evidence that people were fermenting alcoholic drinks in Babylon c. 3000 BC, ancient Egypt c. 3150 BC, pre-Hispanic Mexico c. 2000 BC, and Sudan c. 1500 BC.

The French chemist Louis Pasteur founded zymology, when in 1856 he connected yeast to fermentation. When studying the fermentation of sugar to alcohol by yeast, Pasteur concluded that the fermentation was catalyzed by a vital force, called "ferments", within the yeast cells. The "ferments" were thought to function only within living organisms. "Alcoholic fermentation is an act correlated with the life and organization of the yeast cells, not with the death or putrefaction of the cells", he wrote.

Nevertheless, it was known that yeast extracts can ferment sugar even in the absence of living yeast cells. While studying this process in 1897, Eduard Buchner of Humboldt University of Berlin, Germany, found that sugar was fermented even when there were no living yeast cells in the mixture, by a yeast secreted enzyme complex that he termed *zymase*. In 1907 he received the Nobel Prize in Chemistry for his research and discovery of "cell-free fermentation".

One year earlier, in 1906, ethanol fermentation studies led to the early discovery of NAD^+.

Uses

Food fermentation is the conversion of sugars and other carbohydrates into alcohol or preservative organic acids and carbon dioxide. All three products have found human uses. The production of alcohol is made use of when fruit juices are converted to wine, when grains are made into beer, and when foods rich in starch, such as potatoes, are fermented and then distilled to make spirits such as gin and vodka. The production of carbon dioxide is used to leaven bread. The production of organic acids is exploited to preserve and flavor vegetables and dairy products.

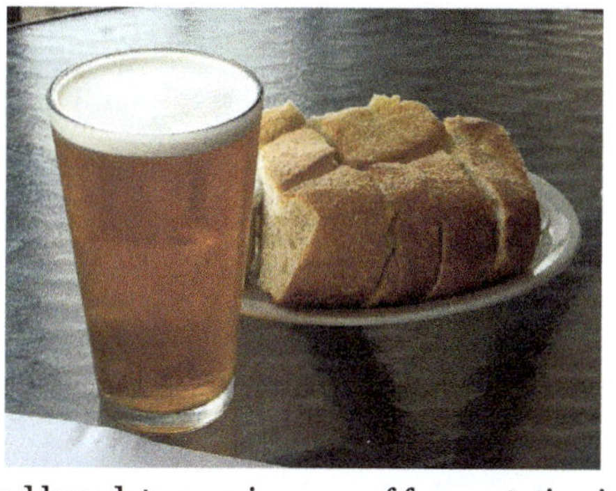

Beer and bread, two major uses of fermentation in food

Food fermentation serves five main purposes: to enrich the diet through development of a diversity of flavors, aromas, and textures in food substrates; to preserve substantial amounts of food through lactic acid, alcohol, acetic acid, and alkaline fermentations; to enrich food substrates with protein, essential amino acids, and vitamins; to eliminate antinutrients; and to reduce cooking time and the associated use of fuel.

Food fermentation is the conversion of sugars and other carbohydrates into alcohol or preservative organic acids and carbon dioxide. All three products have found human uses. The production of alcohol is made use of when fruit juices are converted to wine, when grains are made into beer, and when foods rich in starch, such as potatoes, are fermented and then distilled to make spirits such as gin and vodka. The production of carbon dioxide is used to leaven bread. The production of organic acids is exploited to preserve and flavor vegetables and dairy products.

Food fermentation serves five main purposes: to enrich the diet through development of a diversity of flavors, aromas, and textures in food substrates; to preserve substantial amounts of food through lactic acid, alcohol, acetic acid, and alkaline fermentations; to enrich food substrates with protein, essential amino acids, and vitamins; to eliminate antinutrients; and to reduce cooking time and the associated use of fuel.

Fermented Foods by Region

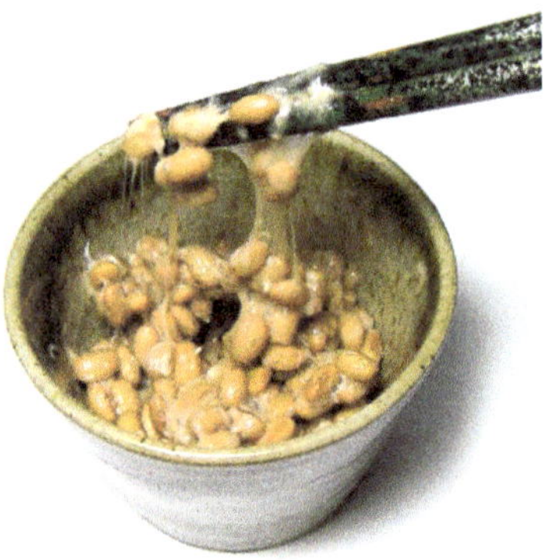

Nattō, a Japanese fermented soybean food

- Worldwide: alcohol(beer, wine), vinegar, olives, yogurt, bread, cheese
- Asia
    - East and Southeast Asia: amazake, atchara, bai-ming, belacan, burong mangga, com ruou, dalok, doenjang, douchi, jeruk, lambanog, kimchi, kombucha, leppet-so, narezushi, miang, miso, nata de coco, nata de pina, natto, naw-mai-dong, oncom, pak-siam-dong, paw-tsaynob, prahok, ruou nep, sake, seokbakji, soju, soy sauce, stinky tofu, szechwan cabbage, tai-tan tsoi, chiraki, tape, tempeh, totkal kimchi, yen tsai, zha cai
    - Central Asia: kumis (mare milk), kefir, shubat (camel milk)
    - South Asia: achar, appam, dosa, dhokla, dahi (yogurt), idli, kaanji, mixed pickle, ngari, hawaichaar, jaand (rice beer), sinki, tongba, paneer
- Africa: fermented millet porridge, garri, hibiscus seed, hot pepper sauce, injera, lamoun makbouss, laxoox, mauoloh, msir, mslalla, oilseed, ogi, ogili, ogiri, iru

- Americas: sourdough bread, cultured milk, chicha, elderberry wine, kombucha, pickling (pickled vegetables), sauerkraut, lupin seed, oilseed, chocolate, vanilla, tabasco, tibicos, pulque, mikyuk (fermented bowhead whale)
- Middle East: kushuk, lamoun makbouss, mekhalel, torshi, boza
- Europe: rakfisk, sauerkraut, pickled cucumber, surströmming, mead, elderberry wine, salami, sucuk, prosciutto, cultured milk products such as quark, kefir, filmjölk, crème fraîche, smetana, skyr, rakı, tupí.
- Oceania: poi, kaanga pirau (rotten corn), sago

Fermented Foods by Type

Bean-based

Cheonggukjang, doenjang, miso, natto, soy sauce, stinky tofu, tempeh, oncom, soybean paste, Beijing mung bean milk, kinama, iru

Dough-based

Proofing (baking technique)

Grain-based

Amazake, beer, bread, choujiu, gamju, injera, kvass, makgeolli, murri, ogi, rejuvelac, sake, sikhye, sourdough, sowans, rice wine, malt whisky, grain whisky, idli, dosa, vodka, boza

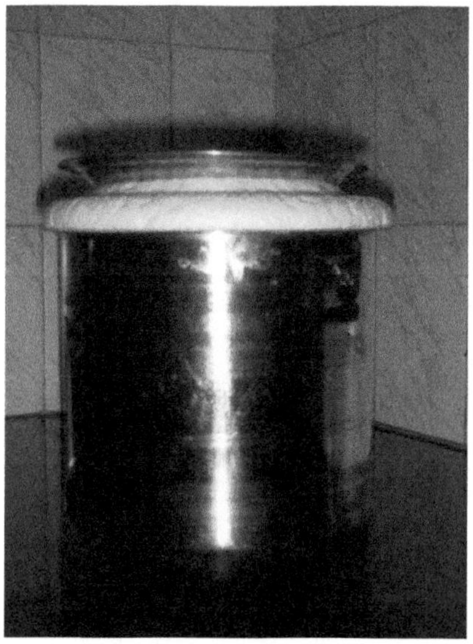

Batter made from rice and lentil (*Vigna mungo*) prepared and fermented for baking idlis and dosas

Vegetable-based

Kimchi, mixed pickle, sauerkraut, Indian pickle, gundruk, tursu

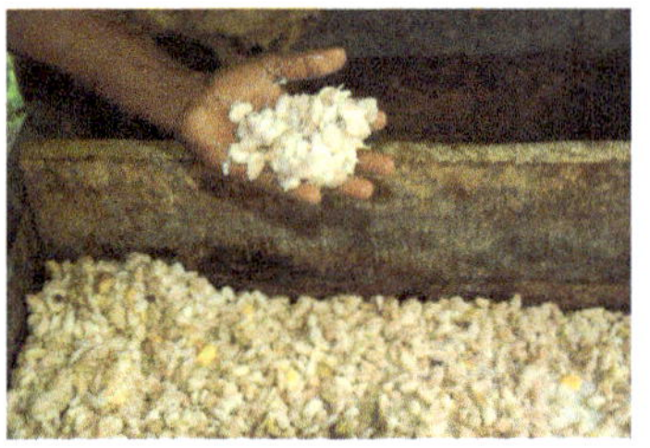

Fermenting cocoa beans

Fruit-based

Wine, vinegar, cider, perry, brandy, atchara, nata de coco, burong mangga, asinan, pickling, vişinată, chocolate, rakı

Honey-based

Mead, metheglin

Dairy-based

Some kinds of cheese also, kefir, kumis (mare milk), shubat (camel milk), cultured milk products such as quark, filmjölk, crème fraîche, smetana, skyr, and yogurt

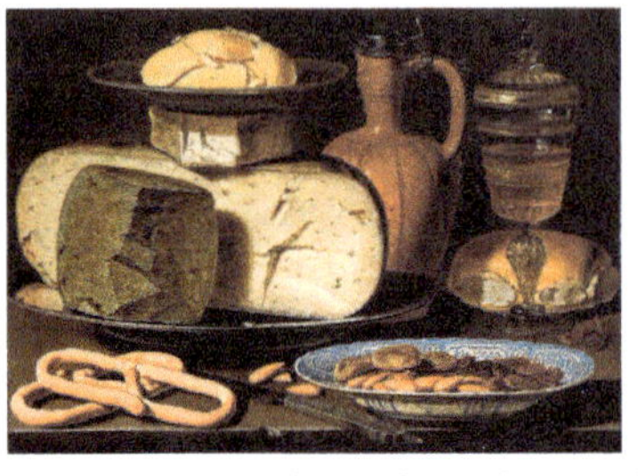

Cheeses in art: *Still Life with Cheeses, Almonds and Pretzels*, Clara Peeters, c. 1615

Fish-based

Bagoong, faseekh, fish sauce, Garum, Hákarl, jeotgal, rakfisk, shrimp paste, surströmming, shidal

Meat-based

Chorizo, salami, sucuk, pepperoni, nem chua, som moo, saucisson

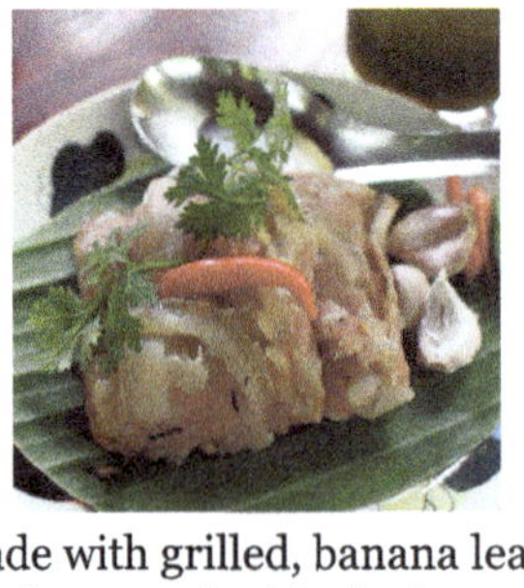

Chin som mok is a northern Thai speciality made with grilled, banana leaf-wrapped pork (both skin and meat) that has been fermented with glutinous rice

Tea-based

Pu-erh tea, Kombucha

Risks

Alaska has witnessed a steady increase of cases of botulism since 1985. It has more cases of botulism than any other state in the United States of America. This is caused by the traditional Eskimo practice of allowing animal products such as whole fish, fish heads, walrus, sea lion, and whale flippers, beaver tails, seal oil, and birds, to ferment for an extended period of time before being consumed. The risk is exacerbated when a plastic container is used for this purpose instead of the old-fashioned, traditional method, a grass-lined hole, as the *Clostridium botulinum* bacteria thrive in the anaerobic conditions created by the air-tight enclosure in plastic.

The World Health Organization has classified pickled foods as possibly carcinogenic, based on epidemiological studies. Other research found that fermented food contains a carcinogenic by-product, ethyl carbamate (urethane). "A 2009 review of the existing studies conducted across Asia concluded that regularly eating pickled vegetables roughly doubles a person's risk for esophageal squamous cell carcinoma."

Food Packaging

Food packaging is packaging for food. A package provides protection, tampering resistance, and special physical, chemical, or biological needs. It may bear a nutrition facts label and other information about food being offered for sale.

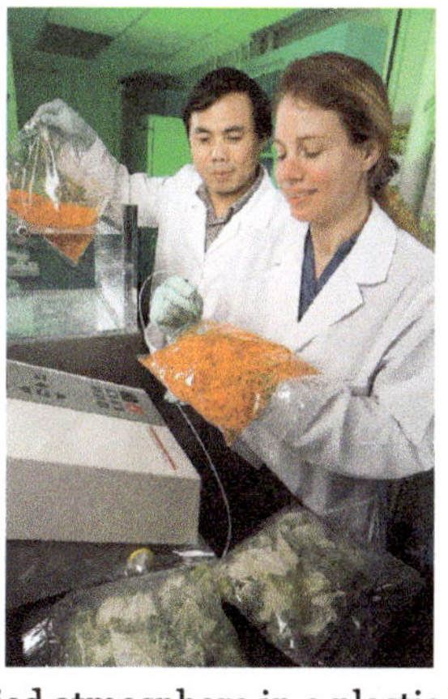

Testing modified atmosphere in a plastic bag of carrots

Functions

Packaging and package labeling have several objectives

- Physical protection - The food enclosed in the package may require protection from, among other things, shock, vibration, compression, temperature, bacteria, etc.

- Barrier protection - A barrier from oxygen, water vapor, dust, etc., is often required. Permeation is a critical factor in design. Some packages contain desiccants or oxygen absorbers to help extend shelf life. Modified atmospheres or controlled atmospheres are also maintained in some food packages. Keeping the contents clean, fresh, and safe for the intended shelf life is a primary function.
- Containment or agglomeration - Small items are typically grouped together in one package to allow efficient handling. Liquids, powders, and granular materials need containment.
- Information transmission - Packages and labels communicate how to use, transport, recycle, or dispose of the package or product. Some types of information are required by governments.
- Marketing - The packaging and labels can be used by marketers to encourage potential buyers to purchase the product. Package design has been an important and constantly evolving phenomenon for several decades. Marketing communications and graphic design are applied to the surface of the package and (in many cases) the point of sale display.
- Security - Packaging can play an important role in reducing the security risks of shipment. Packages can be made with improved tamper resistance to deter tampering and also can have tamper-evident features to help indicate tampering. Packages can be engineered to help reduce the risks of package pilferage; some package constructions are more resistant to pilferage and some have pilfer-indicating seals. Packages may include authentication seals to help indicate that the package and contents are not counterfeit. Packages also can include anti-theft devices, such as dye packs, RFID tags, or electronic article surveillance tags, that can be activated or detected by devices at exit points and require specialized tools to deactivate. Using packaging in this way is a means of retail loss prevention.
- Convenience - Packages can have features which add convenience in distribution, handling, stacking, display, sale, opening, reclosing, use, and reuse.
- Portion control - Single-serving packaging has a precise amount of contents to control usage. Bulk commodities (such as salt) can be divided into packages that are a more suitable size for individual households. It also aids the control of inventory: selling sealed one-liter bottles of milk, rather than having people bring their own bottles to fill themselves.

Types

The above materials are fashioned into different types of food packages and containers such as:

Packaging Type		
Aseptic processing	Primary	Liquid whole eggs or dairy products
Trays	Primary	Portion of fish or meat
Bags	Primary	Potato chips, apples, rice
Boxes	Secondary	Corrugated box of primary packages: box of cereal cartons, frozen pizzas
Cans	Primary	Can of tomato soup
Cartons	Primary	Carton of eggs, milk or juice cartons

Flexible packaging	Primary	Bagged salad
Pallets	Tertiary	A series of boxes on a single pallet used to transport from the manufacturing plant to a distribution center
Wrappers	Tertiary	Used to wrap the boxes on the pallet for transport

Primary packaging is the main package that holds the food that is being processed. Secondary packaging combines the primary packages into one box being made. Tertiary packaging combines all of the secondary packages into one pallet.

Packaging Machines

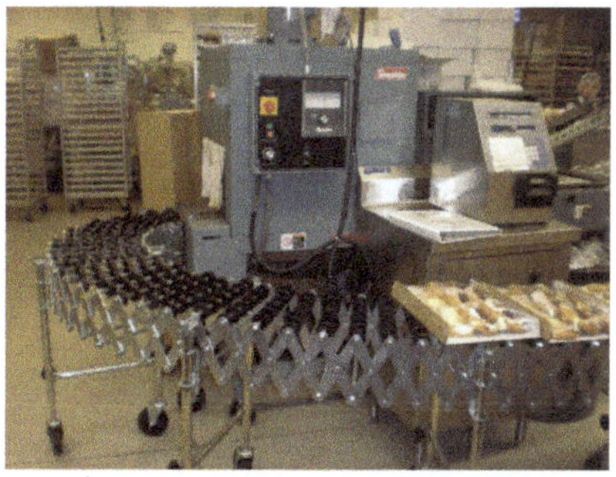

Shrink-wrapping trays of bakery goods

A choice of packaging machinery requires consideration of technical capabilities, labor requirements, worker safety, maintainability, serviceability, reliability, ability to integrate into the packaging line, capital cost, floorspace, flexibility (change-over, materials, etc.), energy usage, quality of outgoing packages, qualifications (for food, pharmaceuticals, etc.), throughput, efficiency, productivity, and ergonomics, at a minimum.

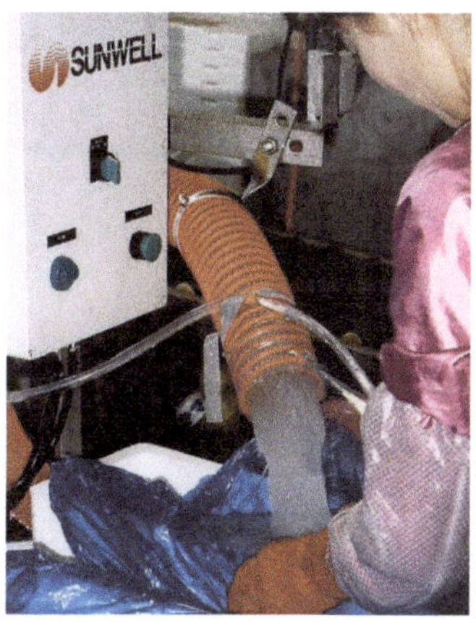

Pumping slurry ice onto fresh fish

Packaging machines may be of the following general types:

- Autocoding label and date verification
- Blister-, skin- and vacuum-packaging machines
- Capping, over-capping, lidding, closing, seaming and sealing machines

- Cartoning machines
- Case and tray forming, packing, unpacking, closing and sealing Machines
- Check weighing machines
- Cleaning, sterilizing, cooling and drying machines
- Conveying and accumulating machines
- Feeding, orienting, and placing machines
- Filling machines for liquid and powdered products
- Package filling and closing Machines
- Form, fill and seal machines
- Inspecting, detecting and checkweighing machines
- Palletizing, depalletizing, and pallet unitizing machines
- Labeling, marking, and other product identification machines
- Wrapping machines
- Converting machines

Reducing Food Packaging

Reduced packaging and sustainable packaging are becoming more frequent. The motivations can be government regulations, consumer pressure, retailer pressure, and cost control. Reduced packaging often saves packaging costs.

In the UK, a Local Government Association survey produced by the British Market Research Bureau compared a range of outlets to buy 29 common food items and found that small local retailers and market traders "produced less packaging and more that could be recycled than the larger supermarkets."

Recycling of Food Packaging

After use, organic matter that is still in the food packaging needs to be separated from the packaging. This may also require rinsing of the food packaging.

Trends in Food Packaging

- Numerous reports industry associations agree that use of smart indicators will increase. There are a number of different indicators with different benefits for food producers, consumers and retailers.
- Temperature recorders are used to monitor products shipped in a cold chain and to help validate the cold chain. Digital temperature data loggers measure and record the temperature

history of food shipments. They sometimes have temperatures displayed on the indicator or have other output (lights, etc.): The data from a shipment can be downloaded (cable, RFID, etc.) to a computer for further analysis. These help identify if there has been temperature abuse of products and can help determine the remaining shelf life. They can also help determine the time of temperature extremes during shipment so corrective measures can be taken.

  - Time temperature indicators integrate the time and temperature experienced by the indicator and adjacent foods. Some use chemical reactions that result in a color change while others use the migration of a dye through a filter media. To the degree that these physical changes in the indicator match the degradation rate of the food, the indicator can help indicate probable food degradation.

- Radio Frequency Identification is applied to food packages for supply chain control and has shown a significant benefit in allowing food producers and retailers create full real time visibility of their supply chain.

- Plastic packaging being used is usually non-biodegradable due to possible interactions with the food. Also, biodegradable polymers often require special composting conditions to properly degrade. Normal sealed landfill conditions do not promote biodegradation. Biodegradable plastics includes biodegradable films and coatings synthesized from organic materials and microbial polymers. Some package materials are edible. For example, pharmaceuticals are sometimes in capsules made of gelatin, starch, potato or other materials. Newer bioplastics, films and products are being developed.

- Barcodes have been used for decades in packaging many products. 2D barcodes used in Autocoding are increasingly applied to food packaging to ensure products are correctly packaged and date coded.

- The ability of a package to fully empty or dispense a viscous food is somewhat dependent on the surface energy of the inner walls of the container. The use of superhydrophobic surfaces is useful but can be further improved by using new lubricant-impregnated surfaces.

Food Safety and Public Health

It is critical to maintain food safety during processing , packaging, storage, logistics (including cold chain), sale, and use. Conformance to applicable regulations is mandatory. Some are country specific such as the US Food and Drug Administration and the US Department of Agriculture; others are regional such as the European Food Safety Authority. Certification programs such as the Global Food Safety Initiative are sometimes used. Food packaging considerations may include: use of hazard analysis and critical control points, verification and validation protocols, Good manufacturing practices, use of an effective quality management system, track and trace systems, and requirements for label content. Special food contact materials are used when the package is in direct contact with the food product. Depending on the packaging operation and the food, packaging machinery often needs specified daily wash-down and cleaning procedures.

Health risks of materials and chemicals used in food packaging need to be carefully controlled. Carcinogens, toxic chemicals, mutagens etc. need to be eliminated from food contact and potential migration into foods.

Food Coloring

Food coloring, or color additive, is any dye, pigment or substance that imparts color when it is added to food or drink. They come in many forms consisting of liquids, powders, gels, and pastes. Food coloring is used both in commercial food production and in domestic cooking. Due to its safety and general availability, food coloring is also used in a variety of non-food applications including cosmetics, pharmaceuticals, home craft projects, and medical devices.

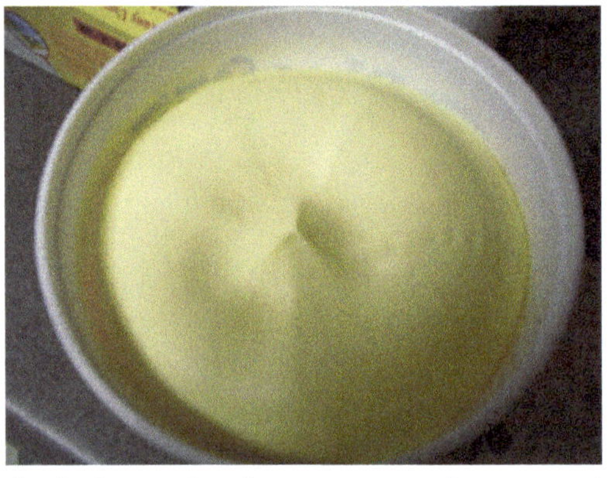

The addition of food coloring, such as beta-carotene, gives margarine its yellow color.

Purpose of Food Coloring

People associate certain colors with certain flavors, and the color of food can influence the perceived flavor in anything from candy to wine. Sometimes the aim is to simulate a color that is perceived by the consumer as natural, such as adding red coloring to glacé cherries (which would otherwise be beige), but sometimes it is for effect, like the green ketchup that Heinz launched in 1999. Color additives are used in foods for many reasons including:

- Offset color loss due to exposure to light, air, temperature extremes, moisture and storage conditions
- Correct natural variations in color
- Enhance colors that occur naturally
- Provide color to colorless and "fun" foods
- Make food more attractive and appetizing, and informative
- Allow consumers to identify products on sight, like candy flavors or medicine dosages
- Food colorants, synthetic

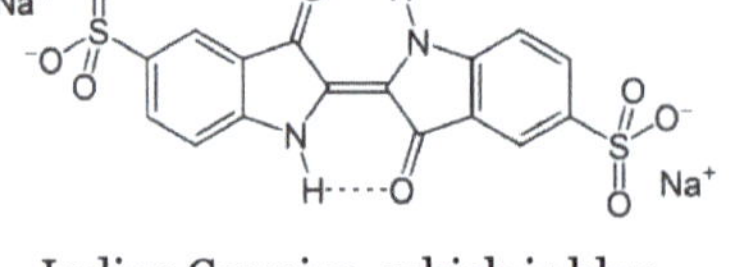

Indigo Carmine, which is blue.

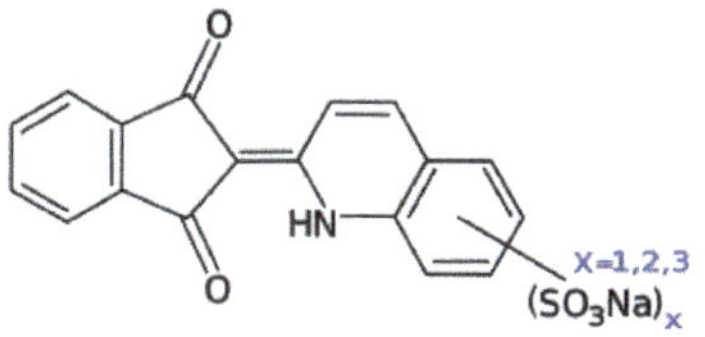

Quinoline Yellow WS, which is yellow.

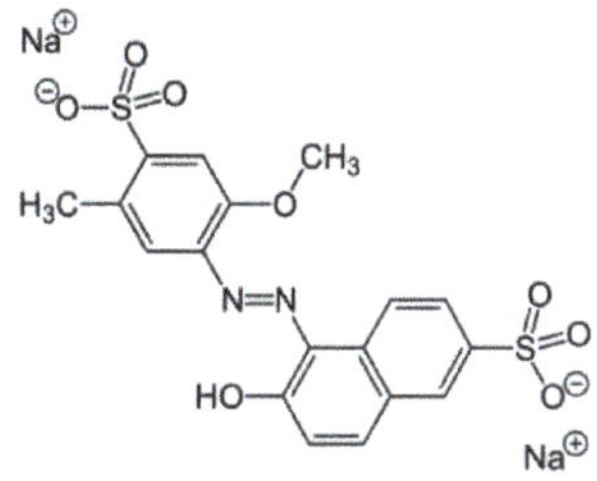

Allura Red AC, which is red.

- Food colorants, natural

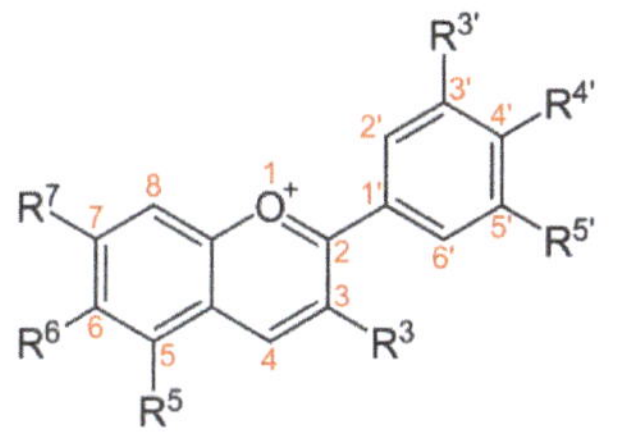

Anthocyanin, a red to blue dye depending on functional groups and pH.

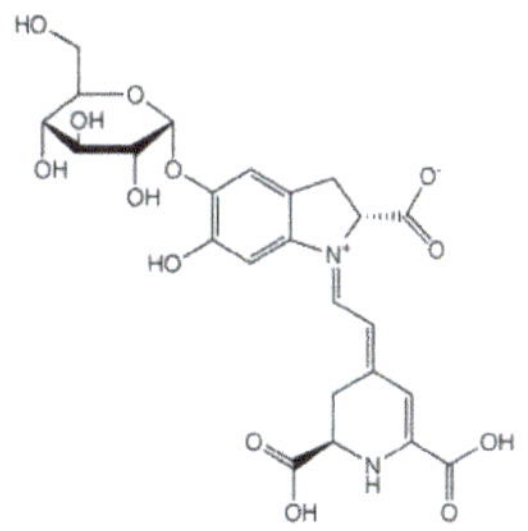

Betanin, a magenta dye, mainly produced from beets.

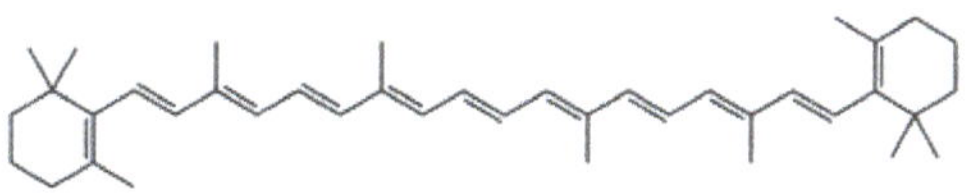

beta-Carotene, a yellow to orange colorant.

Regulation

Past Use and Regulation History

The addition of colorants to foods is thought to have occurred in Egyptian cities as early as 1500 BC, when candy makers added natural extracts and wine to improve the products' appearance. During the Middle Ages, the economy in the European countries was based on agriculture, and the peasants were accustomed to producing their own food locally or trading within the village communities. Under feudalism, aesthetic aspects were not considered, at least not by the vast majority of the generally very poor population. This situation changed with urbanization at the beginning of the Modern Age, when trade emerged—especially the import of precious spices and colors. One of the very first food laws, created in Augsburg, Germany, in 1531, concerned spices or colorants and required saffron counterfeiters to be burned.

With the onset of the industrial revolution, people became dependent on foods produced by others. These new urban dwellers demanded food at low cost. Analytical chemistry was still primitive and regulations few. The adulteration of foods flourished. Heavy metal and other inorganic element-containing compounds turned out to be cheap and suitable to "restore" the color of watered-down milk and other foodstuffs, some more lurid examples being:

- Red lead (Pb_3O_4) and vermillion (HgS) were routinely used to color cheese and confectionery.

- Copper arsenite ($CuHAsO_3$) was used to recolor used tea leaves for resale. It also caused two deaths when used to color a dessert in 1860.

Sellers at the time offered more than 80 artificial coloring agents, some invented for dyeing textiles, not foods.

...Thus, with potted meat, fish and sauces taken at breakfast he would consume more or less Armenian bole, red lead, or even bisulphuret of mercury. At dinner with his curry or cayenne he would run the chance of a second dose of lead or mercury; with pickles, bottled fruit and vegetables he would be nearly sure to have copper administrated to him; and while he partook of bon-bons at dessert, there was no telling of the number of poisonous pigments he might consume. Again his tea if mixed or green, he would certainly not escape without the administration of a little Prussian blue...

Many color additives had never been tested for toxicity or other adverse effects. Historical records show that injuries, even deaths, resulted from tainted colorants. In 1851, about 200 people were poisoned in England, 17 of them fatally, directly as a result of eating adulterated lozenges. In 1856, mauveine, the first synthetic color, was developed by Sir William Henry Perkin and by the turn of the century, unmonitored color additives had spread through Europe and the United States in all sorts of popular foods, including ketchup, mustard, jellies, and wine.

Concerns over food safety led to numerous regulations throughout the world,. German food regulations released in 1882 stipulated the exclusion of dangerous minerals such as arsenic, copper, chromium, lead, mercury and zinc, which were frequently used as ingredients in colorants. In contrast to today, these first laws followed the principle of a negative listing (substances not allowed for use); they were already driven by the main principles of today's food regulations all over the world, since all of these regulations follow the same goal: the protection of consumers from toxic substances and from fraud. In the United States, the Pure Food and Drug Act of 1906 reduced the permitted list of synthetic colors from 700 down to seven. Even with updated food laws, adulteration continued for many years and this, together with more recent adverse press comments on food colors and health, has continued to contribute to consumer concern about color addition to foodstuffs.

In the 20th century, the improvement of chemical analysis and the development of trials to identify the toxic features of substances added to foods led to the replacement of the negative lists by lists of substances allowed to be used for the production and the improvement of foods. This principle is called a positive listing, and almost all recent legislations are based on it. Positive listing implies that substances meant for human consumption have been tested for their safety, and that they have to meet specified purity criteria prior to their approval by the corresponding authorities. In 1962, the first EU directive (62/2645/EEC) approved 36 colorants, of which 20 were naturally derived and 16 were synthetic. This directive did not list which food products the colorants could or could not be used in. At that time, each member state could designate where certain colors could and could not be used. In Germany, for example, quinoline yellow was allowed in puddings and desserts, but tartrazine was not. The reverse was true in France. This was updated in 1989 with 89/107/EEC, which concerned food additives authorized for use in foodstuffs.

Current Regulation

While naturally derived colors are not required to be certified by a number of regulatory bodies throughout the world (including the U.S. FDA), they still need to be approved for use in that country. The FDA lists "color additives exempt from certification" for food in subpart A of the Code of Federal Regulations - Title 21 Part 73. However, this list contains substances which may have synthetic origins, such as nature identical beta-carotene. FDA's permitted colors are classified as subject to certification or exempt from certification, both of which are subject to rigorous safety standards prior to their approval and listing for use in foods.

- Certified colors are synthetically produced and are used widely because they impart an intense, uniform color, are less expensive, and blend more easily to create a variety of hues. There are nine certified color additives approved for use in the United States. Certified food colors generally do not add undesirable flavors to foods.
- Colors that are exempt from certification include pigments derived from natural sources such as vegetables, minerals or animals. Nature derived color additives are typically more expensive than certified colors and may add unintended flavors to foods. Examples of exempt colors include annatto, beet extract, caramel, beta-carotene, turmeric and grape skin extract.

Food colorings are tested for safety by various bodies around the world and sometimes different bodies have different views on food color safety. In the United States, FD&C numbers (which indicate that the FDA has approved the colorant for use in foods, drugs and cosmetics) are given to approved synthetic food dyes that do not exist in nature, while in the European Union, E numbers are used for all additives, both synthetic and natural, that are approved in food applications. The food colors are known by E numbers that begin with a 1, such as E100 (turmeric) or E161b (lutein). The safety of food colors and other food additives in the EU is evaluated by the European Food Safety Authority. Color Directive 94/36/EC, enacted by the European Commission in 1994, outlines permitted natural and artificial colors with their approved applications and limits in different foodstuffs. This is binding to all member countries of the EU. Any changes have to be implemented into their national laws within a given time frame. In non-EU member states, food additives are regulated by their national authorities, which usually, but not in all cases, try to harmonize with the laws adopted by the EU. Most other countries have their own regulations and list of food colors which can be used in various applications, including maximum daily intake limits.

Global Harmonization

Global trade requires harmonization of food regulations on a world-wide basis in order to abolish barriers of trade and to ensure that the economic and nutritional demands of all nations are considered. Since the beginning of the 1960s, JECFA has played an important role in the development of international standards for food additives, not only by its toxicological assessments, which are continuously published by the WHO in a "Technical Report Series", but furthermore by elaborating appropriate purity criteria, which are laid down in the two volumes of the "Compendium of Food Additive Specifications" and their supplements. These specifications are not legally binding but very often serve as a guiding principle, especially in countries where no scientific expert committees have been established.

In order to further regulate the use of these evaluated additives, in 1962 the WHO and FAO created an international commission, the Codex Alimentarius, which is composed of authorities, food industry associations and consumer groups from all over the world. Within the Codex organization, the Codex Committee for Food Additives and Contaminants is responsible for working out recommendations for the application of food additives, the General Standard for Food Additives. In the light of the World Trade Organizations General Agreement on Tariffs and Trade (GATT), the Codex Standard, although not legally binding, influences food color regulations all over the world.

Artificial Coloring

As the 1900s began, a host of synthetic dyes and pigments became available. Originally, these were dubbed `coal-tar' colors because the starting materials were obtained from bituminous coal. Many synthesized dyes were easier and less costly to produce and were superior in coloring properties when compared to naturally derived alternatives of the time.

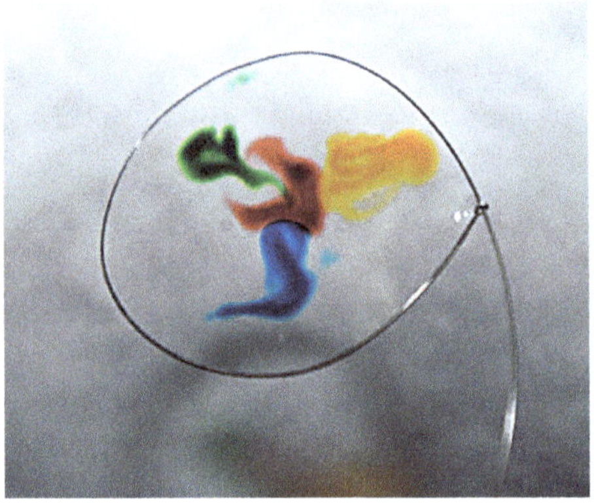

Food coloring spreading on a thin water film in the International Space Station

Also known as "azo-dyes", synthetic colors are generally produced via a two-step chemical synthesis. The first step forms a diazo compound from the reaction of aromatic amines generally formed from nitrosamine and a diazonium compound. The second step couples these diazo compounds with various reactive aromatic hydrocarbons. Due to the π-electrons across the two aromatic sections and the azo-groups, a conjugated system exists that is able to absorb light of specific wavelengths, leading to the color of the compounds (this principle also applies to naturally derived pigments as well).

The attractiveness of the synthetic dyes is that their color, lipophilicity, and other attributes can be engineered by the design of the specific molecule. The color of the dyes can be controlled selecting the number of azo-groups and various substituents. Yellow shades are achieved by using aceto-acetanilide and heterocyclic compounds. Red colors result from the reaction between an aniline derivative (diazo) with a naphthol derivate. A blue results from replacing the aniline derivate with a benzidine derivate. The pair indigo and indigo carmine exhibit the same color, but the former is soluble in lipids, and the latter is water soluble because it has been fitted with sulfonate functional groups.

In The United States

Only seven dyes were initially approved under the U.S. Pure Food and Drug Act of 1906, but several have been delisted and replacements have been found. Some of the food colorings have the abbreviation "FCF" in their names. This stands for "For Coloring Food" (US) or "For Colouring of Food" (UK).

In the United States, manufacturers must get FDA approval for every batch of certified colors produced. FDA personnel evaluate the color's physical appearance and chemically analyze it. Tests include purity (total color content), moisture, residual salts, unreacted intermediates, colored impurities other than the main color (called subsidiary colors), any other specified impurities, and heavy metals (lead, arsenic, and mercury). The results are reviewed for compliance with the identity and specifications described in the listing regulation for the color additive. If the sample is found to meet these requirements, the FDA issues a certificate for the batch that identifies the color additive. For example, a batch of "tartrazine" becomes "FD&C Yellow No. 5."

Current Seven Generally Permitted

In the US, the following seven artificial colorings are generally permitted in food (the most common in bold) as of 2016. The lakes of these colorings are also permitted except the lake of Red No. 3.

- FD&C Blue No. 1 – Brilliant Blue FCF, E133 (blue shade)
- FD&C Blue No. 2 – Indigotine, E132 (indigo shade)
- FD&C Green No. 3 – Fast Green FCF, E143 (turquoise shade)
- FD&C Red No. 3 – Erythrosine, E127 (pink shade, commonly used in glacé cherries)
- FD&C Red No. 40 – Allura Red AC, E129 (red shade)
- FD&C Yellow No. 5 – Tartrazine, E102 (yellow shade)
- FD&C Yellow No. 6 – Sunset Yellow FCF, E110 (orange shade)

Permitted for Limited Use in Foods

Two dyes are allowed by the FDA for limited applications:

- Citrus Red 2 (orange shade) - allowed only to color orange peels.
- Orange B (red shade) - allowed only for use in hot dog and sausage casings (not produced after 1978, but never delisted)

Delisted and Banned in The US

- FD&C Red No. 2 – Amaranth, E123
- FD&C Red No. 4
- FD&C Red No. 32 was used to color Florida oranges.
- FD&C Orange Number 1 was one of the first water-soluble dyes to be commercialized, and one of seven original food dyes allowed under the Pure Food and Drug Act of June 30,

1906.

- FD&C Orange No. 2 was used to color Florida oranges.
- FD&C Yellow No. 1, 2, 3, and 4
- FD&C Violet No. 1

Approved in EU

E numbers 102-143 cover the range of artificial colors. For an overview of currently allowed additives see here . Some artificial dyes approved for food use in the EU include:

- E104: Quinoline Yellow
- E122: Carmoisine
- E124: Ponceau 4R
- E131: Patent Blue V
- E142: Green S

Natural Food Dyes

Carotenoids (E160, E161, E164), chlorophyllin (E140, E141), anthocyanins (E163), and betanin (E162) comprise four main categories of plant pigments grown to color food products. Other colorants or specialized derivatives of these core groups include:

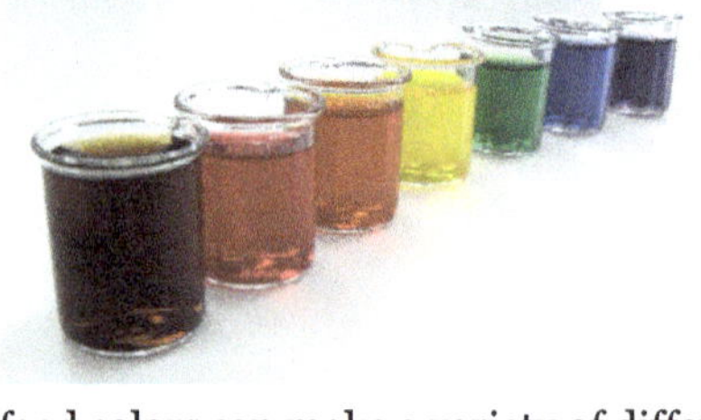

Natural food colors can make a variety of different hues

- Annatto (E160b), a reddish-orange dye made from the seed of the achiote
- Caramel coloring (E150a-d), made from caramelized sugar
- Carmine (E120), a red dye derived from the cochineal insect, *Dactylopius coccus*
- Elderberry juice
- Lycopene (E160d)
- Paprika (E160c)
- Turmeric (E100)

Blue colors are especially rare.

To ensure reproducibility, the colored components of these substances are often provided in highly purified form. For stability and convenience, they can be formulated in suitable carrier materials (solid and liquids). Hexane, acetone, and other solvents break down cell walls in the fruit and vegetables and allow for maximum extraction of the coloring. Traces of these may still remain in the finished colorant, but they do not need to be declared on the product label. These solvents are known as carry-over ingredients.

Dyes and Lakes

Color additives are available for use in food as either "dyes" or lake pigments (commonly known as "lakes").

Dyes dissolve in water, but are not soluble in oil. Dyes are manufactured as powders, granules, liquids or other special purpose forms. They can be used in beverages, dry mixes, baked goods, confections, dairy products, pet foods, and a variety of other products. Dyes also have side effects that lakes lack. Consuming large amounts of dyes can color stools.

Lakes are made by combining dyes with salts (usually aluminum salts) to make insoluble compounds. Lakes tint by dispersion. Lakes are not oil-soluble, but are oil-dispersible. Lakes are more stable than dyes and are ideal for coloring products containing fats and oils or items lacking sufficient moisture to dissolve dyes. Typical uses include coated tablets, cake and doughnut mixes, hard candies and chewing gums, lipsticks, soaps, shampoos, talc, etc.

Other Uses

Because food dyes are generally safer to use than normal artists' dyes and pigments, some artists have used food coloring as a means of making pictures, especially in forms such as body-painting. Red food dye is often used in theatrical blood.

Most artificial food colorings are a type of acid dye, and can be used to dye protein fibers and nylon with the addition of an acid. They are all washfast and most are also lightfast. They will not permanently bond to plant fibers and other synthetics.

Criticism and Health Implications

Widespread public belief that artificial food coloring cause hyperactivity in children originated with Benjamin Feingold a pediatric allergist from California, who proposed in 1973 that salicylates, artificial colors, and artificial flavors cause hyperactivity in children; however, there is no evidence to support broad claims that food coloring causes food intolerance and ADHD-like behavior in children. It is possible that certain food coloring may act as a trigger in those who are genetically predisposed, but the evidence is weak.

After concerns were expressed that food colorings may cause ADHD-like behavior in children, the collective evidence do not support this assertion. The US FDA and other food safety authorities to regularly review the scientific literature, and led the UK Food Standards Agency (FSA) to commission a study by researchers at Southampton University of the effect of a mixture of six food dyes (Tartrazine, Allura Red, Ponceau 4R, Quinoline Yellow WS, Sunset Yellow and Carmoisine (dubbed the "Southampton 6")) on children in the general population. These colorants are found in beverages. The study found “a possible link between the consumption of these artificial colours and a sodium benzoate preservative and increased hyperactivity” in the children; the advisory committee to the FSA that evaluated the study also determined that because of study limitations, the results could not be extrapolated to the general population, and further testing was recommended”. The U.S. FDA did not make changes following the publication of the Southampton study, but following a citizen petition filed by the Center for Science in the Public Interest in 2008, requesting the FDA ban several food additives, the FDA reviewed the available evidence, and still made no changes.

The European regulatory community, with an emphasis on the precautionary principle, required labelling and temporarily reduced the acceptable daily intake (ADI) for the food colorings; the UK FSA called for voluntary withdrawal of the colorings by food manufacturers. However, in 2009 the EFSA re-evaluated the data at hand and determined that “the available scientific evidence does not substantiate a link between the color additives and behavioral effects” for any of the dyes.

Food Technology

Food Technology is a branch of food science that deals with the production processes that make foods.

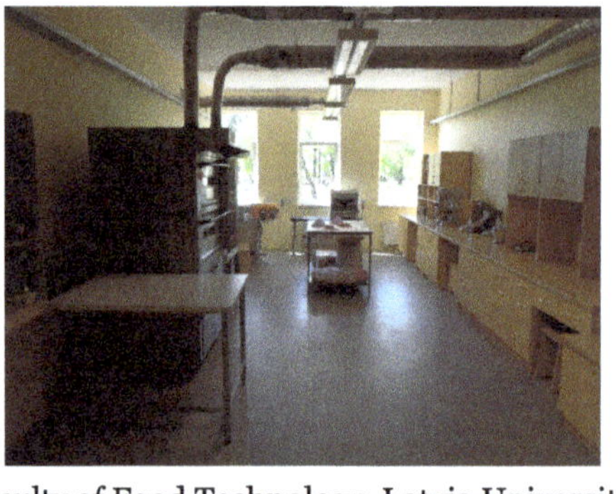

Bakery at the Faculty of Food Technology, Latvia University of Agriculture

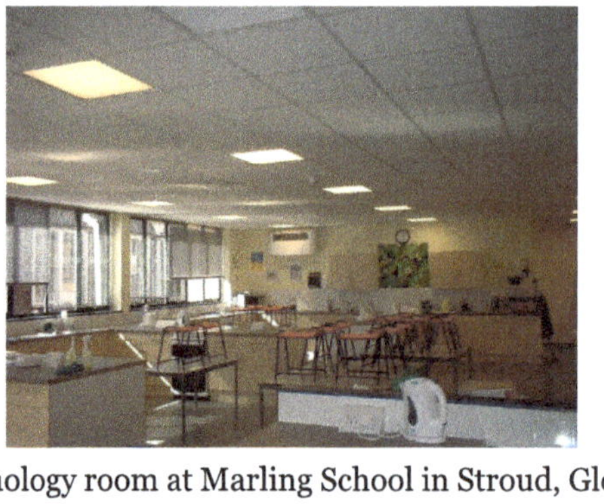

The food technology room at Marling School in Stroud, Gloucestershire

Early scientific research into food technology concentrated on food preservation. Nicolas Appert’s development in 1810 of the canning process was a decisive event. The process wasn’t called canning then and Appert did not really know the principle on which his process worked, but canning has had a major impact on food preservation techniques.

Louis Pasteur's research on the spoilage of wine and his description of how to avoid spoilage in 1864 was an early attempt to apply scientific knowledge to food handling. Besides research into wine spoilage, Pasteur researched the production of alcohol, vinegar, wines and beer, and the souring of milk. He developed pasteurization—the process of heating milk and milk products to destroy food spoilage and disease-producing organisms. In his research into food technology, Pasteur became the pioneer into bacteriology and of modern preventive medicine.

Developments

Developments in food technology have contributed greatly to the food supply and have changed our world. Some of these developments are:

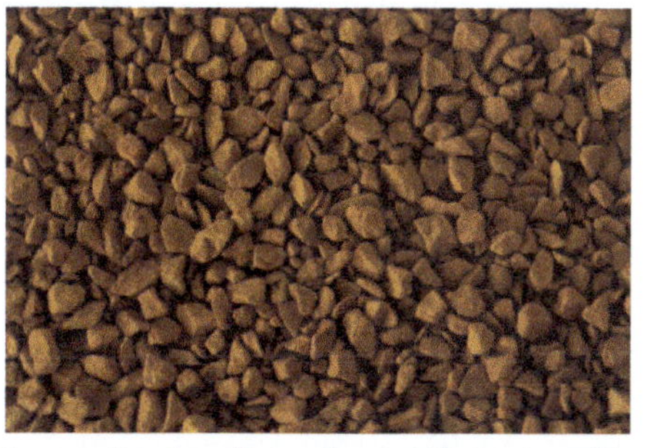

Freeze-dried coffee, a form of instant coffee

- Instantized Milk Powder - D.D. Peebles (U.S. patent 2,835,586) developed the first instant milk powder, which has become the basis for a variety of new products that are rehydratable. This process increases the surface area of the powdered product by partially rehydrating spray-dried milk powder.
- Freeze-drying - The first application of freeze drying was most likely in the pharmaceutical industry; however, a successful large-scale industrial application of the process was the development of continuous freeze drying of coffee.
- High-Temperature Short Time Processing - These processes for the most part are characterized by rapid heating and cooling, holding for a short time at a relatively high temperature and filling aseptically into sterile containers.
- Decaffeination of Coffee and Tea - Decaffeinated coffee and tea was first developed on a commercial basis in Europe around 1900. The process is described in U.S. patent 897,763. Green coffee beans are treated with water, heat and solvents to remove the caffeine from the beans.
- Process optimization - Food Technology now allows production of foods to be more efficient, Oil saving technologies are now available on different forms. Production methods and methodology have also become increasingly sophisticated.

Consumer Acceptance

In the past, consumer attitude towards food technologies was not common talk and was not important in food development. Nowadays the food chain is long and complicated, foods and food technologies are diverse; consequently the consumers are uncertain about the food quality and safety and find it difficult to orient themselves to the subject. That is why consumer acceptance of food technologies is an important question. However, in these days acceptance of food products very often depends on potential benefits and risks associated with the food. This also includes the technology the food is processed with. Attributes like "uncertain", "unknown" or "unfamiliar" are associated with consumers' risk perception and consumer very likely will reject products linked to these attributes. Especially innovative food processing technologies are connected to these characteristics and are perceived as risky by consumers

Acceptance of the different food technologies is very different. Whereas pasteurisation is well recognised, high pressure treatment or even microwaves are perceived as risky very often. In studies done within Hightech Europe project, it was found that traditional technologies were well accepted in contrast to innovative technologies.

Consumers form their attitude towards innovative food technologies by three main factors mechanisms. First, knowledge or beliefs about risks and benefits which are correlated with the technology. Second, attitudes are based on their own experience and third, based on higher order values and beliefs.

Acceptance of innovative technologies can be improved by providing non-emotional and concise information about these new technological processes methods. According to a study made by HighTech project also written information seems to have higher impact than audio-visual information on the consumer in case of sensory acceptance of products processed with innovative food technologies.

Food Additive

Food additives are substances added to food to preserve flavor or enhance its taste and appearance. Some additives have been used for centuries; for example, preserving food by pickling (with vinegar), salting, as with bacon, preserving sweets or using sulfur dioxide as with wines. With the advent of processed foods in the second half of the twentieth century, many more additives have been introduced, of both natural and artificial origin.

Numbering

To regulate these additives, and inform consumers, each additive is assigned a unique number, termed as "E numbers", which is used in Europe for all approved additives. This numbering scheme has now been adopted and extended by the *Codex Alimentarius* Commission to internationally identify all additives, regardless of whether they are approved for use.

E numbers are all prefixed by "E", but countries outside Europe use only the number, whether the additive is approved in Europe or not. For example, acetic acid is written as E260 on products sold in Europe, but is simply known as additive 260 in some countries. Additive 103, alkanet, is not approved for use in Europe so does not have an E number, although it is approved for use in Australia and New Zealand. Since 1987, Australia has had an approved system of labelling for additives in packaged foods. Each food additive has to be named or numbered. The numbers are the same as in Europe, but without the prefix "E".

The United States Food and Drug Administration (FDA) lists these items as "generally recognized as safe" (GRAS); they are listed under both their Chemical Abstracts Service number and FDA regulation under the United States Code of Federal Regulations.

Categories

Food additives can be divided into several groups, although there is some overlap because some additives exert more than one effect. For example, salt is both a preservative as well as a flavor.

Acidulents

confer sour or acid taste. Common acidulents include vinegar, citric acid, tartaric acid, malic acid, fumaric acid, and lactic acid.

Acidity regulators

Acidity regulators are used for controlling the pH of foods for stability or to affect activity of enzymes.

Anticaking agents

Anticaking agents keep powders such as milk powder from caking or sticking.

Antifoaming and foaming agents

Antifoaming agents reduce or prevent foaming in foods. Foaming agents do the reverse.

Antioxidants

Antioxidants such as vitamin C are preservatives by inhibiting the degradation of food by oxygen.

Bulking agents

Bulking agents such as starch are additives that increase the bulk of a food without affecting its taste.

Food coloring

Colorings are added to food to replace colors lost during preparation or to make food look more attractive.

Color retention agents

In contrast to colorings, color retention agents are used to preserve a food's existing color.

Emulsifiers

Emulsifiers allow water and oils to remain mixed together in an emulsion, as in mayonnaise, ice cream, and homogenized milk.

Flavors

Flavors are additives that give food a particular taste or smell, and may be derived from natural ingredients or created artificially.

Flavor enhancers

Flavor enhancers enhance a food's existing flavors. A popular example is monosodium glutamate. Some flavor enhancers have little flavor independent of the food.

Flour treatment agents

Flour treatment agents are added to flour to improve its color or its use in baking.

Glazing agents

Glazing agents provide a shiny appearance or protective coating to foods.

Humectants

Humectants prevent foods from drying out.

Tracer gas

Tracer gas allow for package integrity testing to prevent foods from being exposed to atmosphere, thus guaranteeing shelf life.

Preservatives

Preservatives prevent or inhibit spoilage of food due to fungi, bacteria and other microorganisms.

Stabilizers

Stabilizers, thickeners and gelling agents, like agar or pectin (used in jam for example) give foods a firmer texture. While they are not true emulsifiers, they help to stabilize emulsions.

Sweeteners

Sweeteners are added to foods for flavoring. Sweeteners other than sugar are added to keep the food energy (calories) low, or because they have beneficial effects for diabetes mellitus and tooth decay and diarrhea.

Thickeners

Thickening agents are substances which, when added to the mixture, increase its viscosity without substantially modifying its other properties.

Safety and Regulation

With the increasing use of processed foods since the 19th century, food additives are more widely used. Many countries regulate their use. For example, boric acid was widely used as a food preservative from the 1870s to the 1920s, but was banned after World War I due to its toxicity, as demonstrated in animal and human studies. During World War II, the urgent need for cheap, available food preservatives led to it being used again, but it was finally banned in the 1950s. Such cases led to a general mistrust of food additives, and an application of the precautionary principle led to the conclusion that only additives that are known to be safe should be used in foods. In the United States, this led to the adoption of the Delaney clause, an amendment to the Federal Food, Drug, and Cosmetic Act of 1938, stating that no carcinogenic substances may be used as food additives. However, after the banning of cyclamates in the United States and Britain in 1969, saccharin, the only remaining legal artificial sweetener at the time, was found to cause cancer in rats. Widespread public outcry in the United States, partly communicated to Congress by postage-paid postcards supplied in the packaging of sweetened soft drinks, led to the retention of saccharin, despite its violation of the Delaney clause. However, in 2000, saccharin was later found to only be carcinogenic to rats due to their unique urine chemistry.

Hyperactivity

Periodically, concerns have been expressed about a linkage between additives and hyperactivty, however "no clear evidence of ADHD was provided".

In 2007, Food Standards Australia New Zealand published an official shoppers' guidance with which the concerns of food additives and their labeling are mediated. In the EU it can take 10 years or more to obtain approval for a new food additive. This includes five years of safety testing, followed by two years for evaluation by the European Food Safety Authority and another three years before the additive receives an EU-wide approval for use in every country in the European Union. Apart from testing and analyzing food products during the whole production process to ensure safety and compliance with regulatory standards, Trading Standards officers (in the UK) protect the public from any illegal use or potentially dangerous mis-use of food additives by performing random testing of food products.

There has been significant controversy associated with the risks and benefits of food additives. Natural additives may be similarly harmful or be the cause of allergic reactions in certain individuals. For example, safrole was used to flavor root beer until it was shown to be carcinogenic. Due to the application of the Delaney clause, it may not be added to foods, even though it occurs naturally in sassafras and sweet basil.

Micronutrients

A subset of food additives, micronutrients added in food fortification processes preserve nutrient value by providing vitamins and minerals to foods such as flour, cereal, margarine and milk which normally would not retain such high levels. Preservatives also reduce spoilage from sources such as air, bacteria, fungi, and yeast.

Standardization of Its Derived Products

ISO has published a series of standards regarding the topic and these standards are covered by ICS 67.220.

Science

Many food additives absorb radiation in the ultraviolet and / or visible region of the spectrum. This absorbance can be used to determine the concentration of an additive in a sample using external calibration. However, additives may occur together and the absorbance by one could interfere with the absorbance of another. A prior separation stage is necessary and the additives are first separated by high-pressure liquid chromatography (HPLC) and then determined on-line using a UV and/ or visible light detector.

References

- Saravacos, George D.; Maroulis, Zacharias B. (2011).Food Process Engineering Operations. CRC Press. pp. 198-199. ISBN 1439877858
- Havkin-Frenkel, Daphna; Belanger, Faith C. (2011). Handbook of Vanilla Science and Technology. Chichester, UK: Wiley-Blackwell. pp. 142–145. ISBN 978-1-4051-9325-2.
- Hui YH, Meunier-Goddik L, Josephsen J, Nip WK, Stanfield PS (2004). Handbook of Food and Beverage Fermentation Technology. CRC Press. pp. 27 and passim. ISBN 978-0-8247-5122-7.
- König, J. (2015), "Food colour additives of synthetic origin", in Scotter, Michael J., Colour Additives for Foods and Beverages, Elsevier, pp. 35–60, doi:10.1016/B978-1-78242-011-8.00002-7, ISBN 978-1-78242-011-8
- Tomaska LD and Brooke-Taylor, S. Food Additives - General pp 449-454 in Encyclopedia of Food Safety, Vol 2: Hazards and Diseases. Eds, Motarjemi Y et al. Academic Press, 2013. ISBN 9780123786135
- Hans-Jürgen Bässler und Frank Lehmann : Containment Technology: Progress in the Pharmaceutical and Food Processing Industry. Springer, Berlin 2013, ISBN 978-3642392917
- Assessment of technologies for determining cancer risks from the environment. Darby, Pennsylvania, USA: DIANE publishing. 1981. p. 177. ISBN 1-4289-2437-X.
- Johnson, Paul (2007). "Lobster". Fish Forever: The Definitive Guide to Understanding, Selecting, and Preparing Healthy, Delicious, and Environmentally Sustainable Seafood. John Wiley & Sons. pp. 163–175. ISBN 978-0-7645-8779-5.
- Deshpande, S.S., ed. (2002), "8.5.3 Toxicological Characteristics of Colorants Subject to Certification", Handbook of Food Toxicology, Food Science and Technology, CRC Press, p. 234, ISBN 9780824707606
- Bucci, Luke (1995). Nutrition applied to injury rehabilitation and sports medicine. Boca Raton: CRC Press. p. 151. ISBN 0-8493-7913-X.
- Barrows, Julie N.; Lipman, Arthur L.; Bailey, Catherine J. Cianci, Sebastian, ed. "Color Additives: FDA's Regulatory Process and Historical Perspectives". Food Safety Magazine. No. October/November 2003. Food Safety Magazine. Retrieved 24 July 2016.
- Amchova, Petra; Kotolova, Hana; Ruda-Kucerova, Jana "Health safety issues of synthetic food colorants" Regulatory Toxicology and Pharmacology (2015), 73(3), 914-922.doi:10.1016/j.yrtph.2015.09.026
- Smith, J D; Rajeev Dhiman; Sushant Anand; Ernesto Reza-Garduno; Robert E. Cohen; Gareth H. McKinley; Kripa K. Varanasi (2013). "Droplet mobility on lubricant-impregnated surfaces". Soft Matter. 19 (6): 1972–1980. doi:10.1039/c2sm27032c. Retrieved 22 March 2015.
- Sangani, Rahul; Ghio, Andrew (2013). "Iron, Human Growth, and the Global Epidemic of Obesity". Nutrients. 5 (10): 4231–4249. doi:10.3390/nu5104231. ISSN 2072-6643. PMC 3820071. PMID 24152754.
- Claudio, L (2012). "Our food: packaging & public health". Environ. Health Perspect. 120: A232–7. doi:10.1289/ehp.120-a232. PMC 3385451. PMID 22659036.

5

Food Supplements: An Integrated Study

Dietary supplements are consumed in order to provide nutrients to an individual. Fiber supplements, iron supplements and spirulina are some of the aspects dealt within this text. This chapter elucidates the crucial theories of food supplements.

Dietary Supplement

A dietary supplement is intended to provide nutrients that may otherwise not be consumed in sufficient quantities.

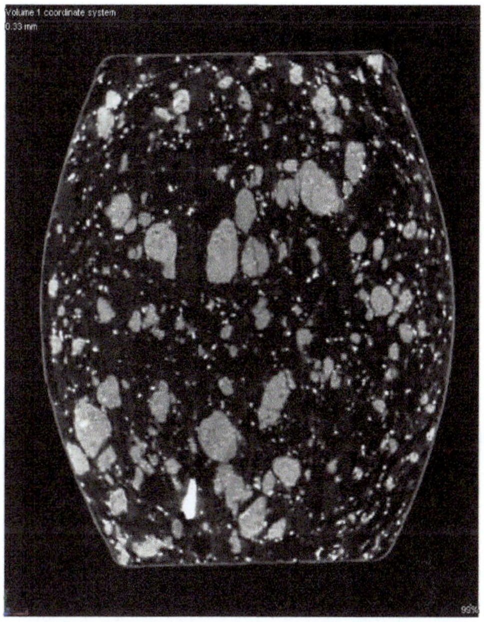

Flight through a CT image stack of a multivitamin tablet "A-Z" by German company Abtei

Supplements as generally understood include vitamins, minerals, fiber, fatty acids, or amino acids, among other substances. U.S. authorities define dietary supplements as foods, while elsewhere they may be classified as drugs or other products.

There are more than 50,000 dietary supplements available. More than half of the U.S. adult population (53% – 55%) consume dietary supplements with most common ones being multivitamins.

These products are not intended to prevent or treat any disease and in some circumstances are dangerous, according to the U.S. National Institutes of Health. For those who fail to consume a balanced diet, the agency says that certain supplements "may have value."

Most supplements should be avoided, and usually people should not eat micronutrients except people with clearly shown deficiency. Those people should first consult a doctor. An exception is vitamin D, which is recommended in Nordic countries due to weak sunlight.

Definition

According to the United States Food and Drug Administration (FDA), dietary supplements are products which are not pharmaceutical drugs, food additives like spices or preservatives, or conventional food, and which also meet any of these criteria:

1. The product is intended to supplement a person's diet, despite it not being usable as a meal replacement.
2. The product is or contains a vitamin, dietary element, herb used for herbalism or botanical used as a medicinal plant, amino acid, any substance which contributes to other food eaten, or any concentrate, metabolite, ingredient, extract, or combination of these things.
3. The product is labeled as a dietary supplement.

In the United States, the FDA has different monitoring procedures for substances depending on whether they are presented as drugs, food additives, food, or dietary supplements. Dietary supplements are eaten or taken by mouth, and are regulated in United States law as a type of food rather than a type of drug. Like food and unlike drugs, no government approval is required to make or sell dietary supplements; the manufacturer checks the safety of dietary supplements but the government does not; and rather than requiring risk–benefit analysis to prove that the product can be sold like a drug, risk–benefit analysis is only used to petition that food or a dietary supplement is unsafe and should be removed from market.

Medical Uses

The intended use of dietary supplements is to ensure that a person gets enough essential nutrients.

Dietary supplements should not be used to treat any disease or as preventive healthcare. An exception to this recommendation is the appropriate use of vitamins.

Dietary supplements are unnecessary if one eats a balanced diet.

Supplements may create harm in several ways, including over-consumption, particularly of minerals and fat-soluble vitamins which can build up in the body. The products may also cause harm related to their rapid absorption in a short period of time, quality issues such as contamination, or by adverse interactions with other foods and medications.

Types

There are many types of dietary supplements.

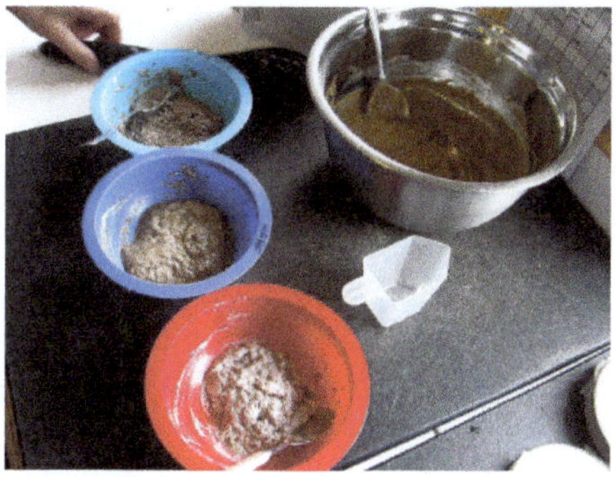

Dietary supplements being mixed into food for pigs

Vitamins

Vitamin is an organic compound required by an organism as a vital nutrient in limited amounts. An organic chemical compound (or related set of compounds) is called a vitamin when it cannot be synthesized in sufficient quantities by an organism, and must be obtained from the diet. Thus, the term is conditional both on the circumstances and on the particular organism. For example, ascorbic acid (vitamin C) is a vitamin for humans, but not for most other animals. Supplementation is important for the treatment of certain health problems but there is little evidence of benefit when used by those who are otherwise healthy.

Dietary Element

Dietary elements, commonly called "dietary minerals" or "minerals", are the chemical elements required by living organisms, other than the four elements carbon, hydrogen, nitrogen, and oxygen present in common organic molecules. The term "dietary mineral" is archaic, as the substances it refers are chemical elements rather than actual minerals.

Herbal Medicine

Herbal medicine is the use of plants for medicinal purposes. Plants have been the basis for medical treatments through much of human history, and such traditional medicine is still widely practiced today. Modern medicine recognizes herbalism as a form of alternative medicine, as the practice of herbalism is not strictly based on evidence gathered using the scientific method. Modern medicine, does, however, make use of many plant-derived compounds as the basis for evidence-tested pharmaceutical drugs, and phytotherapy works to apply modern standards of effectiveness testing to herbs and medicines that are derived from natural sources. The scope of herbal medicine is sometimes extended to include fungal and bee products, as well as minerals, shells and certain animal parts.

Amino Acids and Proteins

Amino acids are biologically important organic compounds composed of amine ($-NH_2$) and carboxylic acid ($-COOH$) functional groups, along with a side-chain specific to each amino acid. The key elements of an amino acid are carbon, hydrogen, oxygen, and nitrogen, though other elements are found in the side-chains of certain amino acids.

Amino acids can be divided into three categories: essential amino acids, non-essential amino acids, and conditional amino acids. Essential amino acids cannot be made by the body, and must be supplied by food. Non-essential amino acids are made by the body from essential amino acids or in the normal breakdown of proteins. Conditional amino acids are usually not essential, except in times of illness, stress, or for someone challenged with a lifelong medical condition.

Essential Fatty Acids

Essential fatty acids, or EFAs, are fatty acids that humans and other animals must ingest because the body requires them for good health but cannot synthesize them. The term "essential fatty acid" refers to fatty acids required for biological processes but does not include the fats that only act as fuel.

Bodybuilding Supplements

Bodybuilding supplements are dietary supplements commonly used by those involved in bodybuilding and athletics. Bodybuilding supplements may be used to replace meals, enhance weight gain, promote weight loss or improve athletic performance. Among the most widely used are vitamin supplements, protein drinks, branched-chain amino acids (BCAA), glutamine, essential fatty acids, meal replacement products, creatine, weight loss products and testosterone boosters. Supplements are sold either as single ingredient preparations or in the form of "stacks" – proprietary blends of various supplements marketed as offering synergistic advantages. While many bodybuilding supplements are also consumed by the general public their salience and frequency of use may differ when used specifically by bodybuilders.

Industry

In 2013, the global market of vitamins, minerals, and nutritional and herbal supplements (VMHS) was valued at $82 billion, with roughly 28 percent of that in the U.S., where sales increased by approximately $6 billion between 2007 and 2012.

The vitamins and dietary supplements sector in the U.S. grew 4% in 2015, to reach US$27.2 billion. The U.S. market was highly competitive in 2015, as no single company accounted for more than a 5% share of value sales.

Controversy

According to University of Helsinki food safety professor Marina Heinonen, more than 90% of dietary supplement health claims are incorrect. In addition, ingredients listed have been found to be different from the contents. For example, Consumer Reports reported unsafe levels of arsenic, cadmium, lead and mercury in several of the protein powders that were tested. Also, the CBC found that protein spiking (the addition of amino acid filler to manipulate analysis) was not uncommon, however many of the companies involved challenged their claim.

Adverse Effects

Among general reasons for harmful effects of dietary supplements are: a) absorption in a short time; b) quality and contamination; and c) enhancing both positive and negative effects at the same time. The number of incidents of liver damage from dietary supplements has tripled in a decade. Most of the products causing that effect were bodybuilding supplements. Some of the victims required liver transplants and some died. A third of the supplements involved contained unlisted steroids. Mild to severe toxicity has occurred on many occasions due to dietary supplements, even when the active ingredients were essential nutrients such as vitamins, minerals or amino acids. This has been a result of adulteration of the product, excessive usage on the part of the consumer, or use by persons at risk for the development of adverse effects. In addition, a number of supplements contain psychoactive drugs, whether of natural or synthetic origin.

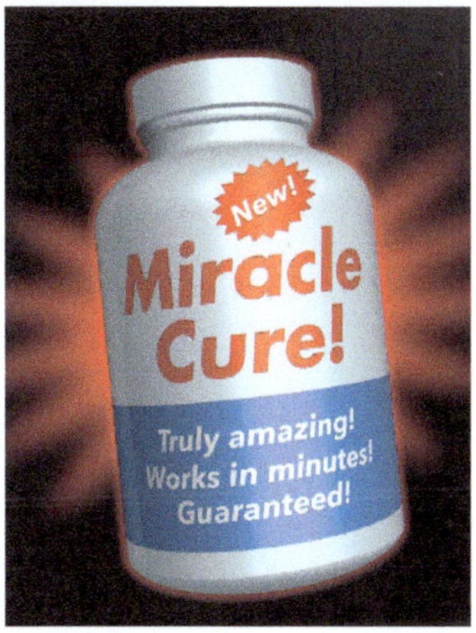

Some products make extraordinary claims and contain active ingredients which may not have been proven effective.

Physical and Chemical Properties

Adulteration in North America

BMC Medicine published a study on herbal supplements in 2013. Most of the supplements studied were of low quality, one third did not contain the active ingredient(s) claimed, and one third contained unlisted substances.

An investigation by the New York Attorney General's office reported in 2015 analyzed 78 bottles of herbal supplements from Walmart, Target, Walgreens and GNC stores in New York State using DNA barcoding, a method used to detect labeling fraud in the seafood industry. Only about 20% contained the ingredient on the label.

Some supplements were contamined by rodent feces and urine.

Only 0.3% of the 55,000 U.S. market dietary supplements have been studied regarding their common side effects.

Society and Culture

Public Health

Work done by scientists in the early 20th century on identifying individual nutrients in food and developing ways to manufacture them raised hopes that optimal health could be achieved and diseases prevented by adding them to food and providing people with dietary supplements; while there were successes in preventing vitamin deficiencies, and preventing conditions like neural tube defects by supplementation and food fortification with folic acid, no targeted supplementation or fortification strategies to prevent major diseases like cancer or cardiovascular diseases have proved successful.

For example, while increased consumption of fruits and vegetables are related to decreases in mortality, cardiovascular diseases and cancers, supplementation with key factors found in fruits and vegetable, like antioxidants, vitamins, or minerals, do not help and some have been found to be harmful in some cases. In general as of 2016, robust clinical data is lacking, that shows that any kind of dietary supplementation does more good than harm for people who are healthy and eating a reasonable diet but there is clear data showing that dietary pattern and lifestyle choices are associated with health outcomes.

As a result of the lack of good data for supplementation and the strong data for dietary pattern, public health recommendations for healthy eating urge people to eat a plant-based diet of whole foods, minimizing processed food, salt and sugar and to get exercise daily, and to abandon Western pattern diets and a sedentary lifestyle.

Legal Regulation

United States

The regulation of food and dietary supplements by the U.S. Food and Drug Administration is governed by various statutes enacted by the United States Congress and interpreted by the U.S. Food and Drug Administration ("FDA"). Pursuant to the Federal Food, Drug, and Cosmetic Act ("the Act") and accompanying legislation, the FDA has authority to oversee the quality of substances sold as food in the United States, and to monitor claims made in the labeling about both the composition and the health benefits of foods.

Substances which the FDA regulates as food are subdivided into various categories, including foods, food additives, added substances (man-made substances which are not intentionally introduced into food, but nevertheless end up in it), and dietary supplements. The specific standards which the FDA exercises differ from one category to the next. Furthermore, the FDA has been granted a variety of means by which it can address violations of the standards for a given category of substances.

Regulation in European Union

The European Union's Food Supplements Directive of 2002 requires that supplements be demonstrated to be safe, both in dosages and in purity. Only those supplements that have been proven to be safe may be sold in the bloc without prescription. As a category of food, food supplements cannot be labeled with drug claims but can bear health claims and nutrition claims.

The dietary supplements industry in the United Kingdom (UK), one of the 28 countries in the bloc, strongly opposed the Directive. In addition, a large number of consumers throughout Europe, including over one million in the UK, and various doctors and scientists, had signed petitions by 2005 against what are viewed by the petitioners as unjustified restrictions of consumer choice.

In 2004, along with two British trade associations, the Alliance for Natural Health (ANH) had a legal challenge to the Food Supplements Directive referred to the European Court of Justice by the High Court in London.

Although the European Court of Justice's Advocate General subsequently said that the bloc's plan to tighten rules on the sale of vitamins and food supplements should be scrapped, he was eventually overruled by the European Court, which decided that the measures in question were necessary and appropriate for the purpose of protecting public health. ANH, however, interpreted the ban as applying only to synthetically produced supplements, and not to vitamins and minerals normally found in or consumed as part of the diet.

Nevertheless, the European judges acknowledged the Advocate General's concerns, stating that there must be clear procedures to allow substances to be added to the permitted list based on scientific evidence. They also said that any refusal to add the product to the list must be open to challenge in the courts.

Research

Effects of most dietary supplements have not been determined in randomized clinical trials and manufacturing is lightly regulated; randomized clinical trials of certain vitamins and antioxidants have found increased mortality rates.

Fibre Supplements

Fibre supplements (or fiber supplements) are considered to be a form of a subgroup of functional dietary fibre, and in the United States are defined by the Institute of Medicine (IOM). According to the IOM, functional fibre "consists of isolated, non-digestible carbohydrates that have beneficial physiological effects in humans".

Fibre supplements are widely available, and can be found in forms such as powders, tablets, and capsules. Consumption of fibre supplements may be for: improving dietary intake, lowering blood cholesterol, alleviating irritable bowel syndrome, reducing the risk of colon cancer, and increasing feelings of satiety.

Excessive fibre intake can lead to fluid imbalance, dehydration, mineral deficiencies, nutrient and drug interactions, and other medical problems.

Rationale for Fibre Supplement Use

The American Dietetic Association recommends that the average adult consume 25 to 38 grams of dietary fibre per day. However, research has shown that the average American only consumes 14 to 15 grams per day. To reach the recommended amount of fibre, consumption of dietary fibre from foods (e.g. plants, vegetables, legumes, and grains) instead of supplements is preferred because they contain additional beneficial nutrients and non-nutritive components (e.g. antioxidants and phytoestrogens). Nevertheless, a fibre supplement may be needed to prevent constipation when food intake is low, which is the case among inactive elderly. A cereal bran such as psyllium seed husk, or a synthetic fiber such as methylcellulose is often used in this case.

Common Fibre Supplements in The Market

Product Name	Soluble / Insoluble	Ingredients	Capsule / Powder
Benefiber	S	natural, manufacturing by-product - wheat dextrin (USA), inulin (Canada)	C/P
Citrucel	S	synthetic - methylcellulose	C/P
FibreSmart	I/S	natural, whole food - flax	C/P
FiberCon	I	synthetic - calcium polycarbophil	C
Fiber Choice	S	natural, manufacturing by-product - inulin	C
Heather's Tummy Fiber	S	natural, whole food - organic acacia senegal	P
Metamucil	I/S	natural, whole food - psyllium	C/P
Natural Brand Psyllium seed husk	I/S	natural, whole food - psyllium	C
PGX	S	natural, manufacturing by-product - glucomannan	C
ReCleanse Fibre Powder	I/S	natural, manufacturing by-product and whole food - inulin/flax	P

S=Soluble, I=Insoluble C=Capsule/Tablet, P=Powder

Fibre Supplement Claims

Blood Cholesterol Reduction

Foods that are high in viscous fibres have been found to lower blood cholesterol by binding with bile acids. In order to compensate for this, cholesterol from the liver may be used to make more bile acids. The products of bacterial fermentation in the colon may also decrease the rate of cholesterol synthesis in the liver.

However, research has produced mixed results with respect to whether fibre supplements are as effective as dietary fibre in reducing blood cholesterol. Two recent studies show nearly opposing results, using fibre-supplemented apple juice containing both the soluble pectin from apples and gum arabic. In the first study, the supplement-enriched juice had no discernible effect on the blood cholesterol levels of 110 hypercholesterolaemic men and women. In the second study, the total and LDL-cholesterol levels of mildly hypercholesterolaemic men were lowered.

In another study, a dietary supplement consisting of both soluble fibre (guar gum, pectin) and insoluble fibre (soy fibre, pea fibre, corn bran) was found to reduce LDL-cholesterol for individuals that have mild to moderate hypercholesterolaemia without reducing HDL-cholesterol or increasing triglycerides.

Supplements containing extracted insoluble fibre may have an effect on blood lipids that most resembles the effects of dietary fibre. In a more recent randomized, double blind clinical study of 58 hypercholesterolaemic volunteers, an extruded carob pulp preparation added to daily diet reduced total and LDL-cholesterol and improved the ratio of HDL:LDL cholesterol in all participants, and also showed a marked reduction in serum cholesterol in the women of the study.

Gastrointestinal Health

Colorectal Cancer

The protective properties of dietary fibre against colorectal cancer are undisputed. However, fibre supplements do not seem to provide the same defensive effect. A study of 1429 men and women over six months showed that a high-fibre cereal (wheat bran) supplement had no protective effect on recurring colorectal adenomas. In addition, no significant improvement in the proportion or features of existing colorectal adenomas was observed.

Diverticular Disease

Diverticulitis is mainly attributed to the low fibre intake typical of the Western diet for which gradual increase dietary fibre over several weeks is common clinical solution. Fibre supplements are again much less effective. One study of 58 men and women with uncomplicated diverticulitis in a double-blind controlled trial concluded that common doses of wheat bran and a psyllium-derived supplement provided relief of constipation only, with no other observable effects.

Irritable Bowel Syndrome

Irritable bowel syndrome (IBS) is a common gastrointestinal ailment for which dietary soluble fibre is often prescribed as part of a therapeutic solution. As a supplement, partially hydrolysed guar gum (PHGG - completely soluble, fully fermentable) has been shown to be quite effective in clinical trials for decreasing IBS symptoms such as abdominal pain and generally improving quality of life for sufferers well beyond treatment. In addition, PHGG has been shown to have prebiotic properties by acidifying bowel contents and increasing gut microflora.

Acacia senegal fiber (gum arabic - completely soluble, fully fermentable) has also been show to have a prebiotic effect in the gut, significantly increasing Bifidobacteria and Lactobacilli after 4 weeks of consumption. Acacia ferments very slowly in the gut, and due to its polymeric nature does not disturb osmotic pressure, so it has a good gastrointestinal tolerance (it has no sudden and painful release of gas, and the total gas production is much lower than with FOS, for instance) and does not present any side effects at dosages up to 50 grams per day. Particularly helpful for IBS is that Acacia senegal behaves as a regulator; it is able to reduce diarrhea and reduce constipation.

Dietary insoluble fiber has long been shown to exacerbate Irritable Bowel Syndrome symptoms.

Weight Management

It has been suggested that the refining of fibre-rich grains has contributed to the obesity epidemic of Western countries. Whole, dietary forms of fibre are more difficult to ingest and absorb than milled and refined food products. This is because dietary fibre may be able to displace available calories and nutrients, requires more time for chewing (thereby slowing intake rate and inducing satiety), and reduces the efficiency of absorption in the small intestine.

Supplemental forms of fibre have been shown to potentially assist weight management by increasing satiety, decreasing the absorption rate of starches and sugars, and binding to lipids in the small intestine thereby reducing serum triglycerides and chylomicron.

Powdered guar gum, a soluble fibre, was shown to be associated with a significantly lower energy intake in obese subjects who ingested a non-restricted diet over one week, when the same participants did not consume the fibre supplement.

A similar reduction of energy intake through fibre supplementation was observed in another study. A dose of guar gum was administered to normal-weight and obese participants. A 10% reduction of energy was observed in the normal subjects, and a 30% reduction of energy for obese subjects. Fibre supplementation has also been indicated to assist compliance to low-calorie diets, as indicated through decreased feelings of hunger and increased ratings of satiety. Other soluble fiber forms such as glucomannan have also been studied in relationship to blood sugar and fat digestion in obese patients.

Safety Considerations

Abruptly adding elevated amounts of fibre to the diet too quickly can lead to intestinal gas, diarrhea, abdominal bloating, cramping, and constipation. It is therefore better to regulate and moderate daily fibre intake. If increased fibre intake is desired, gradually increasing the amount over a few days allows the natural bacteria in the gastrointestinal tract to adjust to the change. Drinking 1- 2 L of water every day can prevent some uncomfortable symptoms by making the stool soft and bulky.

The risk of intestinal obstruction from insoluble fiber in susceptible individuals, fluid imbalance leading to dehydration and mineral deficiencies may increase if more than 50 g of fibre is ingested per day. For this reason, individuals who decide to suddenly double or triple their fibre intake are often advised to double or triple their water intake. In addition, excessive intake of non-fermentable fibre (typically in supplemental form) may lead to mineral deficiencies by reducing the absorption or increasing the excretion of minerals, especially when mineral intake is too low or when mineral needs are increased such as during pregnancy, lactation, or adolescence.

Excessive fibre intake can also contribute to nutrient and drug interactions. For example, antidepressant medications, diabetes medications, carbamazepine, cholesterol-lowering medications and penicillin.

Iron Supplement

Iron supplements are dietary supplements containing iron that can be prescribed by a doctor for a medical reason, or purchased from a vitamin shop, drug store etc. They are primarily used to treat anemia or other iron deficiencies. There are three ways that it can be delivered: orally, intravenously or intramuscularly.

The first iron pills were commonly known as Blaud's pills, which were named after P. Blaud of Beaucaire, the French physician who introduced and started the use of these medications as a treatment for patients with anemia.

Medical Uses

Iron supplements are used to treat iron deficiency and iron-deficiency anemia; parenteral irons can also be used to treat functional iron deficiency, where requirements for iron are greater than the body's ability to supply iron such as in inflammatory states. The main criterion is that other causes of anemia have also been investigated, such as vitamin B_{12}/folate deficiency, drug induced or due to other poisons such as lead, as often the anaemia has more than one underlying cause.

Iron deficiency anemia is classically a microcytic, hypochromic anemia. Generally, in the UK oral preparations are trialled before using parenteral delivery. unless there is the requirement for a rapid response, previous intolerance to oral iron or likely failure to respond. Intravenous iron may decrease the need for blood transfusions however increases the risk of infections when compared to oral iron. A 2015 Cochrane Collaboration review found that daily oral supplementation of iron during pregnancy reduces the risk of maternal anaemia and that effects on infant and on other maternal outcomes are not clear. Another review found that "intermittent regimens (of oral iron supplementation) produced similar maternal and infant outcomes as daily supplementation but were associated with fewer side effects". The quality of evidence was poor, though.

Athletes

There is debate about whether athletes are at an increased risk for iron deficiencies, and whether athletes with low iron, who are not anemic, would benefit from iron supplementation.

Despite these additional sources of iron loss, male athletes have normally been observed to receive adequate amounts of dietary iron at the same levels recommended for the average male. Female athletes, however, have been observed to receive an inadequate supply of iron, but this may be caused more from blood loss from menstruation than from athletic activity. Additionally, pseudo-anemia can be observed in athletes with adequate haemoglobin due to an increase in blood plasma in athletes that dilutes their haemoglobin concentration, making it appear as if they are anemic when they actually have an adequate amount of total haemoglobin.

When an athlete should be recommended to take iron supplements is debated, and should generally be judged on an individual basis. While iron supplementation can be a pragmatic treatment for athletes that are anemic, its effects remain unclear in athletes that are nonanemic. Iron supplementation has not been demonstrated to improve athletic performance in individuals who are nonanemic. For athletes who are nonanemic, however, iron supplementation may function to stave off iron-deficient anemia, as well as prevent excess absorption of toxic metal ions of lead and cadmium. Due to risks associated with differing individual tolerances, drug interactions, and overdosing, iron supplementation should be directed by a medical professional based off a clinical assessment of the athlete's iron parameters and not undertaken as self-medication.

Adverse Effects

Side effects of therapy with oral iron are most often diarrhea or constipation and epigastric abdominal discomfort. Taken after a meal, side effects decrease, but there is an increased risk of interaction with other substances. Side effects are dose-dependent, and the dose may be adjusted.

The patient may notice that his/her stools become black. This is completely harmless, but patients must be warned about this to avoid unnecessary concern. When iron supplements are given in a liquid form, teeth may reversibly discolor (this can be avoided through the use of a straw). Intramuscular injection can be painful, and brown discoloration may be noticed.

Treatments with iron(II) sulfate have higher incidence of adverse events than iron(III)-hydroxide polymaltose complex (IPC) or iron bis-glycinate chelate.

Contraindications

Contraindications often depend on the substance in question. Documented hypersensitivity to any ingredients and anemias without proper work-up (i.e., documentation of iron deficiency) is true of all preparations. Some can be used in iron deficiency, others require iron deficiency anaemia to be present. Some are also contraindicated in rheumatoid arthritis

Iron Supplementation and Infection Risk

Because one of the functions of elevated ferritin (an acute phase reaction protein) in acute infections is thought to be to sequester iron from bacteria, it is generally thought that iron supplementation (which circumvents this mechanism) should be avoided in patients who have active bacterial infections. Replacement of iron stores is seldom such an emergency situation that it cannot wait for any such acute infection to be treated.

Some studies have found that iron supplementation can lead to an increase in infectious disease morbidity in areas where bacterial infections are common. For example, children receiving iron-enriched foods have demonstrated an increased rate in diarrhea overall and enteropathogen shedding. Iron deficiency protects against infection by creating an unfavorable environment for bacterial growth. Nevertheless, while iron deficiency might lessen infections by certain pathogenic diseases, it also leads to a reduction in resistance to other strains of viral or bacterial infections, such as *Salmonella typhimurium* or *Entamoeba histolytica*. Overall, it is sometimes difficult to decide whether iron supplementation will be beneficial or harmful to an individual in an environment that is prone to many infectious diseases; however this is a different question than the question of supplementation in individuals who are already ill with a bacterial infection.

Children living in areas prone for malarial infections are also at risk of developing anemia. It was thought that iron supplementation given to such children could increase the risk of malarial infection in them. A Cochrane systematic review published in 2016 found high quality evidence that iron supplementation does not increase the risk of clinical malaria in children.

Haemochromatosis

Individuals may be genetically predisposed to excessive iron absorption, as is the case with those with HFE hereditary haemochromatosis. Within the general population, 1 out of 400 people has the homozygous form of this genetic trait, and 1 out of every 10 people has its heterozygous form. Neither individuals with the homozygous or heterozygous form should take iron supplements.

Interactions

Non-heme iron forms an insoluble complex with several other drugs, resulting in decreased absorption of both iron and the other drug. Examples include tetracycline, penicillamine, methyldopa, levodopa, bisphosphonates and quinolones. The same can occur with elements in food, such as calcium. Absorption of iron is better at a low pH (i.e. an acidic environment), and absorption is decreased if there is a simultaneous intake of antacids.

Many other substances decrease the rate of non-heme iron absorption. Examples are tannins from foods, such as tea and saw palmetto, phytic acid and roughage. Vegetarians and especially vegans are at increased risk of iron deficiency due to the combination of limited amounts of iron in the diet in a form that is poorly absorbed alongside compounds that further limit absorption.

Taken after a meal, there are fewer side effects but there is also less absorption because of interaction and pH alteration. Generally, an interval of 2–3 hours between the iron intake and that of other drugs seems advisable, but is less convenient for patients and can impact on compliance.

Precautions

Iron overdose has been one of the leading causes of death caused by toxicological agents in children younger than 6 years.

Mortality/Morbidity

Iron poisoning may result in mortality or short-term and long-term morbidity.

Follow-up

Follow-up is needed to ensure compliance and to detect adequate response to therapy. The interval of follow up can widely depend on both the method of administration, and the underlying pathology. For parenteral irons it is recommended that there be a period of 4 weeks before repeating blood test to allow the body to utilise the iron. For oral iron, this can take considerably longer, so waiting 3 months may be appropriate.

Administration

Oral

Iron can be supplemented by the oral route using various pharmacological forms, such as iron(II) sulfate (this is the most common and well studied soluble iron salt, e.g. Feratab, Fer-Iron, Slow-FE,...) and in complex with gluconate, dextran, carbonyl iron, and other salts. Ascorbic acid, vitamin C, significantly increases the absorption of none-heme sources of iron.

Heme iron polypeptide (HIP) (e.g. Proferrin ES and Proferrin Forte) can be used when regular iron supplements such as ferrous sulfate or ferrous fumarate are not tolerated or absorbed. A clinical study demonstrated that HIP increased serum iron levels 23 times greater than ferrous fumarate on a milligram-per-milligram basis.

Another alternative is *ferrous glycine sulfate* or *ferroglycine sulfate*, has less gastrointestinal side-effects than standard preparations such as iron fumarate. It is unusual among oral preparations of iron supplements in that the iron in this preparation has very high oral bioavailability, especially in the liquid formulation. This option should be evaluated before resorting to parenteral therapy. It is especially useful in iron deficiency anemia associated with autoimmune gastritis and *Helicobacter pylori* gastritis, where it generally has satisfactory effect.

Since iron stores in the body are generally depleted, and there is a limit to what the body can process (about 2–6 mg/kg of body mass per day; i.e. for a 100 kg/220 lb man this is equal to a maximum dose of 200–600 mg/per day) without iron poisoning, this is a chronic therapy which may take 3–6 months.

Due to the frequent intolerance of oral iron and the slow improvement, parenteral iron is recommended in many indications.

Parenteral

Parenteral iron therapy (intravenously or intramuscular) is given when oral therapy has failed (not tolerated by the patient), oral absorption is seriously compromised (by illnesses, or when the patient cannot swallow), benefit from oral therapy cannot be expected, or fast improvement is required (for example, prior to elective surgery). Parenteral therapy is more expensive than oral iron preparations and is not suitable during the first trimester of pregnancy.

There are cases where parenteral iron is preferable over oral iron. These are cases where oral iron is not tolerated, where the haemoglobin needs to be increased quickly (e.g. post partum, post operatively, post transfusion), where there is an underlying inflammatory condition (e.g. inflammatory bowel disease) or renal patients, the benefits of parenteral iron far outweigh the risks. In many cases, use of intravenous iron has lower risks of adverse events than a blood transfusion and as long as the patient is stable is a better alternative. Ultimately this always remains a clinical decision based on local guidelines, although National Guidelines are increasingly stipulating IV iron in certain groups of patients.

Soluble iron salts have a significant risk of adverse effects and can cause toxicity due to damage to cellular macromolecules. Delivering iron parenterally has utilised various different molecules to limit this. This has included dextrans, sucrose, carboxymaltose and more recently Isomaltoside 1000.

One formulation of parenteral iron is *iron dextran* which covers the old high molecular weight (trade name *DexFerrum*) and the much safer low molecular iron dextrans (tradenames including Cosmofer and Infed.

Iron sucrose (trade names including *Venofer*) has an occurrence of allergic reactions of less than 1 in 1000. A common side effect is taste changes, especially a metallic taste, occurring in between 1 in 10 and 1 in 100 treated patients. It has a maximum dose of 200 mg on each occasion according to the SPC, but it has been given in doses of 500 mg. Doses can be given up to 3 times a week.

Iron carboxymaltose (trade name *Ferinject*) is a newer formulation of parenteral iron which is dextran free with the shell being fully metabolised in the body to simple sugars. The most common side effect are headaches which occur in 3.3%. It can be given over 15 minutes in doses up to 1,000 mg and has been adopted in many hospitals due to the increased number of patients that can be treated as no test dose is required.

Iron Isomaltoside 1000 (Trade name *Monofer*) is a newer formulation of parenteral iron that has a matrix structure that results in very low levels of free iron and labile iron. It can be given at high doses – 20 mg/kg in a single visit – no upper dose limit. This formulation has the benefit of giving a full iron correction in a single visit.

Iron carboxymaltose and *iron Isomaltoside 1000* both have better safety profiles than older IV preparations, having the ability to be given in larger doses and availing for complete iron replacement in 15–60 minutes.

Airborne (Dietary Supplement)

Airborne is a dietary supplement containing herbal extracts, amino acids, antioxidants, electrolytes, vitamins, and other ingredients marketed to prevent the common cold and improve immune function.

The benefits of its use are uncertain. There are no studies supporting Airborne's effectiveness that meet scientific standards. The former owners were fined by the Federal Trade Commission for deceptive advertising and were the subject of successful class actions.

It was created by schoolteacher Victoria Knight-McDowell in the early 1990s. The website does not list any side effects that one might experience after taking Airborne, aside from "some sensitivity to any of the vitamins or herbal extracts". It is offered for sale over-the-counter in many U.S. retail stores in multiple forms: effervescent tablet, gummy, chewable tablet, lozenge, tablet, or powder.

History

The formula for Airborne was developed by Victoria Knight-McDowell, a former school teacher from Carmel, California. She began brewing herbal and vitamin cocktails in the early 1990s and selling them in tablet form to local drug stores. Later on, Knight-McDowell contracted cartoonist Lloyd Dangle to create Airborne's brand and packaging. In 1997, specialty grocery chain Trader Joe's ordered 300 cases of Airborne tablets to sell, and by 1999 other larger chains, such as Wal-Mart and Rite Aid, began stocking Airborne.

Products

Airborne supplements are available in various flavors like "Zesty Orange", "Very Berry", "Lemon Lime", and "Pink Grapefruit", and in the following forms: effervescent tablets, powder packets, chewable tablets, lozenges, drink mixes, and gummies. The original product was a tablet that was put into water to create a fizzy, effervescent drink.

Testing, Research, and Controversy

Because it is sold as a dietary supplement and not as a drug, current American law allows Airborne to be marketed without prior review and approval of testing results that demonstrate that it provides a medical remedy.

There are no studies supporting Airborne's effectiveness that meet scientific standards. A study by GNG Pharmaceutical Services referenced in the debate over Airborne's effectiveness was sponsored by the Knight-McDowell Labs, manufacturers of Airborne. In February 2006, ABC News discovered that GNG Pharmaceutical Services has no official clinic, scientists, or even doctors. Knight-McDowell Labs later removed all references to the study from their packaging and web site.

A medical report on Airborne addressed some of these concerns, specifically regarding its large amounts of vitamin C:

There are some concerns. First, there is no conclusive evidence that this product or any of its ingredients prevents colds or shortens their duration. Second, the adult tablet contains 1 g of vitamin C, and the directions for use advise taking 1 tablet at the first sign of a cold and repeating the dose every 3 hours as necessary. Vitamin C in doses higher than 1 g increases oxalate and urate excretion and may cause kidney stones. Third, the safety of this herbal extraction combination has not been established. And with herbs and dietary supplements in general, we only have the manufacturers' word on the label for what's in them.

Class Actions and Settlements

The former makers of Airborne had been accused by the FTC of using false advertising in its marketing and making unproven claims that it could help ward off harmful bacteria and germs and help prevent the flu and the common cold.

A class action lawsuit was filed against the former owners of Airborne Health, Inc. (and other defendants) alleging that Airborne falsely advertised certain therapeutic properties, including the ability to cure or prevent the common cold, when marketing products under the Airborne brand name. Defendants denied any wrongdoing or illegal conduct but agreed to settle the litigation.

The Center for Science in the Public Interest (CSPI) participated in the class action lawsuit against Airborne.

On March 4, 2008, the former owners of Airborne Health Inc. agreed to pay $23.3 million to settle the lawsuit.

On August 14, 2008, a press release from the Federal Trade Commission (FTC) stated that the former owners of Airborne Health, Inc. has agreed to pay up to $30 million to settle FTC charges. According to the FTC's complaint:

> "there is no competent and reliable scientific evidence to support the claims made by the defendants that Airborne tablets can prevent or reduce the risk of colds, sickness, or infection; protect against or help fight germs; reduce the severity or duration of a cold; and protect against colds, sickness, or infection in crowded places such as airplanes, offices, or schools."

The FTC complaint also states that the company's former owners and founders, Victoria Knight-McDowell and Thomas John McDowell, "made false claims that Airborne products are clinically proven to treat colds."

Shortly after the settlements, a new management team was brought in to run the company. This management team was led by Marti Morfitt, former CEO and director of CNS, Inc. In October

2009, Airborne was purchased by GF Capital Management and Advisors, LLC, a New York City-based private equity firm. GF Capital said that the entire management team, including CEO Marti Morfitt, would remain intact. In March 2012, Schiff Nutrition acquired Airborne, Inc. In November 2012, Reckitt Benckiser bought Schiff Nutrition for $1.4 billion.

Ingredients

According to the official website, Airborne contains zinc, ginger, *Echinacea* and up to 13 other vitamins, minerals and herbs. Each Airborne product has a different formulation and ingredient list.

The ingredients in most Airborne products include:

- Vitamin A as retinyl palmitate
- Vitamin C (ascorbic acid)
- Vitamin E (as delta-tocopheryl acetate)
- Riboflavin (vitamin B_2)
- Magnesium (as oxide and sulfate);
- Zinc (as sulfate);
- Selenium (as amino acid chelate);
- Manganese (as gluconate);
- Sodium;
- Potassium;
- Herbal extract blend containing: *Lonicera* (flower), *Forsythia* (fruit), *Schizonepeta* (aboveground parts), ginger (dried rhizome), Chinese Vitex (fruit), *Isatis* (root) and *Echinacea* (aboveground parts)
- Amino acids: glutamine (as $_{L}$-glutamine) and lysine (as $_{L}$-lysine HCl);
- Other ingredients: maltodextrin, sorbitol, citric acid, sodium bicarbonate, potassium bicarbonate, orange flavor, mineral oil, acesulfame potassium, and sucralose.

Side Effects

The official website does not list any side effects that one might experience after taking Airborne, aside from "some sensitivity to any of the vitamins or herbal extracts", but people who might be allergic to one of the ingredients of the product are advised to avoid using it or to consult a doctor. Also, people who are taking another type of medication at the same time or who suffer different medical conditions should consult a physician before taking Airborne.

Side effects from vitamin overdoses may occur, especially in patients with kidney failure. In very large doses, vitamin C in kidney-failure patients can cause severe side effects such as oxalate deposits in bone and soft tissues and may interfere with the absorption and metabolism of vitamin B_{12}. High doses of vitamin E may produce headaches, tiredness, double vision, and diarrhea in humans and doses higher than 800 mg may increase blood clotting time, especially for people on blood thinners. Also, magnesium overdose may occur; signs of magnesium toxicity include changes in mental status, nausea, diarrhea, appetite loss, muscle weakness, difficulty breathing, extremely low blood pressure, and irregular heartbeat.

Beano (Dietary Supplement)

Beano is an enzyme-based dietary supplement that is used to reduce gas in the digestive tract, thereby improving digestion and reducing bloating, discomfort, and flatulence caused by gas. It contains the enzyme alpha-galactosidase (α-GAL). It was introduced as a liquid, but that has been discontinued and it is now available only as tablets and strawberry-flavored "Meltaways".

Beano is marketed and distributed by Prestige Brands Holdings, Inc.

Mechanism of Action

Beano contains the enzyme α-GAL, which is derived from the fungus *Aspergillus niger*. The enzyme works in the digestive tract to break down the complex or branching sugars (polysaccharides and oligosaccharides) in foods such as legumes (beans and peanuts) and cruciferous vegetables (cauliflower, broccoli, cabbage, and brussels sprouts, among others). The enzyme breaks those complex sugars into simple sugars, making these foods somewhat more digestible, and reducing intestinal gas.

The polysaccharides and oligosaccharides found in these foods might otherwise pass through the small intestine unaffected. Once in the large intestine, those sugars may be metabolized by intestinal flora, fermenting to produce the gases that cause discomfort.

Two randomized controlled trials show reduction in gas by subjects taking oral α-GAL. Another study indicates it may interfere with the diabetic medication acarbose.

Ingredients

Besides the ingredient α-GAL, Beano tablets also contain a second enzyme that can be used therapeutically, invertase.

History

Beano was developed in 1990 by Alan Kligerman of AkPharma after research into gas-causing vegetables that had begun in 1981. The idea for such a product was proposed at least as early as the 1780s in Benjamin Franklin's essay "A Letter To A Royal Academy". In 1991, Kligerman was awarded the inaugural Ig Nobel Prize in Medicine for inventing Beano.

Its patent is owned by GlaxoSmithKline, which acquired it in 2001 from Block Drug. GlaxoSmithKline sold Beano and 16 other brands to Prestige Brands in 2012.

Beano received a U.S. Patent 5,445,957 on August 29, 1995. The estimated expiration date of this patent is December 5, 2014. As of early 2013, more than four dozen competing products were on the market.

In April 2014, the brand introduced Beano +Dairy Defense

Use in Brewing

Simple sugars are also produced as a consequence of the malting process that eventually produces beer. The complex sugars are not broken down by the yeast, and are eventually consumed by the beer drinker, possibly causing flatulence. Homebrewers have found adding Beano to their brew may produce a beer that has a less malty flavor. The Beano breaks the complex sugars into simple sugars, and these simple sugars are consumed by the yeast, producing alcohol (or some acetic acid in the aerobic reactions in early fermentation).

Spirulina (Dietary Supplement)

Spirulina is a cyanobacterium (blue-green algae) that can be consumed by humans and other animals. There are two species, *Arthrospira platensis* and *Arthrospira maxima.*

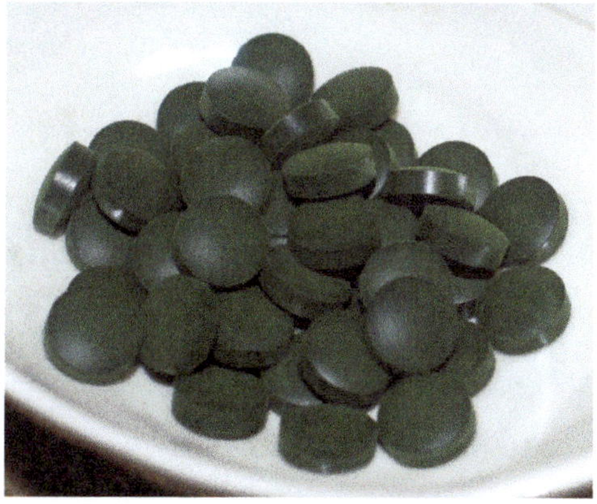

Spirulina tablets

Arthrospira is cultivated worldwide; used as a dietary supplement as well as a whole food; and is also available in tablet, flake and powder form. It is also used as a feed supplement in the aquaculture, aquarium and poultry industries.

Nutrient and Vitamin Content

Protein

Dried spirulina contains about 60% (51–71%) protein. It is a complete protein containing all essential amino acids, with slightly lower amounts of methionine, cysteine, and lysine compared to certain animal-derived products. From a nutritional point of view, spirulina is no better than other protein sources, but is more expensive gram-for-gram and may have adverse interactions when taken with prescribed drugs.

Other Nutrients

Provided in its typical supplement form as a dried powder having 5% water (table), a 100 gram amount of spirulina supplies 290 Calories and is an excellent source (20% or more of the Daily Value, DV) of numerous nutrients, particularly B vitamins (thiamin and riboflavin, 207% and 306% DV, respectively) and dietary minerals, such as iron (219% DV) and manganese (90% DV) (table).

Spirulina's lipid content is 8% by weight (table) providing gamma-linolenic acid, alpha-linolenic acid, linoleic acid, stearidonic acid, eicosapentaenoic acid, docosahexaenoic acid, and arachidonic acid.

Vitamin B_{12} Controversy

Spirulina does not contain vitamin B_{12} naturally and spirulina supplements are not considered to be a reliable source of vitamin B_{12}, as they contain predominantly pseudovitamin B_{12}, which is biologically inactive in humans. Companies that grow and market spirulina have claimed it to be a significant source of B_{12} on the basis of alternative, unpublished assays, although their claims are not accepted by independent scientific organizations. The American Dietetic Association and Dietitians of Canada in their position paper on vegetarian diets state that spirulina cannot be counted on as a reliable source of active vitamin B_{12}. The medical literature similarly advises that spirulina is unsuitable as a source of B_{12}.

Risks

Quality-related Safety and Toxicology

Spirulina is a form of cyanobacterium, some of which are known to produce toxins such as microcystins, BMAA, and others. Some spirulina supplements have been found to be contaminated with microcystins, albeit at levels below the limit set by the Oregon Health Department. Microcystins can cause gastrointestinal disturbances and, in the long term, liver damage. The effects of chronic exposure to even very low levels of microcystins are of concern, because of the potential risk of toxicity to several organ systems and possibly cancer.

These toxic compounds are not produced by spirulina itself, but may occur as a result of contamination of spirulina batches with other toxin-producing blue-green algae. Because spirulina is considered a dietary supplement in the U.S., no active, industry-wide regulation of its production occurs and no enforced safety standards exist for its production or purity. The U.S. National Institutes of Health describes spirulina supplements as "possibly safe", provided they are free of microcystin contamination, but "likely unsafe" (especially for children) if contaminated. Given the lack of regulatory standards in the U.S., some public-health researchers have raised the concern that consumers cannot be certain that spirulina and other blue-green algae supplements are free of contamination.

Heavy-metal contamination of spirulina supplements has also raised concern. The Chinese State Food and Drug Administration reported that lead, mercury, and arsenic contamination was widespread in spirulina supplements marketed in China. One study reported the presence of lead up to 5.1 ppm in a sample from a commercial supplement.

Safety Issues for Certain Target Groups

Like all protein-rich foods, spirulina contains the essential amino acid phenylalanine (2.6-4.1 g/100 g), which should be avoided by people who have phenylketonuria, a rare genetic disorder that prevents the body from metabolizing phenylalanine, which then builds up in the brain, causing damage.

Spirulina contaminated with microcystins has various potential toxicity, especially to children, including liver damage, shock and death.

Animals and Aquaculture

Various studies on spirulina as an alternative feed for animal and aquaculture were done. Spirulina can be fed up to 10% for poultry and less than 4% for Quail. Increase in the *Spirulina* content up to 40g/kg for 16 days in 21-day-old broiler male chicks, resulted in yellow and red coloration of flesh and this may be due to the accumulation of the yellow pigment, zeaxanthin. Pigs, rabbits and lambs can receive up to 10% of the feed and increase in the *Spirulina* content in cattle resulted in increase in milk yield and weight. Spirulina as an alternative feedstock and immune booster for big mouth buffalo, milk fish, cultured striped jack, carp, red sea bream, tilapia, catfish, yellow tail, zebrafish, shrimps and abalone was established and up to 2% *Spirulina* per day in aquaculture feed can be safely recommended.

Toxicological studies of the effects of spirulina consumption on humans and animals, including feeding as much as 800 mg/kg, and replacing up to 60% of protein intake with *Spirulina*, have shown no toxic effects. Fertility, teratogenicity, peri- and postnatal, and multigenerational studies on animals also have found no adverse effects from *Spirulina* consumption.

Etymology and Ecology

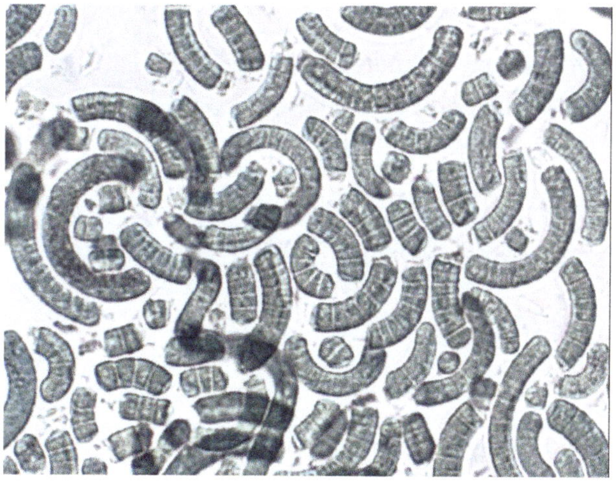

Spirulina powder at 400x, unstained wet mount.

The *maxima* and *plaetensis* species were once classified in the genus *Spirulina*. The common name, *Spirulina*, refers to the dried biomass of *Arthrospira platensis*, which belongs to the oxygenic photosynthetic bacteria that cover the groups Cyanobacteria and Prochlorales. These photosynthetic organisms, Cyanobacteria, were first considered as algae until 1962 and for the first time, these blue green algae were added to prokaryote kingdom and proposed to call these microorganisms as Cyanobacteria where algae is considered to be a very large and diverse group of eukaryotic organisms. This designation was accepted and published in 1974 by the Bergey's Manual of Determinative Bacteriology. Scientifically, there is a quite distinction between *Spirulina* and *Arthrospira* genus. Stizenberger, in 1852 gave the name *Arthrospira* based on the septa presence, helical form and multicellular structure and Gomont in 1892, confirmed aseptate form of the Spirulina genus. Geitler in 1932, reunified both members designating them as Spirulina without considering the septum. The worldwide research on microalgae was carried out in the name of Spirulina, but the original species exploited as food with excellent health properties belongs to genus Arthrospira. This common difference between scientists and customers is difficult to change. These Arthrospira genus, constitute a helical trichomes of varying size and with various degree of coiling including tightly coiled morphology to even straight uncoiled form. The filaments are solitary and reproduce by binary fission and the cells of the trichomes vary from 2 μm to 12 μm and can sometime reach up to 16 μm. Species of the genus Arthrospira have been isolated from alkaline brackish and saline waters in tropical and subtropical regions. Among the various species included in the genus Arthrospira, A. platensis is the most widely distributed and is mainly found in Africa but also in Asia. Arthrospira maxima is believed to be found in California and Mexico. They are now agreed to be in fact *Arthrospira*; nevertheless, and somewhat confusingly, the older term *Spirulina* remains in use for historical reasons.

Arthrospira species are free-floating filamentous cyanobacteria characterized by cylindrical, multicellular trichomes in an open left-hand helix. They occur naturally in tropical and subtropical lakes with high pH and high concentrations of carbonate and bicarbonate. *A. platensis* occurs in Africa, Asia, and South America, whereas *A. maxima* is confined to Central America. Most cultivated spirulina is produced in open channel raceway ponds, with paddle-wheels used to agitate the water. The largest commercial producers of spirulina are located in the United States, Thailand, India, Taiwan, China, Bangladesh, Pakistan, Burma (Myanmar), Greece, and Chile.

Spirulina thrives at a pH around 8.5 and above, which will get more alkaline, and a temperature around 30 °C (86 °F). They are able to make their own food, and do not need a living energy or organic carbon source. In addition, spirulina has to have an ensemble of nutrients to thrive in a home aquarium or pond. A simple nutrient feed for growing it is:

- Baking soda- 16 g/L (61 g/US gal)
- Potassium nitrate- 2 g/L (7.6 g/US gal)
- Sea salt- 1 g/L (3.8 g/US gal)
- Potassium phosphate- 0.1 g/L (0.38 g/US gal)
- Iron sulphate- 0.0378 g/L (0.143 g/US gal)

which can all be found in aquarium or else in the agricultural division, all commonly occurring compounds except for the iron sulphate. The algae has actually been tested and successfully grown in human urine at 1:180 parts. After 7days, 97% of NH_4^+-N, 96.5% of total phosphorus (TP) and 85–98% of urea in the urine (about 120-diluted) were removed by the microalgae under autotrophic culture (30 °C).

Historical Use

Spirulina was a food source for the Aztecs and other Mesoamericans until the 16th century; the harvest from Lake Texcoco and subsequent sale as cakes were described by one of Cortés' soldiers. The Aztecs called it "tecuitlatl".

Spirulina was found in abundance at Lake Texcoco by French researchers in the 1960s, but no reference to its use was made by the Aztecs as a daily food source after the 16th century, probably due to the draining of the surrounding lakes for agricultural and urban development. The topic of the Tecuitlalt, which was earlier discovered in 1520, was not mentioned again until 1940, the French phycologist Pierre Dangeard mentioned about a cake called "*dihe*", consumed by Kanembu tribe, African Lake Chad, Kanem (Chad, Africa). Dangeard studied the "*dihe*" samples and found that it is like a puree of spring form blue algae. Spirulina has also been traditionally harvested in Chad. It is dried into *dihé*, which are used to make broths for meals, and also sold in markets. The spirulina is harvested from small lakes and ponds around Lake Chad.

During 1964 and 1965, the botanist Jean Leonard, during his Belgian Trans-Saharan Expedition, confirmed that *dihe* is made up of *Spirulina* and thus chemical analysis was started on *Spirulina*. During that time, Léonard received a request from Sosa-Texcoco Ltd, Mexico to study a bloom of algae in their sodium hydroxide production facility. As a result, the first systematic and detailed study of the growth requirements and physiology of *Spirulina* was performed. This study, which was a part of Ph.D. thesis by Zarrouk (1966) was the basis for establishing the first large-scale production plant of *Spirulina*. *Spirulina*, in 1967 was established as a "wonderful food source" by the International Association of Applied Microbiology.

The first large-scale spirulina production plant, run by Sosa Texcoco, was established there in the early 1970s.

Research

At present, research is preliminary. According to the U.S. National Institutes of Health, scientific evidence is insufficient to recommend spirulina supplementation for any human condition, and more research is needed to clarify its benefits, if any.

Administration of spirulina has been investigated as a way to control glucose in people with diabetes, but the EFSA rejected those claims in 2013. Live cultures of *Spirulina (Arthospira) sp* grown in open raceway ponds were used for removal of lead from waste water.

Advocates

In 1974, the World Health Organization described spirulina as "an interesting food for multiple reasons, rich in iron and protein, and is able to be administered to children without any risk," considering it "a very suitable food." The United Nations established the Intergovernmental Institution for the use of Micro-algae Spirulina Against Malnutrition in 2003.

In the late 1980s and early 90s, both NASA (CELSS) and the European Space Agency (MELISSA) proposed spirulina as one of the primary foods to be cultivated during long-term space missions.

References

- Robert S. Goodhart; Maurice E. Shils (1980). Modern Nutrition in Health and Disease (6th ed.). Philadelphia: Lea and Febinger. pp. 134–138. ISBN 0-8121-0645-8.
- Fitzgerald M (2014). Diet Cults: The Surprising Fallacy at the Core of Nutrition Fads and a Guide to Healthy Eating for the Rest of US. Pegasus Books. ISBN 978-1-60598-560-2.
- Ross, Ernest; Dominy, Warren (1990). "The nutritional value of dehydrated, blue-green algae (spirulina plantensis) for poultry". Poultry Science. doi:10.3382/ps.0690794. PMID 2114613. Retrieved February 20, 2016.
- Anahad O'Connor (February 3, 2015). "New York Attorney General Targets Supplements at Major Retailers" (the "Well" blog). The New York Times. Retrieved February 3, 2015.
- "What's wrong with herbal remedies They might not contain what they claim—and probably don't work, either". Consumer Reports. February 5, 2015. Retrieved February 7, 2015.
- Peña-Rosas JP, De-Regil LM, Garcia-Casal MN, Dowswell T (2015). "Daily oral iron supplementation during pregnancy.". Cochrane Database Syst Rev. 7: CD0047361. doi:10.1002/14651858.CD004736.pub5. PMID 26198451.
- Siva Kiran RR, Madhu GM, Satyanarayana SV (2015). "Spirulina in combating Protein Energy Malnutrition (PEM) and Protein Energy Wasting (PEW) - A review". Journal of Nutrition Research. 3 (1): 62–79.
- Ali, Md. Shawkat (2014). "Evaluation of the effects of feed attractants (Spirulina and ekangi) on growth performance, feed utilization and body composition of fingerlings of stinging cat fish Heteropneustes fossilis".
- Buono, S; Langellotti, AL; Martello, A; Rinna, F; Fogliano, V (August 2014). "Functional ingredients from microalgae.". Food & Function. 5 (8): 1669–85. doi:10.1039/c4f000125g. PMID 24957182.
- "Charter" (PDF). Intergovernmental Institution for the use of Micro-algae Spirulina Against Malnutrition. 5 March 2003. Retrieved 2 July 2014.
- Katz DL, Meller S (2014). "Can we say what diet is best for health?". Annu Rev Public Health. 35: 83–103. doi:10.1146/annurev-publhealth-032013-182351. PMID 24641555.
- Knight-McDowell, Victoria (30 November 2012). "Breathing New Life into a 142-Year Old Brand". Harvard Business Review. Harvard University. Retrieved 14 September 2013.
- Geffroy, Benjamin; Simon, Olivier (2013). "Effects of a Spirulina platensis-based diet on zebrafish female reproductive performance and larval survival rate" (PDF). Cybium. 37 (1-2): 31–38.
- Chang, Yuanyuan, et al. "Cultivation of Spirulina platensis for biomass production and nutrient removal from synthetic human urine." Applied Energy 102 (2013) C 427-431. doi:10.1016/j.apenergy.2012.07.024
- O'CONNOR, ANAHAD. "Herbal Supplements Are Often Not What They Seem". New York Times. Retrieved 12 November 2013.
- "European Commission website: Food Safety – Labelling & Nutrition – Health & Nutrition Claims". Ec.europa.eu. Retrieved 2012-12-05.
- "Reckitt Benckiser buys Schiff Nutrition in $1.4bn deal". London: The Telegraph. 22 November 2012. Retrieved 30 December 2012.

6

Various Energy Bars and Drinks

Energy bars contain cereals and high-energy food items. They are used as energy sources for particular events like marathons, 100-meter races, and other events. Energy drinks, energy gels and sports drinks are also discussed in the following section. The section serves as a source to comprehend all the numerous energy bars and drinks.

Energy Bar

Energy bars are supplemental bars containing cereals and other high energy foods targeted at people who require quick energy but do not have time for a meal. They are different from energy drinks, which contain caffeine, whereas bars provide food energy.

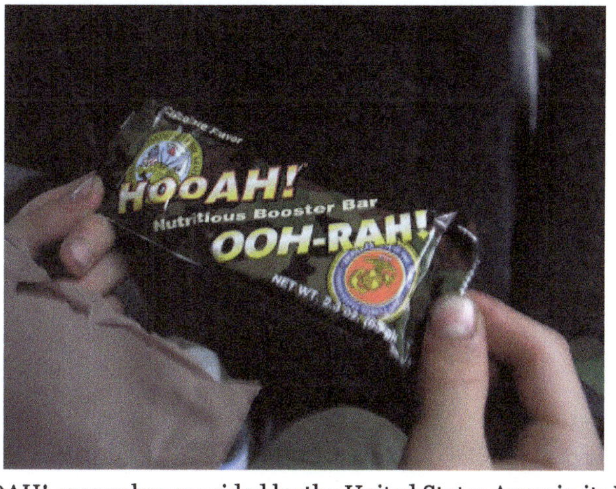

A HOOAH! energy bar provided by the United States Army in its MREs

Nutrition

Energy in food comes from all three main sources: fat, protein, and carbohydrates. A typical energy bar weighs between 45 and 80 g and is likely to supply about 200–300 Cal (840–1,300 kJ), 3–9 g of fat, 7–15 g of protein, and 20–40 g of carbohydrates.

In order to provide energy quickly, most of the carbohydrates are various types of sugars like fructose, glucose, maltodextrin, dextrose and others in various ratios. Use of complex carbohydrate sources like oats and barley is limited and such carbohydrate sources are mostly used in protein bars. Proteins come mostly in the form of fast digesting whey protein. Energy bars generally don't contain sugar alcohols, since these bars, due to type of carbohydrate content, don't require low calorie sweeteners to improve their taste. Fats in energy bars are kept to minimum and their main sources are often cocoa butter and dark chocolate.

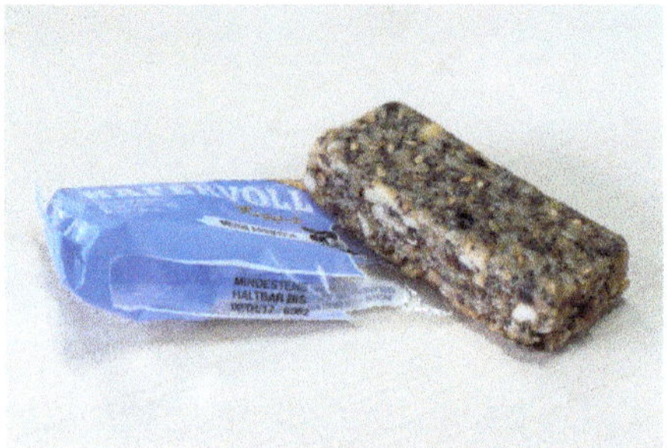

Full Flapjack bars

Usage

Energy bars are used as energy source during athletic events like marathon, triathlon and other events and outdoor activities, where energy expenditure is high, for longer period of time.

Energy Drink

An energy drink is a type of beverage containing stimulant drugs, chiefly caffeine, which is marketed as providing mental and physical stimulation. They may or may not be carbonated and many also contain sugar or other sweeteners, herbal extracts and amino acids. They are a subset of the larger group of energy products, which includes bars and gels, and distinct from sports drinks, which are advertised to enhance sports performance. There are many brands and varieties of energy drinks.

Coffee, tea and other naturally caffeinated beverages are usually not considered energy drinks. Other soft drinks such as cola may contain caffeine, but are also not energy drinks. Some alcoholic beverages, such as Buckfast Tonic Wine, contain caffeine and other stimulants. According to the Mayo Clinic, it is safe for the typical healthy adult to consume a total of 400 mg of caffeine a day. This has been confirmend by a panel of the European Food Safety Authority (ESFA), which also concludes that a caffeine intake of up to 400 mg per day does not raise safety concerns for adults. According to the ESFA this is equivalent to 4 cups of coffee (90 mg each) or 5 standard cans (250 ml) of energy drink (80 mg each).

Energy drinks have the effects caffeine and sugar provide, but there is little or no evidence that the wide variety of other ingredients have any effect. Most of the effects of energy drinks on cognitive performance, such as increased attention and reaction speed, are primarily due to the presence of caffeine. Other studies, however, ascribe those performance improvements to the effects of the combined ingredients. Advertising for energy drinks usually features increased muscle strength and endurance, but there is still no scientific consensus to support these statements. Energy drinks have been associated with health risks, such as an increased rate of alcohol-related injury, and excessive or repeated consumption can lead to cardiac and psychiatric conditions.

Uses

Energy drinks are marketed to provide the benefits among health effects of caffeine along with benefits from the other ingredients they contain. Health experts agree that energy drinks which contain caffeine do provide the effects of caffeine. The consumption of alcohol drinks combined with energy drinks is a common occurrence on many college campuses. The alcohol industry has recently been criticized for marketing cohesiveness of alcohol and energy drinks. The combination of the two in college students is correlated to students experiencing alcohol-related consequences, and several health risks.

There is no good evidence that other ingredients in energy drinks provide further benefits, even though the drinks are frequently advertised in a way that suggests they have unique benefits. The dietary supplements in energy drinks may be purported to provide detoxification, sustain mental process, protect heart health, and reduce muscle fatigue. None of these claims are backed by good evidence, however, the ingredients alone, for example taurine or vitamin B, are scientifically proven to provide positive effects on the metabolism. Various marketing organizations have described energy drinks by saying their beverage "gives you wings", is "scientifically formulated", or that it is a "killer energy brew".

When mixed with alcohol, either as a prepackaged caffeinated alcoholic drink, a mixed drink, or just a beverage consumed around the same time as alcohol, energy drinks are often consumed in social settings.

Variants

Energy Shots

Energy shots are a specialized kind of energy drink. Whereas most energy drinks are sold in cans or bottles, energy shots are usually sold in smaller 50ml bottles. Energy shots can contain the same total amount of caffeine, vitamins or other functional ingredients as their larger versions, and may be considered concentrated forms of energy drinks. The marketing of energy shots generally focuses on their convenience and availability as a low-calorie "instant" energy drink that can be taken in one swallow (or "shot"), as opposed to energy drinks that encourage users to drink an entire can, which may contain 250 calories or more.

Caffeinated Alcoholic Drink

Energy drinks such as Red Bull are often used as mixers with alcoholic beverages, producing mixed drinks such as Vodka Red Bull which are similar to but stronger than rum and coke with respect to the amount of caffeine that they contain. Sometimes this is configured as a bomb shot, such as the Jägerbomb or the *F-Bomb* — Fireball Cinnamon Whisky and Red Bull.

Caffeinated alcoholic drinks are also sold in some countries in a wide variety of formulations. The American products Four Loko and Joose originally combined caffeine and alcohol before caffeinated alcoholic beverages were banned in the U.S. in 2010.

Relaxation Drinks

Several beverages have been marketed in the 2000s as "anti-energy", "chill out", or "relaxation" drinks, including Lava Cola, Slow Cow, Drank, Marley's Mellow Mood, Mary Jane's Relaxing Soda, Chill, Calm, Malava Kava, V.i.B., Take 5, Relax by Rockstar and Jones Gaba. They are growing in popularity, with sales doubling from 2008 to 2010, and expected to more than double again by 2014. They contain ingredients such as theanine and melatonin.

Effects

A health warning on a can of the Austrian Power Horse energy drink: "Consumption of more than two cans in a day may be harmful to your health. Not to be used for pregnant women, breast feeders, children under the age of 16, people with heart disease, high blood pressure, diabetes, allergy to caffeine, and athletes during exercise."

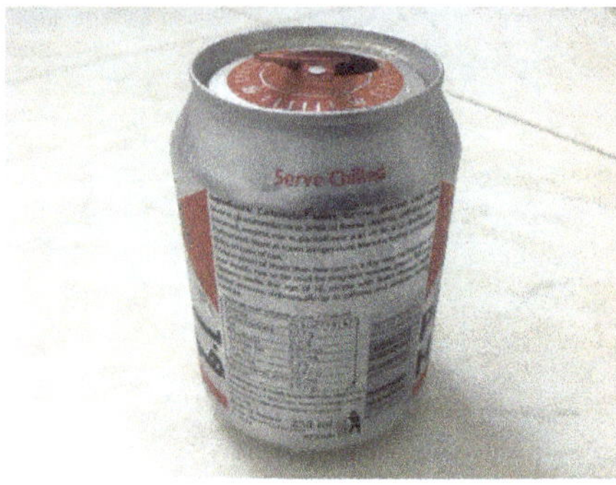

Energy drinks have the effects caffeine and sugar provide, but there is little or no evidence that the wide variety of other ingredients have any effect. Most of the effects of energy drinks on cognitive performance, such as increased attention and reaction speed, are primarily due to the presence of caffeine. Advertising for energy drinks usually features increased muscle strength and endurance, but there is little evidence to support this in the scientific literature.

A caffeine intake of 400 mg per day is considered as safe from the European Food Safety Authority (EFSA). Adverse effects associated with caffeine consumption in amounts greater than 400 mg include nervousness, irritability, sleeplessness, increased urination, abnormal heart rhythms (arrhythmia), and dyspepsia. Consumption also has been known to cause pupil dilation when taken with certain antidepressants or SSRIs. Caffeine dosage is not required to be on the product label for food in the United States, unlike drugs, but some advocates are urging the FDA to change this practice.

Combined use of caffeine and alcohol may increase the rate of alcohol-related injury. Energy drinks can mask the influence of alcohol, and a person may misinterpret their actual level of intoxication. Since caffeine and alcohol are both diuretics, combined use increases the risk of dehydration, and the mixture of a stimulant (caffeine) and depressant (alcohol) sends contradictory messages to the nervous system and can lead to increased heart rate and palpitations. Although people decide to drink energy drinks with alcohol with the intent of counteracting alcohol intoxication, another large majority do so to hide the taste of alcohol. However, in the 2015, the EFSA concluded, that "Consumption of other constituents of energy drinks at concentrations commonly present in such beverages would not affect the safety of single doses of caffeine up to 200 mg." Also the consumption of alcohol, leading to a blood alcohol content of about 0.08%, would, according to the EFSA, not affect the safety of single doses of caffeine up to 200 mg. Up to these levels of intake, caffeine is unlikely to mask the subjective perception of alcohol intoxication.

Excessive or repeated consumption of energy drinks can lead to cardiac problems, such as arrhythmias and heart attacks, and psychiatric conditions such as anxiety and phobias. In Europe, energy drinks containing taurine and caffeine have been associated with the deaths of athletes.

Research suggests that emergency room visits are on the increase. In 2005, there were 1,494 emergency room visits related to energy drink consumption in the United States; whereas, in 2011, energy drinks were linked to 20,783 emergency room visits. During this period of increase, males consumers consistently had a higher likelihood of visiting the emergency room over their female counterparts. Research trends also show that emergency room visits are caused mainly by adverse reactions to the drinks. In 2011, there were 14,042 energy drink-related hospital visits. Misuse and abuse of these caffeinated beverages also cause a significant amount of emergency room visits. By 2011, there were 6,090 visits to the ER due to misuse/abuse of the drinks. In many cases 42% of patients had mixed energy drinks with another stimulant, and in the other 58% of cases the energy drink was the only thing that had been consumed. Several studies suggest that energy drinks may be a gateway drug.

Chemistry

Energy drinks generally contain methylxanthines (including caffeine), B vitamins, carbonated water, and high-fructose corn syrup (for non-diet versions). Other commonly used ingredients are guarana, yerba mate, açaí, and taurine, plus various forms of ginseng, maltodextrin, inositol, carnitine, creatine, glucuronolactone, sucralose and ginkgo biloba.

Supplement Facts

Serving Size 8.0 fl.oz. (240 mL)
Servings Per Container: 2

Amount Per Serving		% Daily Value
Calories	**100**	
Total Carb	**27g**	**9%***
Sugars	27g	†
Riboflavin Vit B2	1.7mg	100%
Niacin Vit B3	20mg	100%
Vitamin B6	2mg	100%
Vitamin B12	6mcg	100%
Sodium	180mg	8%
Taurine	1000mg	†
Panax Ginseng	200mg	†
Energy Blend	2500mg	†
L-Carnitine, Glucose, Caffeine, Guarana, Inositol, Glucuronolactone, Maltodextrin		

*Percent Daily Values are based on a 2000 calorie diet. † Daily Value not established.

A Nutrition facts label for an energy drink.

Some energy drink manufacturers do not report how much caffeine their products contain. One survey found that various energy drinks had 6–242 milligrams (mg) of caffeine per serving. In comparison, an 8 US fluid ounces (240 ml) cup of coffee contains 100 mg of caffeine and 12 US fluid ounces (350 ml) of Coca-Cola Classic contains 35 mg of caffeine. Consumer Reports expected that the caffeine content of a beverage should be within 20% of what the label claims, but product testing on United States energy drinks found that the caffeine levels of some energy drinks vary beyond that range. A major producer of energy drinks in the United States explained that they do not report caffeine levels because "there is no legal or commercial business requirement to do so, and also because our products are completely safe, and the actual numbers are not meaningful to most consumers." Scientific groups and consumer organizations have requested more disclosure in ingredient lists.

The sugar in non-diet energy drinks is food energy that can be utilized by the human body.

Frequency of Use

Globally, energy drinks are typically attractive to young people. Approximately 66 percent of consumers are between the ages of 13 and 35 years, with males being approximately 65 percent of the market. A 2008 statewide Patient Poll conducted by the Pennsylvania Medical Society's Institute for Good Medicine found that: 20 percent of respondents aged between 21 and 30 had used energy drinks in high school or college to stay awake longer to study, or to write a paper; and 70 percent of respondents knew someone who had used an energy drink to stay awake longer to study or work.

US research by Packaged Facts in 2012 showed that consumers aged between 18 and 34 years, men, Hispanics, Pacific region residents and adults with children in the household were the demographic groups that were using the highest amounts of energy drinks.

History

Energy drinks were an active subset of the early soft drink industry; Pepsi, for instance, was originally marketed as an energy booster. Coca-Cola's name was derived from its two active ingredients, both known stimulants: coca leaves and kola nuts (a source of caffeine). Fresh coca leaves were replaced by "spent" ones in 1904 because of concerns over the use of cocaine in food products; the federal lawsuit *United States v. Forty Barrels and Twenty Kegs of Coca-Cola* pressured The Coca-Cola Company into reducing the amount of caffeine in its formula by 1916. These developments brought an end to the first wave of energy drinks.

In the UK, Lucozade Energy was originally introduced in 1929 as a hospital drink for "aiding the recovery;" in the early 1980s, it was promoted as an energy drink for "replenishing lost energy." One of the first post-*Forty Barrels* energy drinks introduced in America was Dr. Enuf. Its origins date back to 1949, when a Chicago businessman named William Mark Swartz was urged by co-workers to formulate a soft drink fortified with vitamins as an alternative to sugar sodas full of empty calories. He developed an "energy booster" drink containing B vitamins, caffeine and cane sugar. After placing a notice in a trade magazine seeking a bottler, he formed a partnership with Charles Gordon of Tri-City Beverage to produce and distribute the soda. Dr. Enuf is still being manufactured in Johnson City, Tennessee and sold sparsely throughout the nation.

In Japan, the energy drink dates at least as far back as the early 1960s, with the launch of the Lipovitan brand. However, in Japan, most of the products of this kind bear little resemblance to soft drinks, and are sold instead in small brown glass medicine bottles, or cans styled to resemble such containers. These "eiyō dorinku" (literally, "nutritional drinks") are marketed primarily to *salarymen*. Bacchus-F, a South Korean drink closely modeled after Lipovitan, also appeared in the early 1960s and targets a similar demographic.

In 1985, Jolt Cola was introduced in the United States. Its marketing strategy centered on the drink's caffeine content, billing it as a means to promote wakefulness. The drink's initial slogan read: "All the sugar and twice the caffeine."

In 1995, PepsiCo launched Josta, the first energy drink introduced by a major US beverage company (one that had interests outside energy drinks), but Pepsi discontinued the product in 1999. Pepsi would later return to the energy drink market with the AMP brand.

In Europe, energy drinks were pioneered by the Lisa company and a product named "Power Horse", before Dietrich Mateschitz, an Austrian entrepreneur, introduced the Red Bull product, a worldwide bestseller in the 21st century. Mateschitz developed Red Bull based on the Thai drink Krating Daeng, itself based on Lipovitan. Red Bull became the dominant brand in the US after its introduction in 1997, with a market share of approximately 47% in 2005.

In New Zealand and Australia, the leading energy drink product in those markets, V, was introduced by Frucor Beverages. The product now represents over 60% of market in New Zealand and Australia.

UK supermarkets have launched their own brands of energy drinks, sold at lower prices than the major soft drink manufacturers, that are mostly produced by Canadian beverage maker Cott. Tesco supermarkets sell "Kx" (formerly known as "Kick"), Sainsbury's sell "Blue Bolt" and Asda sell "Blue Charge"—all three drinks are sold in 250-milliliter cans and 1-liter bottles—while Morrison's sell "Source" in 250-milliliter cans. Cott sells a variety of other branded energy drinks to independent retailers in various containers.

Since 2002, there has been a growing trend for packaging energy drinks in bigger cans. In many countries, including the US and Canada, there is a limitation on the maximum caffeine per serving in energy drinks, so manufacturers include a greater amount of caffeine by including multiple servings per container. Popular brands such as Red Bull, Hype Energy Drinks and Monster have increased the amount of ounces per can.

The energy shot product, an offshoot of the energy drink, was launched in the US with products such as "5-Hour Energy," which was first released onto the market in 2004. A consumer health analyst explained in a March 2014 media article: "Energy shots took off because of energy drinks. If you're a white collar worker, you're not necessarily willing to down a big Monster energy drink, but you may drink an energy shot."

In 2007, energy drink powders and effervescent tablets were introduced, whereby either can be added to water to create an energy drink.

Energy drinks are also popular as drink mixers—Red Bull and vodka is a popular combination. In the US, a product called "Four Loko" formerly mixed beer with caffeine, while Kahlua is a coffee-flavored alcoholic beverage.

On August 14, 2012, the word "energy drink" was listed for the first time in the Merriam-Webster's Collegiate Dictionary.

Sales

Market research firm Euromonitor calculated that the global energy drink market was worth US$3.8 billion in 1999 and this value grew to US$27.5 billion in 2013.

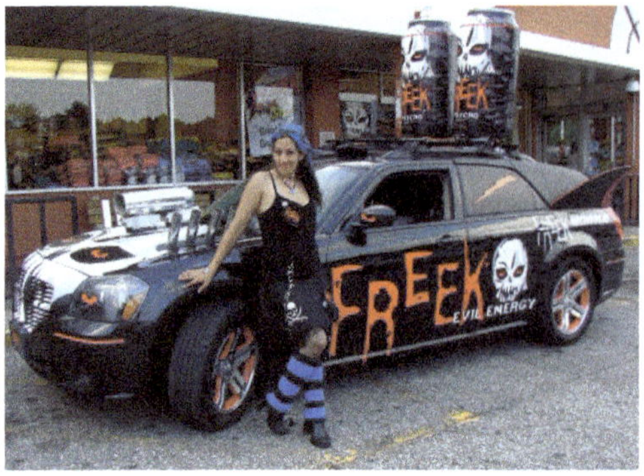

a model advertises an energy drink

In 2000, the US energy drink market was worth US$350 million and data from the Packaged Facts company shows that the industry grew by 60 percent between 2008 and 2012 in the US—by 2012 total US sales were over US$12.5 Billion. Red Bull and Monster were the two best-selling brands in 2012, accounting for nearly 80% of US energy drink sales, and the energy shot market is worth over US$1 billion in 2014.

Regulation

The energy drink Red Bull did not get market approval in France after the death of an 18-year-old Irish athlete, Ross Cooney, who died within hours after playing a basketball game and consuming four cans of the product. This market approval was challenged in the European Court of Justice in 2004, and consequently lifted. Norway did not allow Red Bull for a time, although this restriction has recently been relaxed. In May 2009 it became legal to sell in Norway. The Norwegian version has reduced B-vitamin B6. The United Kingdom investigated the drink, but only issued a warning against its consumption by children and pregnant women.

In 2009, Colombia, under the Ministry of Social Protection, prohibited the sale and commercialization of energy drinks to minors under the age of 14 under resolution 4150 of 2009.

In November 2012, President Ramzan Kadyrov of Chechnya (Russian Federation) ordered his government to develop a bill banning the sale of energy drinks, arguing that as a form of "intoxicating drug", such drinks were "unacceptable in a Muslim society". Kadyrov cited reports of one death and 530 hospital admissions in 2012 due to "poisoning" from the consumption of such drinks. A similar view was expressed by Gennady Onishchenko, Chief Sanitary Inspector of Russia.

In 2009, a school in Hove, England requested that local shops refrain from selling energy drinks to students. Headteacher Malvina Sanders added that "This was a preventative measure, as all research shows that consuming high-energy drinks can have a detrimental impact on the ability of young people to concentrate in class." The school negotiated for their local branch of the Tesco supermarket to display posters asking students not to purchase the products. Similar measures were taken by a school in Oxted, England, which banned students from consuming drinks and sent letters to parents.

Some countries have certain restrictions on the sale and manufacture of energy drinks. In Australia and New Zealand, energy drinks are regulated under the Australia New Zealand Food Standards Code; limiting the caffeine content of 'formulated caffeinated beverages' (energy drinks) at

320 mg/L (9.46 mg/oz) and soft-drinks at 145 mg/L (4.29 mg/oz). Mandatory caffeine labeling is issued for all food products containing guarana in the country, and Australian energy drink labels warn consumers to drink no more than two cans per day.

On June 7, 2012, the parliament of Latvia approved changes in the legislation of sale of consumable goods, to prohibit sale of energy drinks to persons under the age of 18.

As of 2013 in the United States some energy drinks, including Monster Energy and Rockstar Energy, were reported to be rebranding their products as beverages rather than as dietary supplements. As beverages they would be relieved of F.D.A. reporting requirements with respect to deaths and injuries and can be purchased with food stamps, but must list ingredients on the can.

In May 2014 Lithuania became the first state in the world to explicitly ban selling energy drinks to minors below 18 years of age, effective November. An energy drink is described as any beverage containing at least 150 mg/L of caffeine.

Ban on Caffeinated Alcoholic Beverages

Some places ban the sale of prepackaged caffeinated alcoholic beverages, which can be described as energy drinks containing alcohol. In response to these bans, the marketers can change the formula of their products.

Energy Gel

Energy gels are carbohydrate gels that provide energy for exercise and promote recovery, commonly used in endurance events such as running, cycling, and triathlons. Energy gels are also referred to as endurance gels, sports gels, nutritional gels, and carbohydrate gels. They come in small, single-serve plastic packets. Each packet has a strip with a small notch at the top that can be peeled off to reveal an opening through which the gel can be consumed.

History

Sports energy gels emerged in the United Kingdom in 1986 as a "convenient, prewrapped, portable" way to deliver carbohydrates during endurance events. Gels have a gooey texture and are sometimes referred to as "goo" generically. The gel Leppin Squeezy was distributed at the Hawaii Ironman Triathlon in 1988. Once considered a "cult product in clear packaging", energy gel products are now marketed in fancy packaging and come in a variety of flavors. The energy gel market grew during the 1990s, as professional athletes began endorsing products. Manufacturers generally encourage the consumption of multiple packets, with water, when participating in endurance events. Individual packets typically cost between 99 cents and $1.29 (as reported by the *St. Petersburg Times* in 2003).

Nutritional Behavior

Once consumed, the carbohydrates found in the gels are absorbed into the blood to supply the body with calories and nutrients to fuel exercise activity by helping to delay muscular fatigue, raise blood sugar levels, and enhance performance. Most energy gels have no fat, fiber, or protein, so they can be digested quickly. They contain mainly sugars and maltodextrins, which make them similar to sports drinks without the water. Since simple carbohydrates slow down gastric emptying and can cause gastrointestinal distress in athletes, there are attempts to create new categories of energy gels made with complex, long chain carbohydrates and/or fat. Spring gel is an example of a gel with low sugar, low glycemic index carbohydrate content with the addition of fat and Vespa-power is an example of a gel made with fat. Some gels, such as e-Gel, also come with added electrolytes. There are also gels with extras such as ginseng and other herbs, amino acids, vitamins, and Coenzyme Q10. Caffeine can be found in some gels as well. Examples of common energy gels are GU, PowerBar Gel, and Clif Shot.

Use

The recommended use of an energy gel is 15 minutes before starting and 30–45 minutes after starting the endurance exercise. The first gel prior to exercise may be skipped in favor of a high carbohydrate snack instead. Energy gels are then to be used every 30–45 minutes during exercise. The notch can be peeled off at the top and an intake of energy gel is recommended to be followed with a drink of water to avoid risk of dehydration. This is especially important for gels with high simple carbohydrate content. These gels create hyperosmolar gastric content which prevents carbohydrate absorption and gastrointestinal distress. For this reason, energy gels with low sugar content are frequently called “hydrogels”. The exact intake of the gel varies for every athlete depending on their metabolism, body weight, and fitness level.

Sports Drink

Sports drinks are beverages whose stated purpose is to help athletes replace water, electrolytes, and energy after training or competition, though their efficacy for that purpose has been questioned, particularly after exercise.

Categories of Sport Drinks

Sports drinks can be split into three major types:

- Isotonic sport drinks contain similar concentrations of salt and sugar as in the human body.
- Hypertonic sport drinks contain a higher concentration of salt and sugar than the human body.
- Hypotonic sport drinks contain a lower concentration of salt and sugar than the human body.

Most sports drinks are approximately isotonic, having between 4 and 5 heaped teaspoons of sugar per five ounce (13 and 19 grams per 250ml) serving.

Purpose and Effectiveness

Athletes actively training and competing lose water and electrolytes by sweating, and expending energy. However, Robert Robergs, an exercise physiologist at the University of New Mexico who studied Gatorade, said that unless someone is exercising or competing in a sporting event for longer than 90 minutes, there is no reason to drink something with excess sugar and electrolytes. The Australian Institute of Sport states that excessive salt supplementation during exercise may lead to "gastrointestinal problems or cause further impairment of fluid balance" and may cause salt-induced cramps.

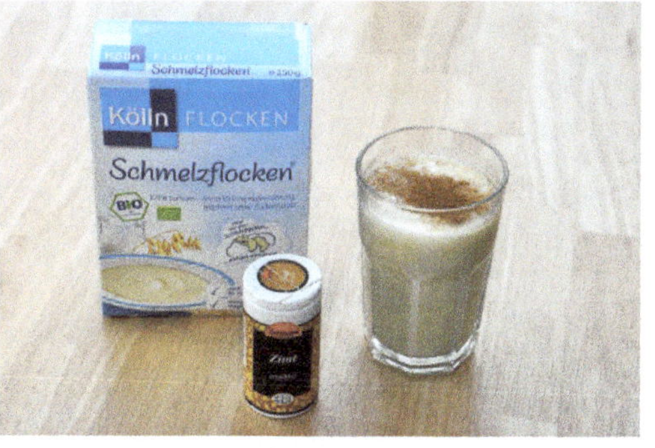

Sport drink made with processed oats, cinnamon, orange juice and milk

Sodium in drinks might help to avoid hyponatraemia (low sodium), but only after sustaining athletic activity for more than four hours; a sports drink containing sodium may be appropriate for recovery from intense and prolonged training or competition.

A stated purpose of sports drinks, which provide many calories of energy from sugars, is to improve performance and endurance. In an analysis by Matthew Thompson and colleagues from the Oxford Centre for Evidence Based Medicine, of 431 marketing claims of performance enhancement, most cited no evidence. 174 sources were cited for GlaxoSmithKline's Lucozade; of them, Thompson found only three studies of high quality with a low risk of bias. The rigorous studies that did show improved endurance were "of limited relevance to most people because the tests were on elite athletes". Thompson said that, for the vast majority of people, drinking such products "could completely counteract exercising more, playing football more, going to the gym more".

The drinks are marketed as soft drinks. In response to the Oxford analysis, a soft drinks industry spokesman claimed "By helping people participating in sport to perform better and to recover more quickly, sports drinks can encourage people to exercise more".

An effect of drinking sports drinks with carbohydrates without prolonged exercise is weight gain. A study presented at the Obesity Society's Obesity 2012 scientific meeting found people in their teens gained 3.5 pounds (1.6 kg) over two years for every bottle of sports drink consumed per day. The leading author of the study, Alison Field of Harvard Medical School, said she was surprised to find that "Sports drinks have an even stronger relationship than sugared sodas with weight gain".

History

In the 19th and early 20th century, athletes occasionally drank beer of low alcohol content replenishing water, minerals and energy in the body. As the water is boiled during the brewing process and thus sterilized, the beer was safer option than water from an unknown source. However, it is studied that even a low dose of ethanol decreases endurance performance: it inhibits liver glucose output during exercise, and also impairs psychomotor skills such as reaction time, hand-eye coordination and balance.

References

- Ronald Hamowy (2007), Government and public health in America (illustrated ed.), Edward Elgar Publishing, pp. 140–141, ISBN 978-1-84542-911-9
- Fred W. Sauceman (1 March 2009). The Place Setting: Timeless Tastes of the Mountain South, from Bright Hope to Frog Level. Mercer University Press. pp. 89–. ISBN 978-0-88146-140-4.
- Petit A, Karila L, Lejoyeux M (2015). "[Abuse of energy drinks: does it pose a risk?].". Presse Med. 44 (3): 261–70. doi:10.1016/j.lpm.2014.07.029. PMID 25622514.
- Smith, Leesa (3 September 2014). "'My heart just hit the floor': A mother's pain after her son died from drinking FOUR energy drinks daily... as a doctor warns no more than two caffeinated beverages per day". Daily Mail Australia. Retrieved 3 September 2014.
- Mora-Rodriguez R, Pallarés JG (2014). "Performance outcomes and unwanted side effects associated with energy drinks.". Nutr Rev. 72 Suppl 1: 108–20. doi:10.1111/nure.12132. PMID 25293550.
- Meier, Barry (1 January 2013). "Energy Drinks Promise Edge, but Experts Say Proof Is Scant". The New York Times. New York: NYTC. ISSN 0362-4331. Retrieved 26 September 2014.
- Hoare, Peter (January 9, 2014). "5 Awesome Drinks You Can Make With Fireball Cinnamon Whisky". Food & drinks. MTV. Retrieved June 17, 2014.
- Pennsylvania Medical Society (19 September 2008). "Energy Drinks "" Busting Your Health for the Buzz". Newswise. Newswise, Inc. Retrieved 27 March 2014.
- Roberto A. Ferdman (26 March 2014). "The American energy drink craze in two highly caffeinated charts". Quartz. Retrieved 27 March 2014.
- Clare O'Connor (8 February 2012). "The Mystery Monk Making Billions With 5-Hour Energy". Forbes. Forbes LLC. Retrieved 27 March 2014.
- Blake, Judith (November 19, 2004). "A new fuel for athletes: energy gels". The Baltimore Sun. Tribune Company. ISSN 1930-8965. Retrieved January 23, 2014.
- Consumer Reports (December 2012). "Energy Drinks – Caffeine Levels". consumerreports.org. Retrieved 26 September 2014.
- Barry Meier (March 19, 2013). "In a New Aisle, Energy Drinks Sidestep Some Rules". The New York Times. Retrieved March 20, 2013.
- Klineman, Jeffrey (2008-04-30). ""Little competition: energy shots aim for big" profits". Bevnet.com. Retrieved 2013-05-24.
- Jennifer Nelson, M.S.; Katherine Zeratsky (2010-03-06). "Relaxation drinks: Does calm come in a can?". Mayo Clinic. Retrieved 2011-07-20.
- FDA (November 3, 2010). "List of Manufacturers of Caffeinated Alcoholic Beverages". U.S. Food and Drug Administration. Retrieved 11 November 2010.
- Zezima, Katie (October 26, 2010). "A Mix Attractive to Students and Partygoers". The New York Times. Retrieved November 11, 2010.

7

Significant Aspects of Nutrition and Food Science

The significant aspects of nutrition and food sciences are examined in this chapter. The study of the interactions of biological and non-biological components of food items is known as food chemistry. Other facets elucidated are food engineering, food microbiology, molecular gastronomy and malnutrition. The topics discussed in the text are of great importance to broaden the existing knowledge on nutrition and food science.

Food Chemistry

Food chemistry is the study of chemical processes and interactions of all biological and non-biological components of foods. The biological substances include such items as meat, poultry, lettuce, beer, and milk as examples. It is similar to biochemistry in its main components such as carbohydrates, lipids, and protein, but it also includes areas such as water, vitamins, minerals, enzymes, food additives, flavors, and colors. This discipline also encompasses how products change under certain food processing techniques and ways either to enhance or to prevent them from happening. An example of enhancing a process would be to encourage fermentation of dairy products with microorganisms that convert lactose to lactic acid; an example of preventing a process would be stopping the browning on the surface of freshly cut Red Delicious apples using lemon juice or other acidulated water.

History of Food Chemistry

The scientific approach to food and nutrition arose with attention to agricultural chemistry in the works of J. G. Wallerius, Humphry Davy, and others. For example, Davy published *Elements of Agricultural Chemistry, in a Course of Lectures for the Board of Agriculture* (1813) in the United Kingdom which would serve as a foundation for the profession worldwide, going into a fifth edition. Earlier work included that by Carl Wilhelm Scheele who isolated malic acid from apples in 1785.

In 1874 the Society of Public Analysts was formed, with the aim of applying analytical methods to the benefit of the public. Its early experiments were based on bread, milk and wine.

It was also out of concern for the quality of the food supply, mainly food adulteration and contamination issues that would first stem from intentional contamination to later with chemical food additives by the 1950s. The development of colleges and universities worldwide, most notably in the United States, would expand food chemistry as well with research of the dietary substances, most notably the Single-grain experiment during 1907-11. Additional research by Harvey W. Wiley at the United States Department of Agriculture during the late 19th century would play a key factor in the creation of the United States Food and Drug Administration in 1906. The American Chemical Society would establish their Agricultural and Food Chemistry Division in 1908 while the Institute of Food Technologists would establish their Food Chemistry Division in 1995.

Food chemistry concepts are often drawn from rheology, theories of transport phenomena, physical and chemical thermodynamics, chemical bonds and interaction forces, quantum mechanics and reaction kinetics, biopolymer science, colloidal interactions, nucleation, glass transitions and freezing/disordered or noncrystalline solids, and thus has Food Physical Chemistry as a foundation area.

Water in Food Systems

A major component of food is water, which can encompass anywhere from 50% in meat products to 95% in lettuce, cabbage, and tomato products. It is also an excellent place for bacterial growth and food spoilage if it is not properly processed. One way this is measured in food is by water activity which is very important in the shelf life of many foods during processing. One of the keys to food preservation in most instances is reduce the amount of water or alter the water's characteristics to enhance shelf-life. Such methods include dehydration, freezing, and refrigeration This field encompasses the *"physiochemical principles of the reactions and conversions that occur during the manufacture, handling, and storage of foods"*.

Carbohydrates

Comprising 75% of the biological world and 80% of all food intake for human consumption, the most common known human carbohydrate is Sucrose. The simplest version of a carbohydrate is a monosaccharide which possesses the properties of carbon, hydrogen, and oxygen in a 1:2:1 ratio under a general formula of $C_nH_{2n}O_n$ where n is a minimum of 3. Glucose is an example of a monosaccharide as is fructose. Combine them in the picture shown to the right and you have sucrose, one of the more common sugar products around.

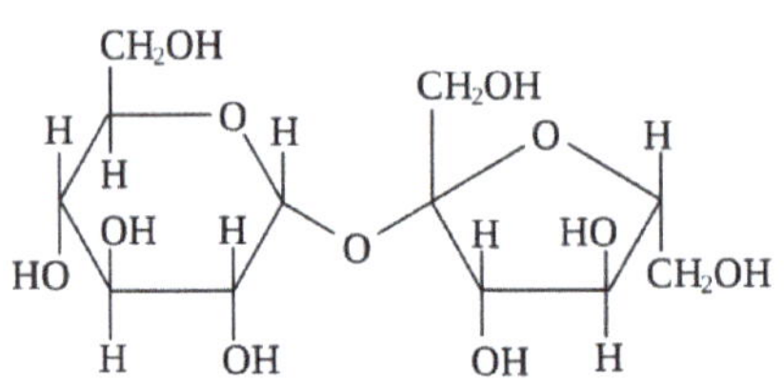

Sucrose: ordinary table sugar and probably the most familiar carbohydrate.

A chain of monosaccharides form to make a polysaccharide. Such polysaccharides include pectin, dextran, agar, and xanthan.

Sugar content is commonly measured in degrees brix.

Lipids

The term lipid comprises a diverse range of molecules and to some extent is a catchall for relatively water-insoluble or nonpolar compounds of biological origin, including waxes, fatty acids (including essential fatty acids), fatty-acid derived phospholipids, sphingolipids, glycolipids and terpenoids, such as retinoids and steroids. Some lipids are linear aliphatic molecules, while others have ring structures. Some are aromatic, while others are not. Some are flexible, while others are rigid.

Most lipids have some polar character in addition to being largely nonpolar. Generally, the bulk of their structure is nonpolar or hydrophobic ("water-fearing"), meaning that it does not interact well with polar solvents like water. Another part of their structure is polar or hydrophilic ("water-loving") and will tend to associate with polar solvents like water. This makes them amphiphilic molecules (having both hydrophobic and hydrophilic portions). In the case of cholesterol, the polar group is a mere -OH (hydroxyl or alcohol).

Lipids in food include the oils of such grains as corn, soybean, from animal fats, and are parts of many foods such as milk, cheese, and meat. They also act as vitamin carriers as well.

Food Proteins

Proteins compose over 50% of the dry weight of an average living cell and are very complex macromolecules. They also play a fundamental role in the structure and function of cells. Consisting mainly of carbon, nitrogen, hydrogen, oxygen, and some sulfur, they also may contain iron, copper, phosphorus, or zinc.

In food, proteins are essential for growth and survival and vary depending upon a person's age and physiology (e.g., pregnancy). Protein is commonly obtained from animal sources: eggs, milk, and meat. Nuts, grains and legumes provide vegetable sources of protein, and protein combining of vegetable sources is used to achieve complete protein nutritional quotas from vegetables.

Protein sensitivity as food allergy is detected with the ELISA test.

Enzymes

Enzymes are biochemical catalysts used in converting processes from one substance to another. They are also involved in reducing the amount of time and energy required to complete a chemical process. Many aspects of the food industry use catalysts, including baking, brewing, dairy, and fruit juices, to make cheese, beer, and bread.

Vitamins

Vitamins are nutrients required in small amounts for essential metabolic reactions in the body. These are broken down in nutrition as either water-soluble (Vitamin C) or fat-soluble (Vitamin E). An adequate supply of vitamins can prevent diseases such as beriberi, anemia, and scurvy while an overdose of vitamins can produce nausea and vomiting or even death.

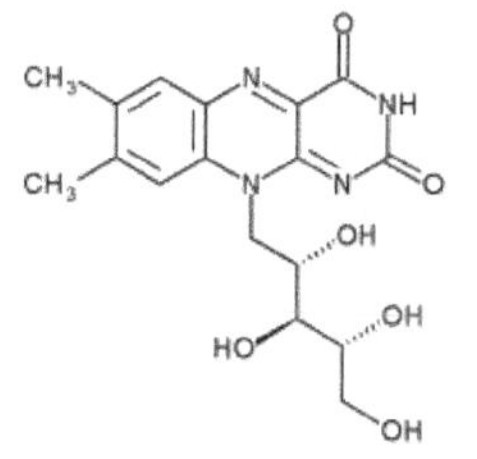

Riboflavin (Vitamin B_2), water-soluble.

Minerals

Dietary minerals in foods are large and diverse with many required to function while other trace elements can be hazardous if consumed in excessive amounts. Bulk minerals with a Reference Daily Intake (RDI, formerly Recommended Daily Allowance (RDA)) of more than 200 mg/day are calcium, magnesium, and potassium while important trace minerals (RDI less than 200 mg/day) are copper, iron, and zinc. These are found in many foods, but can also be taken in dietary supplements.

Color

Food coloring is added to change the color of any food substance. It is mainly for sensory analysis purposes. It can be used to simulate the natural color of a product as perceived by the customer, such as red dye (like FD&C Red No.40 Allura Red AC) to ketchup or to add unnatural colors to a product like Kellogg's Froot Loops. Caramel is a natural food dye; the industrial form, caramel coloring, is the most widely used food coloring and is found in foods from soft drinks to soy sauce, bread, and pickles.

Flavors

Flavor in food is important in how food smells and tastes to the consumer, especially in sensory analysis. Some of these products occur naturally like salt and sugar, but flavor chemists (called a "flavorist") develop many of these flavors for food products. Such artificial flavors include methyl salicylate which creates the wintergreen odor and lactic acid which gives milk a tart taste.

Food Additives

Food additives are substances added to food for preserving flavors, or improving taste or appearance. The processes are as old as adding vinegar for pickling or as an emulsifier for emulsion mixtures like mayonnaise. These are generally listed by "E number" in the European Union or GRAS ("generally recognized as safe") by the United States Food and Drug Administration.

Branch of Food Chemistry

Food Physical Chemistry

Food physical chemistry is considered to be a branch of Food chemistry concerned with the study of both physical and chemical interactions in foods in terms of physical and chemical principles applied to food systems, as well as the applications of physical/chemical techniques and instrumentation for the study of foods. This field encompasses the *"physiochemical principles of the reactions and conversions that occur during the manufacture, handling, and storage of foods"*

Food physical chemistry concepts are often drawn from rheology, theories of transport phenomena, physical and chemical thermodynamics, chemical bonds and interaction forces, quantum mechanics and reaction kinetics, biopolymer science, colloidal interactions, nucleation, glass transitions and freezing, disordered/noncrystalline solids.

Techniques utilized range widely from dynamic rheometry, optical microscopy, electron microscopy, AFM, light scattering, X-ray diffraction/neutron diffraction, to MRI, spectroscopy (NMR,

FT-NIR/IR, NIRS, ESR and EPR, CD/VCD, Fluorescence, FCS, HPLC, GC-MS, and other related analytical techniques.

Understanding food processes and the properties of foods requires a knowledge of physical chemistry and how it applies to specific foods and food processes. Food physical chemistry is essential for improving the quality of foods, their stability and food product development. Because food science is a multi-disciplinary field, food physical chemistry is being developed through interactions with other areas of food chemistry and food science, such as: food analytical chemistry, food process engineering/food processing, food and bioprocess technology, food extrusion, food quality control, food packaging, food biotechnology and food microbiology.

Topics in Food Physical Chemistry

The following are examples of topics in food physical chemistry that are of interest to both food industry and food science:

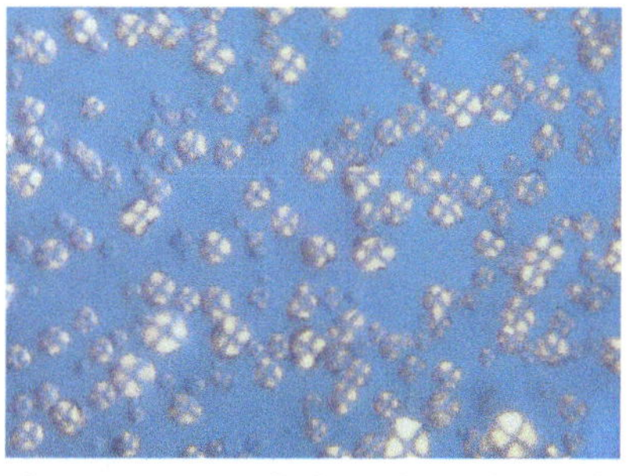

Starch, 800x magnified, under polarized light

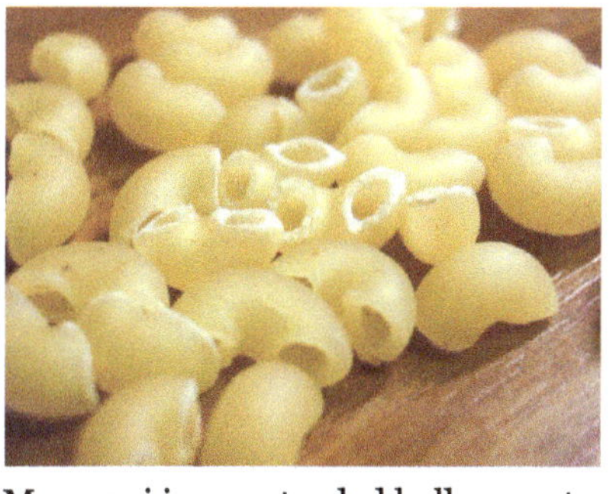

Macaroni is an extruded hollow pasta.

- Water in foods
    - Local structure in liquid water
    - Micro-crystallization in ice cream emulsions
- Dispersion and surface-adsorption processes in foods
- Water and protein activities
- Food hydration and shelf-life
- Hydrophobic interactions in foods

- Hydrogen bonding and ionic interactions in foods
- Disulfide bond breaking and formation in foods
- Food dispersions
- Structure-functionality in foods
- Food micro- and nano- structure
- Food gels and gelling mechanisms
- Cross-linking in foods
- Starch gelatinization and retrogradation
- Physico-chemical modification of carbohydrates
- Physico-chemical interactions in food formulations
- Freezing effects on foods and freeze concentration of liquids
- Glass transition in wheat gluten and wheat doughs
- Drying of foods and crops
- Rheology of wheat doughs, cheese and meat
- Rheology of extrusion processes
- Food enzyme kinetics
- Immobilized enzymes and cells
- Microencapsulation
- Carbohydrates structure and interactions with water and proteins
- Maillard browning reactions
- Lipids structures and interactions with water and food proteins
- Food proteins structure, hydration and functionality in foods
- Food protein denaturation
- Food enzymes and reaction mechanisms
- Vitamin interactions and preservation during food processing
- Interaction of salts and minerals with food proteins and water
- Color determinations and food grade coloring
- Flavors and sensorial perception of foods

- Properties of food additives

Related Fields

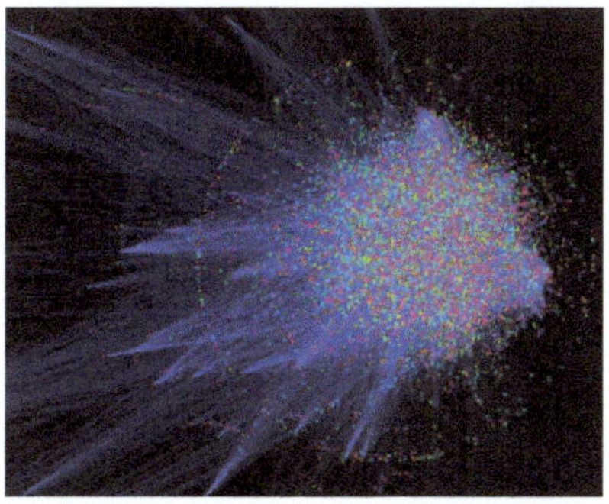

Visualisation of the human interactome network topology with the blue lines between proteins (represented as points) showing protein-protein interactions.

- Food chemistry
- Food physics and Rheology
- Biophysical chemistry
- Physical chemistry
    - Spectroscopy-applied
    - Intermolecular forces
    - Nanotechnology and nanostructures
- Chemical physics
    - Molecular dynamics
    - Surface chemistry and Van der Waals forces
    - Chemical reactions and Reaction chemistry
- Quantum chemistry
    - Quantum genetics
    - Molecular models of DNA and Molecular modelling of proteins and viruses
- Bioorganic chemistry
- Polymer chemistry
- Biochemistry and Biological chemistry
    - Enzymology
    - Protein–protein interactions

    - Biomembranes
- Complex system biology
    - Integrative biology
    - Mathematical biophysics
    - Systems biology
    - Genomics, Proteomics, Interactomics, Structural bioinformatics and Cheminformatics
- Food technology, Food engineering, Food safety and Food biotechnology
    - Agricultural biotechnology
        -
            - Immobilized cells and enzymes
            - Microencapsulation of food additives and vitamins, etc.
- Chemical engineering
- Plant biology and Crop sciences
- Animal sciences

Techniques Gallery: High-Field Nmr, Cars (Raman Spectroscopy), Fluorescence Confocal Microscopy and Hyperspectral Imaging

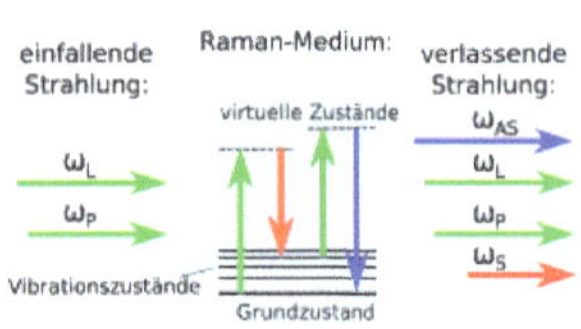

CARS Raman Spectroscopy

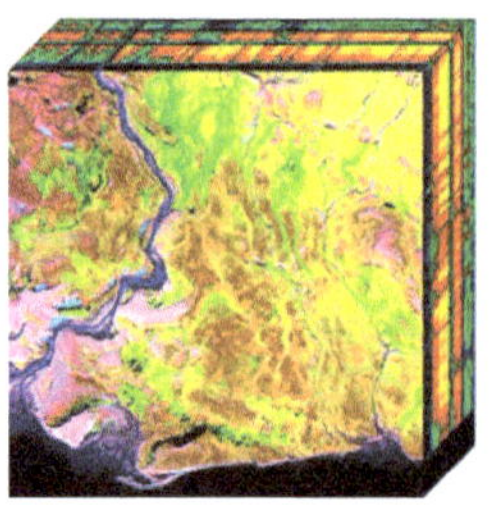

Hyperspectral Imaging Cube

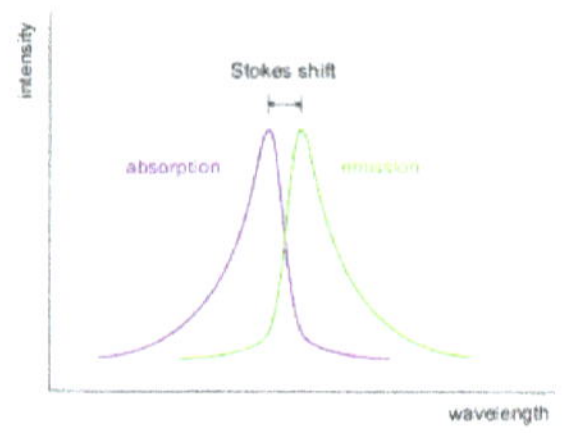

Stoks and anti-Stokes shifts

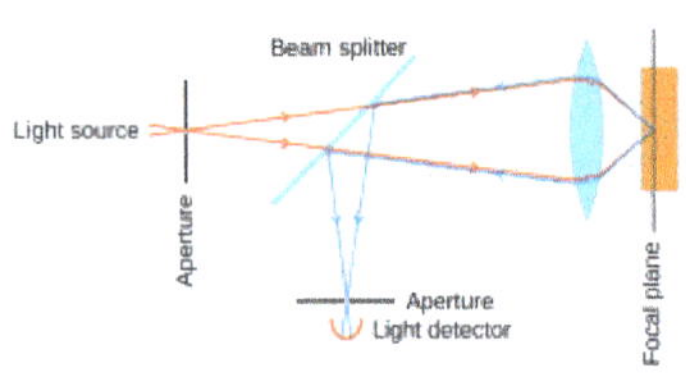

Confocal Imaging Principle

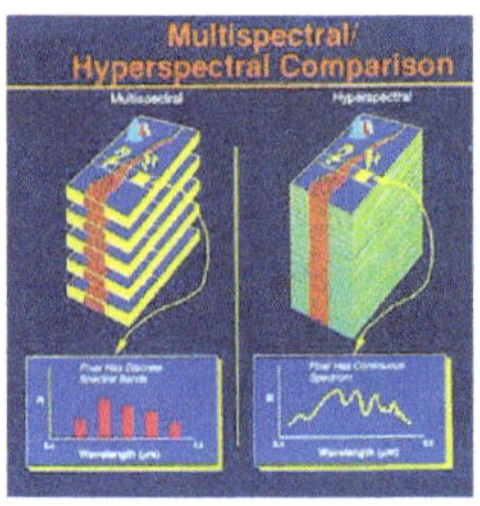

Multi-spectral Imaging principle

Food Engineering

Food engineering is a multidisciplinary field of applied physical sciences which combines science, microbiology, and engineering education for food and related industries. Food engineering includes, but is not limited to, the application of agricultural engineering, mechanical engineering and chemical engineering principles to food materials. Food engineers provide the technological knowledge transfer essential to the cost-effective production and commercialization of food products and services. Physics, chemistry, and mathematics are fundamental to understanding and engineering products and operations in the food industry.

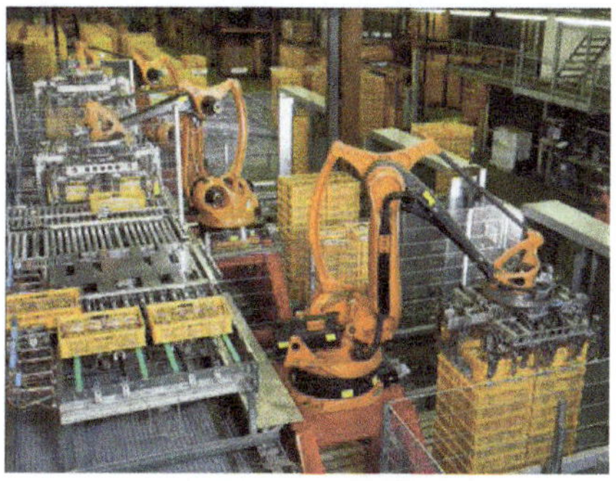

Bread factory in Germany

Food engineering encompasses a wide range of activities. Food engineers are employed in food processing, food machinery, packaging, ingredient manufacturing, instrumentation, and control. Firms that design and build food processing plants, consulting firms, government agencies, pharmaceutical companies, and health-care firms also employ food engineers. Specific food engineering activities include:

- drug/food products;
- design and installation of food/biological/pharmaceutical production processes;
- design and operation of environmentally responsible waste treatment systems;
- marketing and technical support for manufacturing plants.

Topics in Food Engineering

In the development of food engineering, one of the many challenges is to employ modern tools, technology, and knowledge, such as computational materials science and nanotechnology, to develop new products and processes. Simultaneously, improving quality, safety, and security remain critical issues in food engineering study. New packaging materials and techniques are being developed to provide more protection to foods, and novel preservation technology is emerging. Additionally, process control and automation regularly appear among the top priorities identified in food engineering. Advanced monitoring and control systems are developed to facilitate automation and flexible food manufacturing. Furthermore, energy saving and minimization of environmental problems continue to be important food engineering issues, and significant progress is being made in waste management, efficient utilization of energy, and reduction of effluents and emissions in food production.

Typical topics include:

- Advances in classical unit operations in engineering applied to food manufacturing
- Progresses in the transport and storage of liquid and solid foods
- Developments in heating, chilling and freezing of foods
- Advanced mass transfer in foods
- New chemical and biochemical aspects of food engineering and the use of kinetic analysis
- New techniques in dehydration, thermal processing, non-thermal processing, extrusion, liquid food concentration, membrane processes and applications of membranes in food processing
- Shelf-life, electronic indicators in inventory management, and sustainable technologies in food processing
- Modern packaging, cleaning, and sanitation technologies.
- Development of sensors systems for quality and safety assessment

Food Microbiology

Food microbiology is the study of the microorganisms that inhabit, create, or contaminate food, including the study of microorganisms causing food spoilage. "Good" bacteria, however, such as probiotics, are becoming increasingly important in food science. In addition, microorganisms are essential for the production of foods such as cheese, yogurt, bread, beer, wine and, other fermented foods.

Food Safety

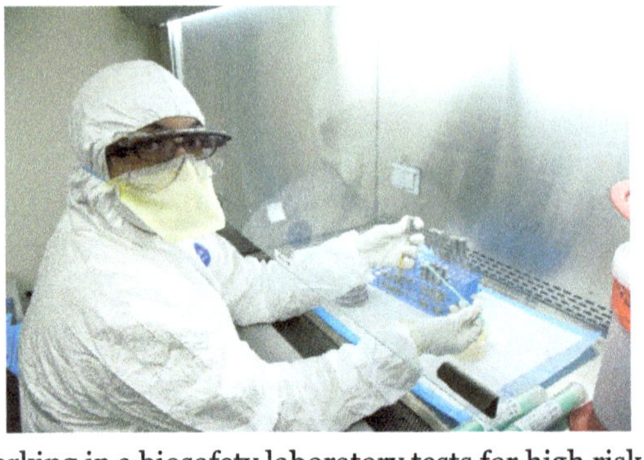

A microbiologist working in a biosafety laboratory tests for high risk pathogens in food.

Food safety is a major focus of food microbiology. Pathogenic bacteria, viruses and toxins produced by microorganisms are all possible contaminants of food. However, microorganisms and their products can also be used to combat these pathogenic microbes. Probiotic bacteria, including those that produce bacteriocins, can kill and inhibit pathogens. Alternatively, purified bacteriocins such as nisin can be added directly to food products. Finally, bacteriophages, viruses that only infect bacteria, can be used to kill bacterial pathogens. Thorough preparation of food, including proper cooking, eliminates most bacteria and viruses. However, *toxins produced* by contaminants may not be liable to change to non-toxic forms by heating or cooking the contaminated food.

Fermentation

Fermentation is one of the methods to preserve food and alter its quality. Yeast, especially *Saccharomyces cerevisiae*, is used to leaven bread, brew beer and make wine. Certain bacteria, including lactic acid bacteria, are used to make yogurt, cheese, hot sauce, pickles, fermented sausages and dishes such as kimchi. A common effect of these fermentations is that the food product is less hospitable to other microorganisms, including pathogens and spoilage-causing microorganisms, thus extending the food's shelf-life. Some cheese varieties also require molds to ripen and develop their characteristic flavors.

Microbial Biopolymers

Several microbially produced polymers are used in the food industry.

Alginate

Alginates can be used as thickening agents. Although listed here under the category 'Microbial polysaccharides', commercial alginates are currently only produced by extraction from brown seaweeds such as *Laminaria hyperborea* or *L. japonica*.

Poly-γ-glutamic Acid

Poly-γ-glutamic acid (γ-PGA) produced by various strains of *Bacillus* has potential applications as a thickener in the food industry.

Food Authenticity

It is important to be able to detect microorganisms in food, in particular pathogenic microorganisms or genetically modified microorganisms.

Food Testing

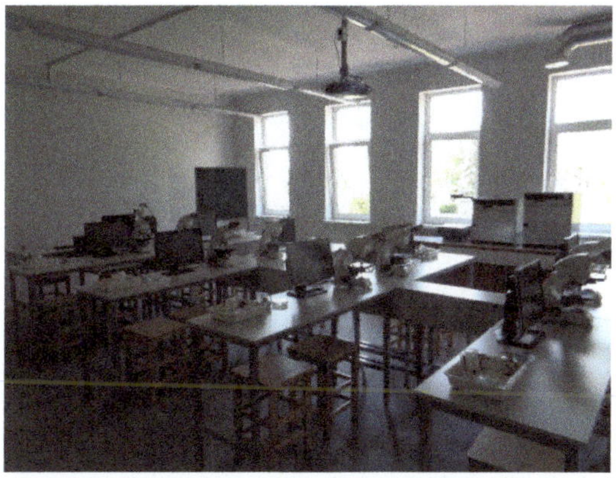

Food microbiology laboratory at the Faculty of Food Technology, Latvia University of Agriculture.

To ensure safety of food products, microbiological tests such as testing for pathogens and spoilage organisms are required. This way the risk of contamination under normal use conditions can be examined and food poisoning outbreaks can be prevented. Testing of food products and ingredients is important along the whole supply chain as possible flaws of products can occur at every stage of production. Apart from detecting spoilage, microbiological tests can also determine germ content, identify yeasts and molds, and salmonella. For salmonella, scientists are also developing rapid and portable technologies capable of identifying unique variants of Salmonella .

Polymerase Chain Reaction (PCR) is a quick and inexpensive method to generate numbers of copies of a DNA fragment at a specific band ("PCR (Polymerase Chain Reaction)," 2008). For that reason, scientists are using PCR to detect different kinds of viruses or bacteria, such as HIV and anthrax based on their unique DNA patterns. Various kits are commercially available to help in food pathogen nucleic acids extraction, PCR detection, and differentiation. The detection of bacterial strands in food products is very important to everyone in the world, for it helps prevent the occurrence of food borne illness. Therefore, PCR is recognized as a DNA detector in order to amplify and trace the presence of pathogenic strands in different processed food.

Molecular Gastronomy

Molecular gastronomy is a subdiscipline of food science that seeks to investigate the physical and chemical transformations of ingredients that occur in cooking. Its program includes three axes, as cooking was recognized to have three components, which are social, artistic and technical. Molecular cuisine is a modern style of cooking, and takes advantage of many technical innovations from the scientific disciplines.

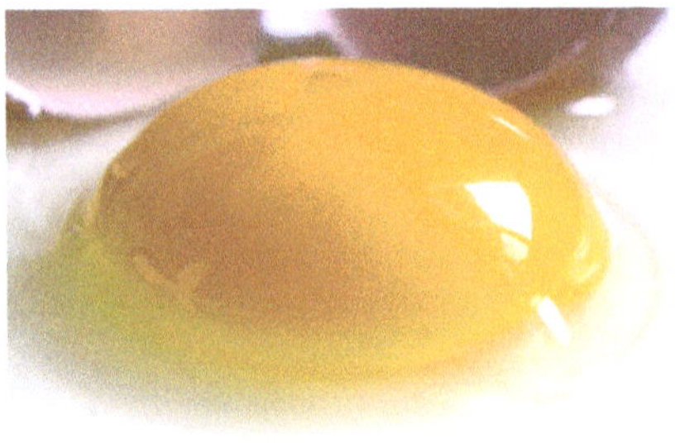

Molecular gastronomy includes the study of how different cooking temperatures affect eggs, and their viscosity, their surface tension, and different ways of introducing air into them.

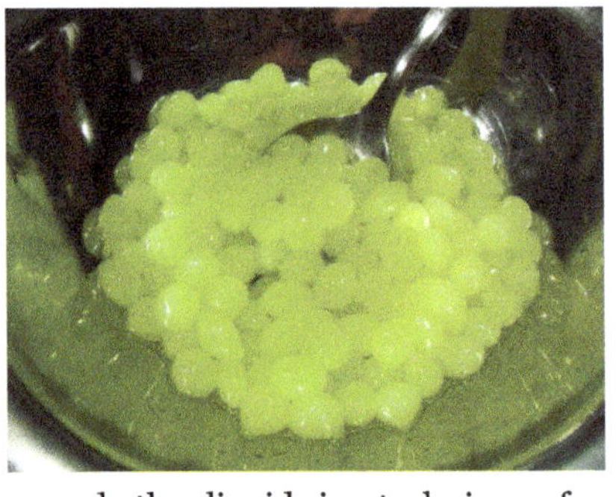

Spherification of juices and other liquids is a technique of molecular gastronomy

The term "molecular gastronomy" was coined in 1988 by late Oxford physicist Nicholas Kurti and the French INRA chemist Hervé This. Some chefs associated with the term choose to reject its use, preferring other terms such as multi sensory cooking, modernist cuisine, culinary physics, and experimental cuisine.

History

There are many branches of food science that study different aspects of food, such as safety, microbiology, preservation, chemistry, engineering and physics. Until the advent of molecular gastronomy, there was no formal discipline dedicated to studying the chemical processes of cooking in the home and in restaurants - as opposed to food preparation for the mass market. Food science has mostly been concerned with industrial food production and while the disciplines may overlap with each other to varying degrees, they are considered separate areas of investigation.

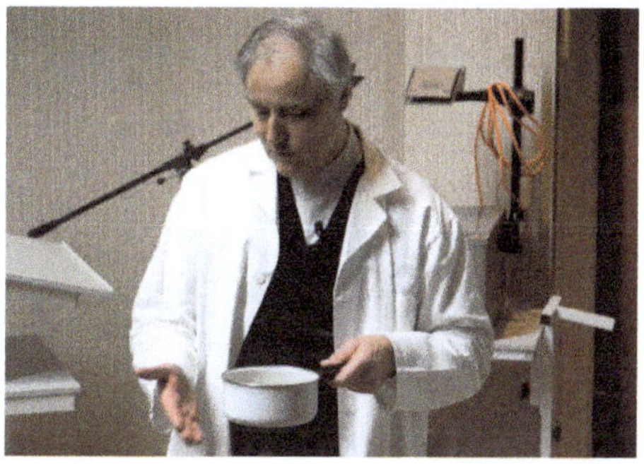

Internationally renowned French chemist and cook Hervé This, known as "The Father of Molecular Gastronomy"

Though many disparate examples of the scientific investigation of cooking exist throughout history, the creation of the discipline of molecular gastronomy was intended to bring together what had previously been fragmented and isolated investigation into the chemical and physical processes of cooking into an organized discipline within food science to address what the other disciplines within food science either do not cover, or cover in a manner intended for scientists rather than cooks. These mere investigations into the scientific process of cooking have unintentionally evolved into a revolutionary practice that is now prominent in today's culinary world.

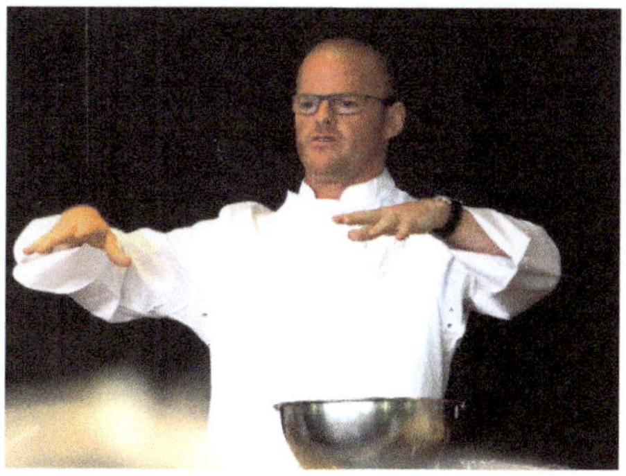

Heston Blumenthal dislikes the term 'molecular gastronomy', believing it makes the practice sound "complicated" and "elitist."

The term "molecular and physical gastronomy" was coined in 1988 by Hungarian physicist Nicholas Kurti and French physical chemist Hervé This. In 1992, it became the title for a set of workshops held in Erice, Italy (originally titled "Science and Gastronomy") that brought together scientists and professional cooks for discussions about the science behind traditional cooking preparations. Eventually, the shortened term "Molecular Gastronomy" also became the name of the scientific discipline co-created by Kurti and This, based on exploring the science behind traditional cooking methods.

Kurti and This have been the co-directors of the "Molecular and Physical Gastronomy" meetings in Erice and had considered the creation of a formal discipline around the subjects discussed in the meetings. The American food science writer Harold McGee, was invited for the first Workshop. After Kurti's death in 1998, the name of the Erice workshops was changed by This to "The International Workshop on Molecular Gastronomy 'N. Kurti'". This remained the sole director of the subsequent workshops from 1999 through 2004 and continues his research in the field of Molecular Gastronomy today.

University of Oxford physicist Nicholas Kurti was an enthusiastic advocate of applying scientific knowledge to culinary problems. He was one of the first television cooks in the UK, hosting a black and white television show in 1969 entitled "The Physicist in the Kitchen" where he demonstrated techniques such as using a syringe to inject hot mince pies with brandy in order to avoid disturbing the crust. That same year, he held a presentation for the Royal Society of London (also entitled "The Physicist in the Kitchen") in which he is often quoted to have stated:

> " I think it is a sad reflection on our civilization that while we can and do measure the temperature in the atmosphere of Venus we do not know what goes on inside our soufflés. "

—Nicholas Kurti

During the presentation Kurti demonstrated making meringue in a vacuum chamber, the cooking of sausages by connecting them across a car battery, the digestion of protein by fresh pineapple juice and a reverse baked alaska - hot inside, cold outside — cooked in a microwave oven. Kurti was also an advocate of low temperature cooking, repeating 18th century experiments by the English scientist Benjamin Thompson by leaving a 2 kg (4.4 lb) lamb joint in an oven at 80 °C (176 °F). After 8.5 hours, both the inside and outside temperature of the lamb joint were around 75 °C (167 °F), and the meat was tender and juicy. Together with his wife, Giana Kurti, Nicholas Kurti edited an anthology on food and science by fellows and foreign members of the Royal Society.

Hervé This started collecting "culinary precisions" (old kitchen wives' tales and cooking tricks) in the early 1980s and started testing these precisions to see which ones held up; his collection now numbers some 25,000. In 1995, he also has received a PhD in Physical Chemistry of Materials for which he wrote his thesis on "La gastronomie moléculaire et physique" (molecular and physical gastronomy), served as an adviser to the French minister of education, lectured internationally, and was invited to join the lab of Nobel Prize winning molecular chemist Jean-Marie Lehn. This has published several books in French, four of which have been translated into English, including *Molecular Gastronomy: Exploring the Science of Flavor*, *Kitchen Mysteries: Revealing the Science of Cooking*, *Cooking: The Quintessential Art*, and *Building a Meal: From Molecular Gastronomy to Culinary Constructivism*. He currently publishes a series of essays in French and hosts free monthly seminars on molecular gastronomy at the INRA in France. He gives free and public seminars on molecular gastronomy any month, and once a year, he gives a public and free course on molecular gastronomy. Hervé This also authors a website and a pair of blogs on the subject in French and publishes monthly collaborations with French chef Pierre Gagnaire on Gagnaire's website.

Though she is rarely credited, the origins of the Erice workshops (originally entitled "Science and Gastronomy") can be traced back to the cooking teacher Elizabeth Cawdry Thomas who studied at Le Cordon Bleu in London and ran a cooking school in Berkeley, California. The one-time wife of a physicist, Thomas had many friends in the scientific community and an interest in the science of cooking. In 1988 while attending a meeting at the Ettore Majorana Center for Scientific Culture in Erice, Thomas had a conversation with Professor Ugo Valdrè of the University of Bologna who agreed with her that the science of cooking was an undervalued subject and encouraged her to organize a workshop at the Ettore Majorana Center. Thomas eventually approached the director of the Ettore Majorana center, physicist Antonino Zichichi who liked the idea. Thomas and Valdrè approached Kurti to be the director of the workshop. By Kurti's invitation, noted food science writer Harold McGee and French Physical Chemist Hervé This became the co-organizers of the workshops, though McGee stepped down after the first meeting in 1992.

Up until 2001, The International Workshop on Molecular Gastronomy "N. Kurti" (IWMG) was named the "International Workshops of Molecular and Physical Gastronomy" (IWMPG). The first meeting was held in 1992 and the meetings have continued every few years thereafter until the most recent in 2004. Each meeting encompassed an overall theme broken down into multiple sessions over the course of a few days.

The focus of the workshops each year were as follows:

- 1992 - First Meeting
- 1995 - Sauces, or dishes made from them
- 1997 - Heat in cooking
- 1999 - Food flavors - how to get them, how to distribute them, how to keep them
- 2001 - Textures of Food: How to create them?
- 2004 - Interactions of food and liquids

Examples of sessions within these meetings have included:

- Chemical Reactions in Cooking
- Heat Conduction, Convection and Transfer
- Physical aspects of food/liquid interaction
- When liquid meets food at low temperature
- Solubility problems, dispersion, texture/flavour relationship
- Stability of flavour

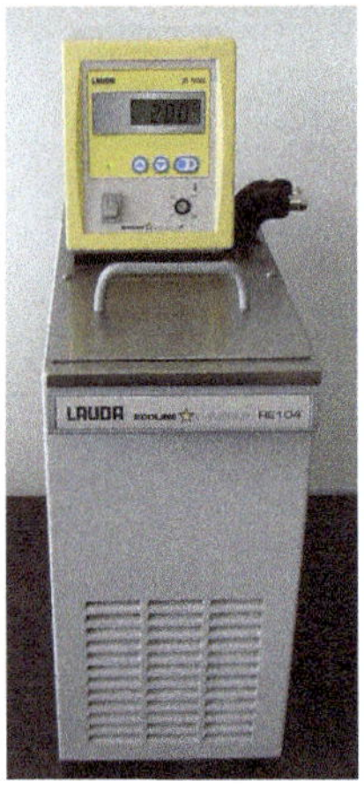

Heated bath used for low temperature cooking

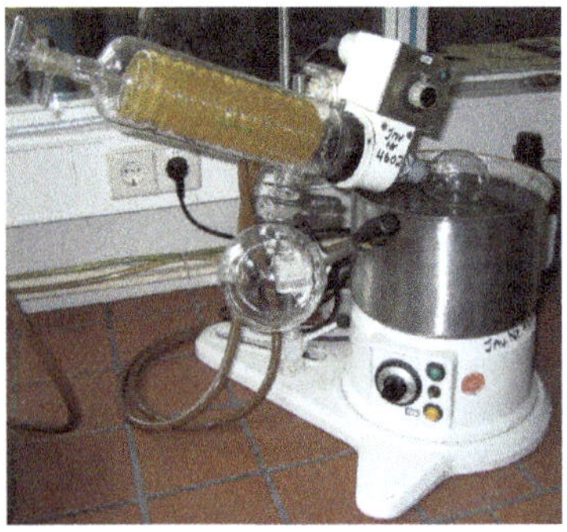

Rotary evaporator used in the preparation of distillates and extracts

Precursors

The idea of using techniques developed in chemistry to study food is not a new one, for instance the discipline of food science has existed for many years. Kurti and This acknowledged this fact and though they decided that a new, organized and specific discipline should be created within food science that investigated the processes in regular cooking (as food science was primarily concerned with the nutritional properties of food and developing methods to process food on an industrial scale), there are several notable examples throughout history of investigations into the science of everyday cooking recorded as far as back to 18th century.

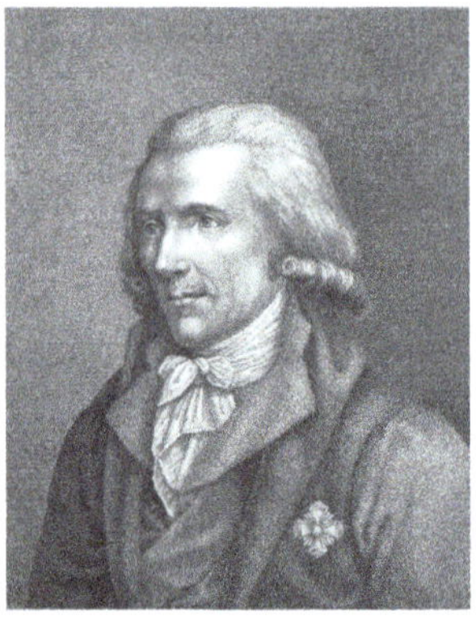

Benjamin Thompson, Count Rumford (1753–1814) was one of the early pioneers in the science of food & cooking.

Professors Evelyn G. Halliday and Isabel T. Noble

In 1943 the University of Chicago Press published a book entitled *Food Chemistry and Cookery* by the then University of Chicago Associate Professor of Home Economics Evelyn G. Halliday and University of Minnesota Associate Professor of Home Economics Isabel T Noble. In the foreword of the 346 page book the authors state that, "The main purpose of this book is to give an understanding of the chemical principles upon which good practices in food preparation and preservation are based."

The book includes chapters such as "The Chemistry of Milk", "The Chemistry of Baking Powders and Their Use in Baking", "The Chemistry of Vegetable Cookery" and "Determination of Hydrogen Ion Concentration" and contains numerous illustrations of lab experiments including such things as a *Distillation Apparatus for Vegetable Samples* and a *Pipette for Determining the Relative Viscosity of Pectin Solutions*. The professors had previously published *The Hows and Whys of Cooking* in 1928.

Professor Belle Lowe of Iowa State College (1886–1961)

In 1932 the academic Belle Lowe, then the professor of Food and Nutrition at Iowa State College, published a book entitled *Experimental Cookery: From The Chemical And Physical Standpoint* which became a standard textbook for home economics courses across the United States. The book is an exhaustively researched look into the science of everyday cooking referencing hundreds of sources and including many experiments. At a length of over 600 pages with section titles such as "The Relation Of Cookery To Colloidal Chemistry", "Coagulation Of Proteins", "The Factors Affecting The Viscosity Of Cream And Ice Cream", "Syneresis", "Hydrolysis Of Collagen" and "Changes In Cooked Meat And The Cooking Of Meat", the volume rivals or exceeds the scope of many other books on the subject, at a much earlier date.

Belle Lowe was born near Utica, Missouri on February 7, 1886. She graduated from Chillicothe High School and then received a teaching certificate (1907) from the Kirksville State Normal School in Kirksville, Missouri. She also received a Ph. B. (1911) and an M.S. (1934) from the University of Chicago. In 1957, Lowe received an honorary Ph.D. from Iowa State College (University). In addition to "Experimental Cookery", she published numerous articles on the subject of the science of cooking. She died in 1961.

According to Hervé:

In the second century BC, the anonymous author of a papyrus kept in London used a balance to determine whether fermented meat was lighter than fresh meat. Since then, many scientists have been interested in food and cooking. In particular, the preparation of meat stock—the aqueous solution obtained by thermal processing of animal tissues in water—has been of great interest. It was first mentioned in the fourth century BC by Roman *Apicius* (André (ed), 1987), and recipes for stock preparation appear in classic texts (La Varenne, 1651; Menon, 1756; Carême & Plumerey, 1981) and most French culinary books. Chemists have been interested in meat stock preparation and, more generally, food preparation since the eighteenth century (Lémery, 1705; Geoffrey le Cadet, 1733; Cadet de Vaux, 1818; Darcet, 1830). Antoine-Laurent de Lavoisier is perhaps the most famous among them—in 1783, he studied the processes of stock preparation by measuring density to evaluate quality (Lavoisier, 1783). In reporting the results of his experiments, Lavoisier wrote, "Whenever one considers the most familiar objects, the simplest things, it's impossible not to be surprised to see how our ideas are vague and uncertain, and how, as a consequence, it is important to fix them by experiments and facts" (author's translation). Of course, Justus von Liebig should not be forgotten in the history of culinary science (von Liebig, 1852) and stock was not his only concern. Another important figure was Benjamin Thompson, later knighted Count Rumford, who studied culinary transformations and made many proposals and inventions to improve them, for example by inventing a special coffee pot for better brewing. There are too many scientists who have contributed to the science of food preparation to list here. — Hervé This, 2006

Marie-antoine Carême (1784–1833)

The concept of molecular gastronomy was perhaps presaged by Marie-Antoine Carême, one of the most famous French chefs, who said in the early 19th century that when making a food stock "the broth must come to a boil very slowly, otherwise the albumin coagulates, hardens; the water, not having time to penetrate the meat, prevents the gelatinous part of the osmazome from detaching itself."

Objectives

The objectives of molecular gastronomy, as defined by Hervé This, are:

Current Objectives

Looking for the mechanisms of culinary transformations and processes (from a chemical and physical point of view) in three areas:

1. the social phenomena linked to culinary activity
2. the artistic component of culinary activity
3. the technical component of culinary activity

Original Objectives

The original fundamental objectives of molecular gastronomy were defined by This in his doctoral dissertation as:

1. Investigating culinary and gastronomical proverbs, sayings and old wives' tales
2. Exploring existing recipes
3. Introducing new tools, ingredients and methods into the kitchen
4. Inventing new dishes
5. Using molecular gastronomy to help the general public understand the contribution of science to society

However, This later recognized points 3, 4 and 5 as being not entirely scientific endeavours (more application of technology and educational), and has since revised the primary objectives of molecular gastronomy.

Examples

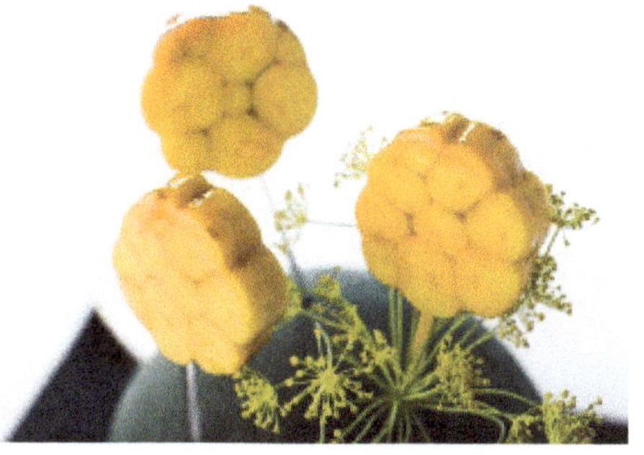

Adam Melonas's signature preparation is an edible floral center piece named the "Octopop": a very low temperature cooked octopus fused using transglutaminase, dipped into an orange and saffron carrageenan gel and suspended on dill flower stalks

Example Areas of Investigation

- How ingredients are changed by different cooking methods
- How all the senses play their own roles in our appreciation of food
- The mechanisms of aroma release and the perception of taste and flavor
- How and why we evolved our particular taste and flavor sense organs and our general food likes and dislikes
- How cooking methods affect the eventual flavor and texture of food ingredients
- How new cooking methods might produce improved results of texture and flavor
- How our brains interpret the signals from all our senses to tell us the "flavor" of food
- How our enjoyment of food is affected by other influences, our environment, our mood, how it is presented, who prepares it, etc.

Eponymous Recipes

New dishes named after famous scientists include:

- Gibbs - infusing vanilla pods in egg white with sugar, adding olive oil and then microwave cooking. Named after physicist Josiah Willard Gibbs (1839–1903).
- Vauquelin - using orange juice or cranberry juice with added sugar when whipping eggs to increase the viscosity and to stabilize the foam, and then microwave cooking. Named after Nicolas Vauquelin (1763–1829), one of Lavoisier's teachers.
- Baumé - soaking a whole egg for a month in alcohol to create a coagulated egg. Named after the French chemist Antoine Baumé (1728–1804).

As A Style of Cooking

The term *molecular gastronomy* was originally intended to refer only to the scientific investigation of cooking, though it has been adopted by a number of people and applied to cooking itself or to describe a style of cuisine.

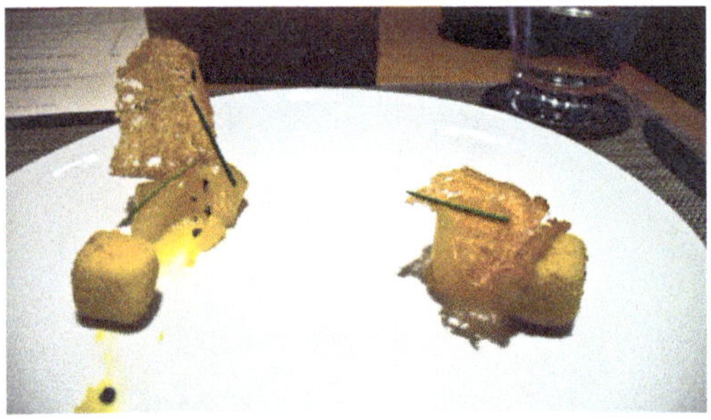

A molecular gastronomy rendition of eggs Benedict served by wd~50 in New York City. The cubes are deep-fried Hollandaise sauce.

In the late 1990s and early 2000s, the term started to be used to describe a new style of cooking in which some chefs began to explore new possibilities in the kitchen by embracing science, research, technological advances in equipment and various natural gums and hydrocolloids produced by the commercial food processing industry. It has since been used to describe the food and cooking of a number of famous chefs, though many of them do not accept the term as a description of their style of cooking.

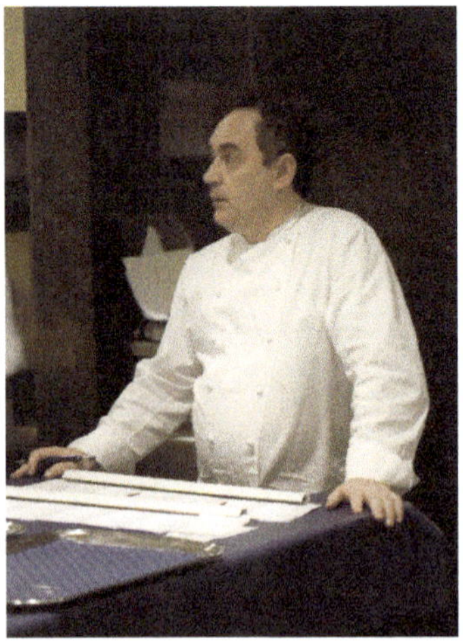

Ferran Adrià of El Bulli, prefers the term 'deconstructivist' to describe his style of cooking.

Other names for the style of cuisine practiced by these chefs include:

- Avant-garde cuisine
- Culinary constructivism
- Cocina de vanguardia - term used by Ferran Adrià
- Emotional cuisine
- Experimental cuisine

- Forward-thinking movement - term used at Grant Achatz's Alinea
- Kitchen science
- Modern cuisine
- Modernist cuisine, which shares its name with a cookbook, and which is endorsed by Ferran Adrià of El Bulli and David Chang
- Molecular cuisine
- Molecular cooking
- New cuisine
- New cookery
- Nueva cocina
- Progressive cuisine
- Techno-emotional cuisine—term preferred by elBulli research and development chef Ferran Adrià
- Technologically forward cuisine
- Vanguard cuisine
- Techno-cuisine

No singular name has ever been applied in consensus, and the term "molecular gastronomy" continues to be used often as a blanket term to refer to any and all of these things - particularly in the media. Ferran Adrià hates the term "molecular gastronomy" and prefers 'deconstructivist' to describe his style of cooking. A 2006 open letter by Ferran Adria, Heston Blumenthal, Thomas Keller and Harold McGee published in *The Times* used no specific term, referring only to "a new approach to cooking" and "our cooking".

Chefs

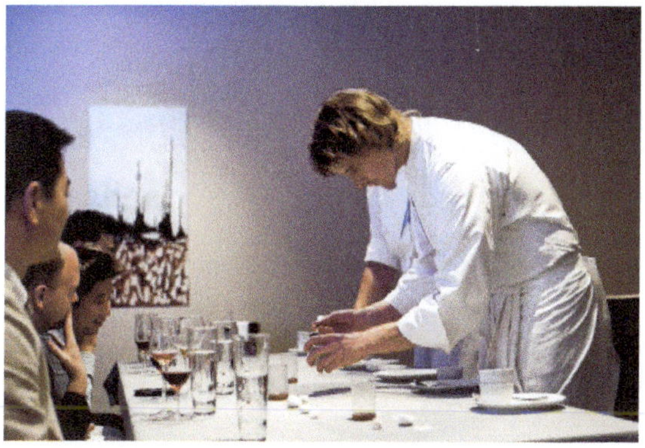

Grant Achatz (photo: plating a dish at Alinea) is the leading American chef in molecular gastronomy shown here plating the dessert pictured above.

Chefs who are often associated with molecular gastronomy because of their embrace of science include Heston Blumenthal, Grant Achatz, Ferran Adrià, José Andrés, Sat Bains, Richard Blais, Marcel Vigneron, Sean Brock, Homaro Cantu, Michael Carlson, Wylie Dufresne, Pierre Gagnaire, Adam Melonas, Kevin Sousa, and Laurent Gras.

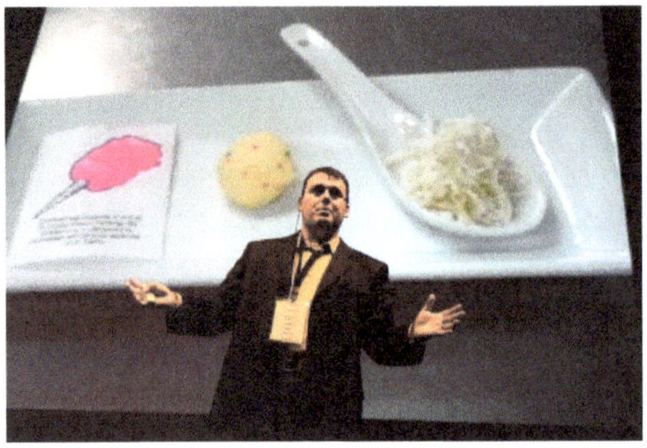

Homaro Cantu of Moto Restaurant was a molecular gastronomer

Despite their central role in the popularisation of science based cuisine, both Adria and Blumenthal have expressed their frustration with the common mis-classification of their food and cooking as "molecular gastronomy", On 10 December 2006 Heston Blumenthal and Harold McGee published a 'Statement on the "New Cookery" in the Observer in order to summarise what they saw as the central tenets of modern cuisine. Ferran Adria of El Bulli and Thomas Keller of the French Laundry and Per Se signed up to this and together released a joint statement in 2006 clarifying their approach to cooking, stating that the term "molecular gastronomy" was coined in 1992 for a single workshop that did not influence them, and that the term does not describe any style of cooking.

In February 2011, Nathan Myhrvold published the *Modernist Cuisine*, which led many chefs to further classify molecular gastronomy versus modernist cuisine. Myhrvold believes that his cooking style should not be called molecular gastronomy.

Techniques, Tools and Ingredients

- Carbon dioxide source, for adding bubbles and making foams
- Foams can also be made with an immersion blender
- Liquid nitrogen, for flash freezing and shattering
- Ice cream maker, often used to make unusual flavors, including savory
- Anti-griddle, for cooling and freezing
- Thermal immersion circulator for sous-vide (low temperature cooking)
- Food dehydrator
- Centrifuge
- Maltodextrin - can turn a high-fat liquid into a powder

- Sugar substitutes
- Enzymes
- Lecithin - an emulsifier and non-stick agent
- Hydrocolloids such as starch, gelatin, pectin and natural gums - used as thickening agents, gelling agents, emulsifying agents and stabilizers, sometimes needed for foams
- Transglutaminase - a protein binder, called meat glue
- Spherification - a caviar-like effect
- Syringe, for injecting unexpected fillings
- Edible paper made from soybeans and potato starch, for use with edible fruit inks and an inkjet printer
- Aromatic accompaniment: gases trapped in a bag, a serving device, or the food itself; an aromatic substance presented as a garnish or creative serveware; or a smell produced by burning
- Presentation style is often whimsical or avant-garde, and may include unusual serviceware
- Unusual flavor combinations (food pairings) are favored, such as combining savory and sweet
- Using ultrasound to achieve more precise cooking times

Malnutrition

Malnutrition or malnourishment is a condition that results from eating a diet in which nutrients are either not enough or are too much such that the diet causes health problems. It may involve calories, protein, carbohydrates, vitamins or minerals. Not enough nutrients is called undernutrition or undernourishment while too much is called overnutrition. Malnutrition is often used specifically to refer to undernutrition where there is not enough calories, protein, or micronutrients. If undernutrition occurs during pregnancy, or before two years of age, it may result in permanent problems with physical and mental development. Extreme undernourishment, known as starvation, may have symptoms that include: a short height, thin body, very poor energy levels, and swollen legs and abdomen. People also often get infections and are frequently cold. The symptoms of micronutrient deficiencies depend on the micronutrient that is lacking.

Undernourishment is most often due to not enough high-quality food being available to eat. This is often related to high food prices and poverty. A lack of breastfeeding may contribute, as may a number of infectious diseases such as: gastroenteritis, pneumonia, malaria, and measles, which increase nutrient requirements. There are two main types of undernutrition: protein-energy malnutrition and dietary deficiencies. Protein-energy malnutrition has two severe forms: marasmus (a lack of protein and calories) and kwashiorkor (a lack of just protein). Common micronutrient deficiencies include: a lack of iron, iodine, and vitamin A. During pregnancy, due to the body's increased need, deficiencies may become more common. In some developing countries, overnutrition in the form of obesity is beginning to present within the same communities as undernutrition. Other causes of malnutrition include anorexia nervosa and bariatric surgery.

Efforts to improve nutrition are some of the most effective forms of development aid. Breastfeeding can reduce rates of malnutrition and death in children, and efforts to promote the practice increase the rates of breastfeeding. In young children, providing food (in addition to breastmilk) between six months and two years of age improves outcomes. There is also good evidence supporting the supplementation of a number of micronutrients to women during pregnancy and among young children in the developing world. To get food to people who need it most, both delivering food and providing money so people can buy food within local markets are effective. Simply feeding students at school is insufficient. Management of severe malnutrition within the person's home with ready-to-use therapeutic foods is possible much of the time. In those who have severe malnutrition complicated by other health problems, treatment in a hospital setting is recommended. This often involves managing low blood sugar and body temperature, addressing dehydration, and gradual feeding. Routine antibiotics are usually recommended due to the high risk of infection. Longer-term measures include: improving agricultural practices, reducing poverty, improving sanitation, and the empowerment of women.

There were 793 million undernourished people in the world in 2015 (13% of the total population). This is a reduction of 216 million people since 1990 when 23% were undernourished. In 2012 it was estimated that another billion people had a lack of vitamins and minerals. In 2013, protein-energy malnutrition was estimated to have resulted in 469,000 deaths—down from 510,000 deaths in 1990. Other nutritional deficiencies, which include iodine deficiency and iron deficiency anemia, result in another 84,000 deaths. In 2010, malnutrition was the cause of 1.4% of all disability adjusted life years. About a third of deaths in children are believed to be due to undernutrition, although the deaths are rarely labelled as such. In 2010, it was estimated to have contributed to about 1.5 million deaths in women and children, though some estimate the number may be greater than 3 million. An additional 165 million children were estimated to have stunted growth from malnutrition in 2013. Undernutrition is more common in developing countries. Certain groups have higher rates of undernutrition, including women—in particular while pregnant or breastfeeding—children under five years of age, and the elderly. In the elderly, undernutrition becomes more common due to physical, psychological, and social factors.

Definitions

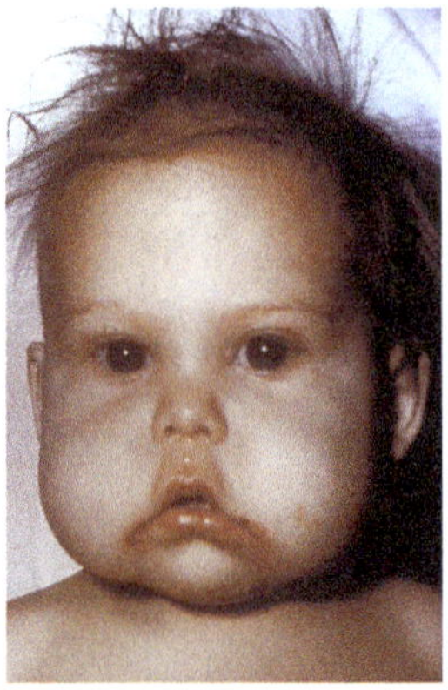

Child in the United States with signs of Kwashiorkor, a dietary protein deficiency.

Unless specifically mentioned otherwise, the term malnutrition refers to undernutrition for the remainder of this article. Malnutrition can divided in two different types, SAM and MAM. SAM is refers to children with severe acute malnutrition. MAM refers to moderate acute malnutrition.

Undernutrition and Overnutrition

Malnutrition is caused by eating a diet in which nutrients are *not enough* or are *too much* such that it causes health problems. It is a category of diseases that includes undernutrition and overnutrition. Overnutrition can result in obesity and being overweight. In some developing countries, overnutrition in the form of obesity is beginning to present within the same communities as undernutrition.

However, the term malnutrition is commonly used to refer to undernutrition only. This applies particularly to the context of development cooperation. Therefore, "malnutrition" in documents by the World Health Organization, UNICEF, Save the Children or other international non-governmental organizations (NGOs) usually is equated to undernutrition.

Protein-energy Malnutrition

Undernutrition is sometimes used as a synonym of protein–energy malnutrition (PEM). While other include both micronutrient deficiencies and protein energy malnutrition in its definition. It differs from calorie restriction in that calorie restriction may not result in negative health effects. The term hypoalimentation means underfeeding.

The term "severe malnutrition" or "severe undernutrition" is often used to refer specifically to PEM. PEM is often associated with micronutrient deficiency. Two forms of PEM are kwashiorkor and marasmus, and they commonly coexist.

Kwashiorkor

Kwashiorkor ('displaced child') is mainly caused by inadequate protein intake resulting in a low concentration of amino acids. The main symptoms are edema, wasting, liver enlargement, hypoalbuminaemia, steatosis, and possibly depigmentation of skin and hair. Kwashiorkor is identified by swelling of the extremities and belly, which is deceiving of actual nutritional status.

Marasmus

Marasmus ('to waste away') is caused by an inadequate intake of protein and energy. The main symptoms are severe wasting, leaving little or no edema, minimal subcutaneous fat, severe muscle wasting, and non-normal serum albumin levels. Marasmus can result from a sustained diet of inadequate energy and protein, and the metabolism adapts to prolong survival. It is traditionally seen in famine, significant food restriction, or more severe cases of anorexia. Conditions are characterized by extreme wasting of the muscles and a gaunt expression.

Undernutrition, Hunger

Undernutrition encompasses stunted growth (stunting), wasting, and deficiencies of essential vitamins and minerals (collectively referred to as micronutrients). The term hunger, which describes a feeling of discomfort from not eating, has been used to describe undernutrition, especially in reference to food insecurity.

Definition by Gomez

In 1956, Gómez and Galvan studied factors associated with death in a group of malnourished (undernourished) children in a hospital in Mexico City, Mexico and defined categories of malnutrition: first, second, and third degree. The degrees were based on weight below a specified percentage of median weight for age. The risk of death increases with increasing degree of malnutrition. An adaptation of Gomez's original classification is still used today. While it provides a way to compare malnutrition within and between populations, the classification has been criticized for being "arbitrary" and for not considering overweight as a form of malnutrition. Also, height alone may not be the best indicator of malnutrition; children who are born prematurely may be considered short for their age even if they have good nutrition.

Degree of PEM	% of desired body weight for age and sex
	Normal 90%-100%
Mild: Grade I (1st degree)	75%-89%
Moderate: Grade II (2nd degree)	60%-74%
Severe: Grade III (3rd degree)	<60%
SOURCE:"Serum Total Protein and Albumin Levels in Different Grades of Protein Energy Malnutrition"	

Definition by Waterlow

John Conrad Waterlow established a new classification for malnutrition. Instead of using just weight for age measurements, the classification established by Waterlow combines weight-for-height (indicating acute episodes of malnutrition) with height-for-age to show the stunting that results from chronic malnutrition. One advantage of the Waterlow classification over the Gomez classification is that weight for height can be examined even if ages are not known.

Degree of PEM	**Stunting (%) Height for age**	**Wasting (%) Weight for height**
Normal: Grade 0	>95%	>90%
Mild: Grade I	87.5-95%	80-90%
Moderate: Grade II	80-87.5%	70-80%
Severe: Grade III	<80%	<70%
SOURCE: "Classification and definition of protein-calorie malnutrition." by Waterlow, 1972		

These classifications of malnutrition are commonly used with some modifications by WHO.

Effects

Malnutrition increases the risk of infection and infectious disease, and moderate malnutrition weakens every part of the immune system. For example, it is a major risk factor in the onset of active tuberculosis. Protein and energy malnutrition and deficiencies of specific micronutrients (including iron, zinc, and vitamins) increase susceptibility to infection. Malnutrition affects HIV transmission by increasing the risk of transmission from mother to child and also increasing replication of the virus. In communities or areas that lack access to safe drinking water, these additional health risks present a critical problem. Lower energy and impaired function of the brain also represent the downward spiral of malnutrition as victims are less able to perform the tasks they need to in order to acquire food, earn an income, or gain an education.

Vitamin-deficiency-related diseases (such as scurvy and rickets).

Hypoglycemia (low blood sugar) can result from a child not eating for 4 to 6 hours. Hypoglycemia should be considered if there is lethargy, limpness, convulsion, or loss of consciousness. If blood sugar can be measured immediately and quickly, perform a finger or heel stick.

Signs

In those with malnutrition some of the signs of dehydration differ. Children; however, may still be interested in drinking, have decreased interactions with the world around them, have decreased urine output, and may be cool to touch.

Site	Sign
Face	Moon face (kwashiorkor), simian facies (marasmus)
Eye	Dry eyes, pale conjunctiva, Bitot's spots (vitamin A), periorbital edema
Mouth	Angular stomatitis, cheilitis, glossitis, spongy bleeding gums (vitamin C), parotid enlargement
Teeth	Enamel mottling, delayed eruption
Hair	Dull, sparse, brittle hair, hypopigmentation, flag sign (alternating bands of light and normal color), broomstick eyelashes, alopecia
Skin	Loose and wrinkled (marasmus), shiny and edematous (kwashiorkor), dry, follicular hyperkeratosis, patchy hyper- and hypopigmentation, erosions, poor wound healing
Nail	Koilonychia, thin and soft nail plates, fissures or ridges
Musculature	Muscles wasting, particularly in the buttocks and thighs
Skeletal	Deformities usually a result of calcium, vitamin D, or vitamin C deficiencies
Abdomen	Distended - hepatomegaly with fatty liver, ascites may be present
Cardiovascular	Bradycardia, hypotension, reduced cardiac output, small vessel vasculopathy
Neurologic	Global development delay, loss of knee and ankle reflexes, poor memory
Hematological	Pallor, petechiae, bleeding diathesis
Behavior	Lethargic, apathetic
Source: "Protein Energy Malnutrition"	

Cognitive Development

Protein-calorie malnutrition can cause cognitive impairments. For humans, "critical period varies from the final third of gestation to the first 2 years of life". Iron deficiency anemia in children under two years of age likely affects brain function acutely and probably also chronically. Folate deficiency has been linked to neural tube defects.

Malnutrition in the form of iodine deficiency is "the most common preventable cause of mental impairment worldwide." "Even moderate deficiency, especially in pregnant women and infants, lowers intelligence by 10 to 15 I.Q. points, shaving incalculable potential off a nation's development. The most visible and severe effects — disabling goiters, cretinism and dwarfism — affect a tiny minority, usually in mountain villages. But 16 percent of the world's people have at least mild goiter, a swollen thyroid gland in the neck."

Causes

Major causes of malnutrition include poverty and food prices, dietary practices and agricultural productivity, with many individual cases being a mixture of several factors. Clinical malnutrition, such as in cachexia, is a major burden also in developed countries. Various scales of analysis also have to be considered in order to determine the sociopolitical causes of malnutrition. For example, the population of a community may be at risk if the area lacks health-related services, but on a smaller scale certain households or individuals may be at even higher risk due to differences in income levels, access to land, or levels of education.

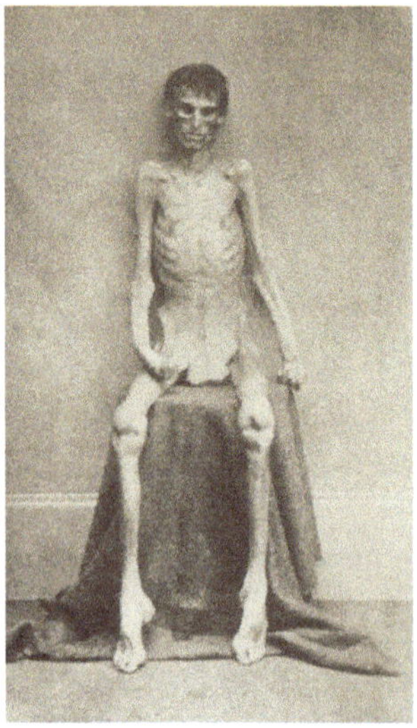

Union Army soldier on his release from Andersonville prison, 1865

Diseases

Malnutrition can be a consequence of health issues such as gastroenteritis or chronic illness, especially the HIV/AIDS pandemic. Diarrhea and other infections can cause malnutrition through decreased nutrient absorption, decreased intake of food, increased metabolic requirements, and direct nutrient loss. Parasite infections, in particular intestinal worm infections (helminthiasis), can also lead to malnutrition. A leading cause of diarrhea and intestinal worm infections in children in developing countries is lack of sanitation and hygiene.

People may become malnourished due to abnormal nutrient loss (due to diarrhea or chronic illness) or increased energy expenditure (secondary malnutrition).

Dietary Practices

Undernutrition

A lack of adequate breastfeeding leads to malnutrition in infants and children, associated with the deaths of an estimated one million children annually. Illegal advertising of breast milk substitutes continues three decades after its 1981 prohibition under the *WHO International Code of Marketing Breast Milk Substitutes*.

Deriving too much of one's diet from a single source, such as eating almost exclusively corn or rice, can cause malnutrition. This may either be from a lack of education about proper nutrition, or from only having access to a single food source.

It is not just the total amount of calories that matters but specific nutritional deficiencies such as vitamin A deficiency, iron deficiency or zinc deficiency can also increase risk of death.

Overnutrition

Overnutrition caused by overeating is also a form of malnutrition. In the United States, more than half of all adults are now overweight — a condition that, like hunger, increases susceptibility to disease and disability, reduces worker productivity, and lowers life expectancy. Overeating is much more common in the United States, where for the majority of people, access to food is not an issue. Many parts of the world have access to a surplus of non-nutritious food, in addition to increased sedentary lifestyles. Yale psychologist Kelly Brownell calls this a "toxic food environment" where fat and sugar laden foods have taken precedence over healthy nutritious foods.

The issue in these developed countries is choosing the right kind of food. More fast food is consumed per capita in the United States than in any other country. The reason for this mass consumption of fast food is its affordability and accessibility. Often fast food, low in cost and nutrition, is high in calories and heavily promoted. When these eating habits are combined with increasingly urbanized, automated, and more sedentary lifestyles, it becomes clear why weight gain is difficult to avoid.

Not only does obesity occur in developed countries, problems are also occurring in developing countries in areas where income is on the rise. Overeating is also a problem in countries where hunger and poverty persist. In China, consumption of high-fat foods has increased while consumption of rice and other goods has decreased.

Overeating leads to many diseases, such as heart disease and diabetes, that may result in death.

Poverty and Food Prices

In Bangladesh, poor socioeconomic position was associated with chronic malnutrition since it inhibits purchase of nutritious foods such as milk, meat, poultry, and fruits. As much as food shortages may be a contributing factor to malnutrition in countries with lack of technology, the FAO (Food and Agriculture Organization) has estimated that eighty percent of malnourished children living in the developing world live in countries that produce food surpluses. The economist Amartya Sen observed that, in recent decades, famine has always been a problem of food distribution and/or poverty, as there has been sufficient food to feed the whole population of the world. He states that malnutrition and famine were more related to problems of food distribution and purchasing power.

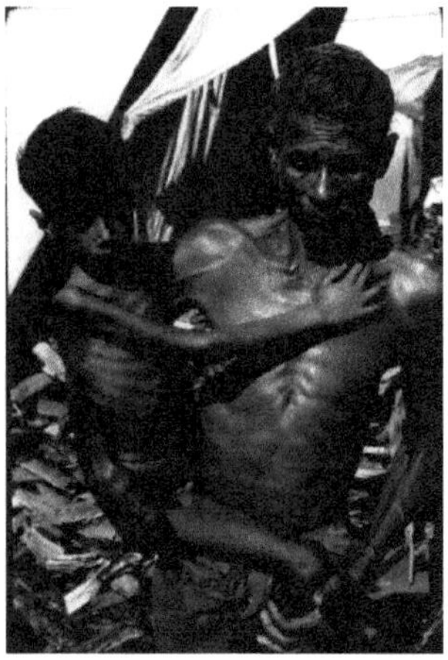

A child with extreme malnutrition

It is argued that commodity speculators are increasing the cost of food. As the real estate bubble in the United States was collapsing, it is said that trillions of dollars moved to invest in food and primary commodities, causing the 2007–2008 food price crisis.

The use of biofuels as a replacement for traditional fuels and raises the price of food. The United Nations special rapporteur on the right to food, Jean Ziegler proposes that agricultural waste, such as corn cobs and banana leaves, rather than crops themselves be used as fuel.

Agricultural Productivity

Local food shortages can be caused by a lack of arable land, adverse weather, lower farming skills such as crop rotation, or by a lack of technology or resources needed for the higher yields found in modern agriculture, such as fertilizers, pesticides, irrigation, machinery and storage facilities. As a result of widespread poverty, farmers cannot afford or governments cannot provide the resources necessary to improve local yields. The World Bank and some wealthy donor countries also press nations that depend on aid to cut or eliminate subsidized agricultural inputs such as fertilizer, in the name of free market policies even as the United States and Europe extensively subsidized their own farmers. Many, if not most, farmers cannot afford fertilizer at market prices, leading to low agricultural production and wages and high, unaffordable food prices. Reasons for the unavailability of fertilizer include moves to stop supplying fertilizer on environmental grounds, cited as the obstacle to feeding Africa by the Green Revolution pioneers Norman Borlaug and Keith Rosenberg.

Future Threats

There are a number of potential disruptions to global food supply that could cause widespread malnutrition.

Climate change is of importance to food security, with 95 percent of all malnourished peoples living in the relatively stable climate region of the sub-tropics and tropics. According to the latest IPCC reports, temperature increases in these regions are "very likely." Even small changes in temperatures can lead to increased frequency of extreme weather conditions. Many of these have great impact on agricultural production and hence nutrition. For example, the 1998–2001 central Asian drought brought about an 80 percent livestock loss and 50 percent reduction in wheat and barley crops in Iran. Similar figures were present in other nations. An increase in extreme weather such as drought in regions such as Sub-Saharan Africa would have even greater consequences in terms of malnutrition. Even without an increase of extreme weather events, a simple increase in temperature reduces the productivity of many crop species, also decreasing food security in these regions.

Colony collapse disorder is a phenomenon where bees die in large numbers. Since many agricultural crops worldwide are pollinated by bees, this represents a threat to the supply of food.

An epidemic of wheat stem rust caused by race Ug99 is currently spreading across Africa and into Asia and, it is feared, could wipe out more than 80 percent of the world's wheat crops.

Prevention

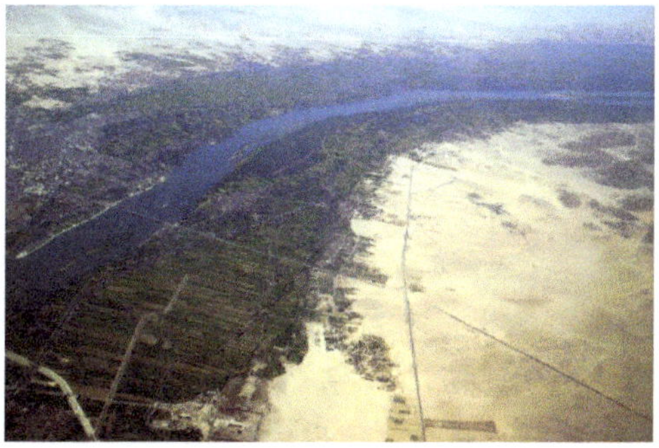

Irrigation canals have opened dry desert areas of Egypt to agriculture.

Food Security

The effort to bring modern agricultural techniques found in the West, such as nitrogen fertilizers and pesticides, to Asia, called the Green Revolution, resulted in decreases in malnutrition similar to those seen earlier in Western nations. This was possible because of existing infrastructure and institutions that are in short supply in Africa, such as a system of roads or public seed companies that made seeds available. Investments in agriculture, such as subsidized fertilizers and seeds, increases food harvest and reduces food prices. For example, in the case of Malawi, almost five million of its 13 million people used to need emergency food aid. However, after the government changed policy and subsidies for fertilizer and seed were introduced against World Bank strictures, farmers produced record-breaking corn harvests as production leaped to 3.4 million in 2007 from 1.2 million in 2005, making Malawi a major food exporter. This lowered food prices and increased wages for farm workers. Such investments in agriculture are still needed in other African countries like the Democratic Republic of the Congo. The country has one of the highest prevalence of malnutrition even though it is blessed with great agricultural potential John Ulimwengu explains in his article for D+C. Proponents for investing in agriculture include Jeffrey Sachs, who has championed the idea that wealthy countries should invest in fertilizer and seed for Africa's farmers.

New technology in agricultural production also has great potential to combat undernutrition. By improving agricultural yields, farmers could reduce poverty by increasing income as well as open up area for diversification of crops for household use. The World Bank itself claims to be part of the solution to malnutrition, asserting that the best way for countries to succeed in breaking the cycle of poverty and malnutrition is to build export-led economies that will give them the financial means to buy foodstuffs on the world market.

Breastfeeding

As of 2016 is estimated that about 821,000 deaths of children less than five years old could be prevented globally per year through more widespread breastfeeding.

Fortified Foods

Manufacturers are trying to fortify everyday foods with micronutrients that can be sold to consumers such as wheat flour for Beladi bread in Egypt or fish sauce in Vietnam and the iodization of salt.

For example, flour has been fortified with iron, zinc, folic acid and other B vitamins such as thiamine, riboflavin,niacin and vitamin B12.

World Population

Restricting population size is a proposed solution. Thomas Malthus argued that population growth could be controlled by natural disasters and voluntary limits through "moral restraint." Robert Chapman suggests that an intervention through government policies is a necessary ingredient of curtailing global population growth. However, there are many who believe that the world has more than enough resources to sustain its population. Instead, these theorists point to unequal distribution of resources and under- or unutilized arable land as the cause for malnutrition problems. For example, Amartya Sen advocates that, "no matter how a famine is caused, methods of breaking it call for a large supply of food in the public distribution system. This applies not only to organizing rationing and control, but also to undertaking work programmes and other methods of increasing purchasing power for those hit by shifts in exchange entitlements in a general inflationary situation."

Food Sovereignty

One suggested policy framework to resolve access issues is termed food sovereignty—the right of peoples to define their own food, agriculture, livestock, and fisheries systems, in contrast to having food largely subjected to international market forces. Food First is one of the primary think tanks working to build support for food sovereignty. Neoliberals advocate for an increasing role of the free market.

Health Facilities

Another possible long term solution would be to increase access to health facilities to rural parts of the world. These facilities could monitor undernourished children, act as supplemental food distribution centers, and provide education on dietary needs. These types of facilities have already proven very successful in countries such as Peru and Ghana.

Global Initiatives

In April 2012, the Food Assistance Convention was signed, the world's first legally binding international agreement on food aid. The May 2012 Copenhagen Consensus recommended that efforts to combat hunger and malnutrition should be the first priority for politicians and private sector philanthropists looking to maximize the effectiveness of aid spending. They put this ahead of other priorities, like the fight against malaria and AIDS.

The main global policy to reduce hunger and poverty are the Sustainable Development Goals. In particular Goal 2: Zero hunger sets globally agreed targets to end hunger, achieve food security and improved nutrition and promote sustainable agriculture. The partnership Compact2025, led by IFPRI with the involvement of UN organisations, NGOs and private foundations develops and disseminates evidence-based advice to politicians and other decision-makers aimed at ending hunger and undernutrition in the coming 10 years, by 2025.

The EndingHunger campaign is an online communication campaign aimed at raising awareness of the hunger problem. It has many worked through viral videos depicting celebrities voicing their anger about the large number of hungry people in the world. Another initiative focused on improving the hunger situation by improving nutrition is the Scaling up Nutrition movement (SUN). Started in 2010 this movement of people from governments, civil society, the United Nations, donors, businesses and researchers, publishes a yearly progress report on the changes in their 55 partner countries.

Management

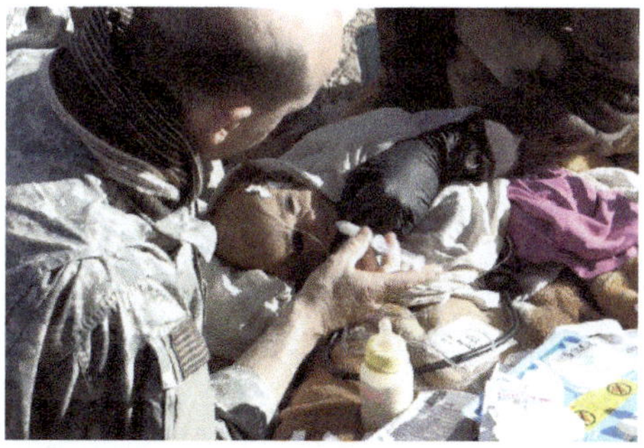

A malnourished Afghan child being treated by a medical team.

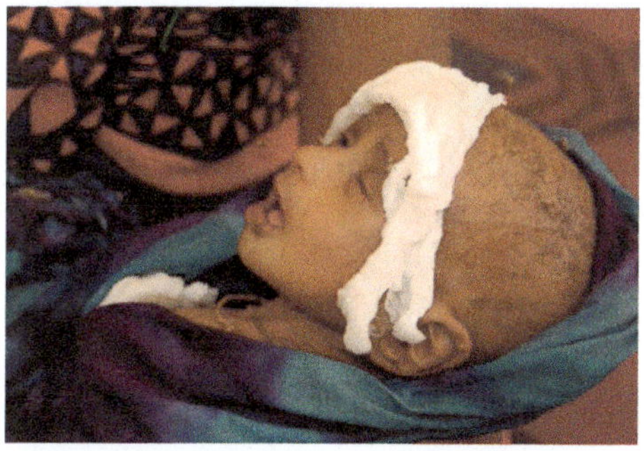

A Somali boy receiving treatment for malnourishment at a health facility.

In response to child malnutrition, the Bangladeshi government recommends ten steps for treating severe malnutrition. They are to prevent or treat dehydration, low blood sugar, low body temperature, infection, correct electrolyte imbalances and micronutrient deficiencies, start feeding cautiously, achieve catch-up growth, provide psychological support, and prepare for discharge and follow-up after recovery.

Among those patients who are hospitalized, nutritional support improves protein, colorie intake and weight.

Food

The evidence for benefit of supplementary feeding is poor. This is due to the small amount of research done on this treatment.

Specially formulated foods do however appear useful in those from the developing world with moderate acute malnutrition. In young children with severe acute malnutrition it is unclear if ready-to-use therapeutic food differs from a normal diet. They may have some benefits in humanitarian emergencies as they can be eaten directly from the packet, do not require refrigeration or mixing with clean water, and can be stored for years.

In those who are severely malnourished, feeding too much too quickly can result in refeeding syndrome. This can result regardless of route of feeding and can present itself a couple of days after eating with heart failure, dysrhythmias and confusion that can result in death.

Micronutrients

Treating malnutrition, mostly through fortifying foods with micronutrients (vitamins and minerals), improves lives at a lower cost and shorter time than other forms of aid, according to the World Bank. The Copenhagen Consensus, which look at a variety of development proposals, ranked micronutrient supplements as number one.

In those with diarrhea, once an initial four-hour rehydration period is completed, zinc supplementation is recommended. Daily zinc increases the chances of reducing the severity and duration of the diarrhea, and continuing with daily zinc for ten to fourteen days makes diarrhea less likely recur in the next two to three months.

In addition, malnourished children need both potassium and magnesium. This can be obtained by following the above recommendations for the dehydrated child to continue eating within two to three hours of starting rehydration, and including foods rich in potassium as above. Low blood potassium is worsened when base (as in Ringer's/Hartmann's) is given to treat acidosis without simultaneously providing potassium. As above, available home products such as salted and unsalted cereal water, salted and unsalted vegetable broth can be given early during the course of a child's diarrhea along with continued eating. Vitamin A, potassium, magnesium, and zinc should be added with other vitamins and minerals if available.

For a malnourished child with diarrhea from any cause, this should include foods rich in potassium such as bananas, green coconut water, and unsweetened fresh fruit juice.

Diarrhea

The World Health Organization (WHO) recommends rehydrating a severely undernourished child who has diarrhea relatively slowly. The preferred method is with fluids by mouth using a drink called oral rehydration solution (ORS). The oral rehydration solution is both slightly sweet and slightly salty and the one recommended in those with severe undernutrition should have half the usual sodium and greater potassium. Fluids by nasogastric tube may be use in those who do not drink. Intravenous fluids are recommended only in those who have significant dehydration due to their potential complications. These complications include congestive heart failure. Over time, ORS developed into ORT, or oral rehydration therapy, which focused on increasing fluids by supplying salts, carbohydrates, and water. This switch from type of fluid to amount of fluid was crucial in order to prevent dehydration from diarrhea.

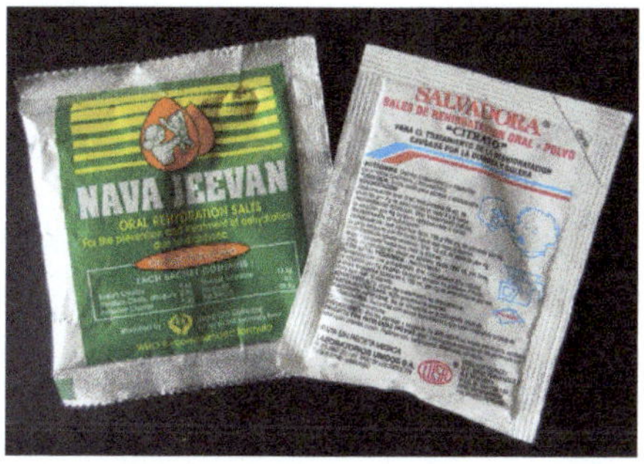

Examples of commercially available oral rehydration salts (Nepal on left, Peru on right).

Breast feeding and eating should resume as soon as possible. Drinks such as soft drinks, fruit juices, or sweetened teas are not recommended as they contain too much sugar and may worsen diarrhea. Broad spectrum antibiotics are recommended in all severely undernourished children with diarrhea requiring admission to hospital.

To prevent dehydration readily available fluids, preferably with a modest amount of sugars and salt such as vegetable broth or salted rice water, may be used. The drinking of additional clean water is also recommended. Once dehydration develops oral rehydration solutions are preferred. As much of these drinks as the person wants can be given, unless there are signs of swelling. If vomiting occurs, fluids can be paused for 5–10 minutes and then restarting more slowly. Vomiting rarely prevents rehydration as fluid are still absorbed and the vomiting rarely last long. A severely malnourished child with what appears to be dehydration but who has not had diarrhea should be treated as if they have an infection.

For babies a dropper or syringe without the needle can be used to put small amounts of fluid into the mouth; for children under 2, a teaspoon every one to two minutes; and for older children and adults, frequent sips directly from a cup. After the first two hours, rehydration should be continued at the same or slower rate, determined by how much fluid the child wants and any ongoing diarrheal loses. After the first two hours of rehydration it is recommended that to alternate between rehydration and food.

In 2003, WHO and UNICEF recommended a reduced-osmolarity ORS which still treats dehydration but also reduced stool volume and vomiting. Reduced-osmolarity ORS is the current standard ORS with reasonably wide availability. For general use, one packet of ORS (glucose sugar, salt, potassium chloride, and trisodium citrate) is added to one liter of water; however, for malnourished children it's recommended that one packet of ORS be added to two liters of water along with an extra 50 grams of sucrose sugar and some stock potassium solution.

Malnourished children have an excess of body sodium. Recommendations for home remedies agree with one liter of water (34 oz.) and 6 teaspoons sugar and disagree regarding whether it's then one teaspoon of salt added or only 1/2, with perhaps most sources recommending 1/2 teaspoon of added salt to one liter water.

Low Blood Sugar

Hypoglycemia, whether known or suspected, can be treated with a mixture of sugar and water. If the child is conscious, the initial dose of sugar and water can be given by mouth. If the child is unconscious, give glucose by intravenous or nasogastric tube. If seizures occur after despite glucose, rectal diazepam is recommended. Blood sugar levels should be re-checked on two hour intervals.

Hypothermia

Hypothermia can occur. To prevent or treat this, the child can be kept warm with covering including of the head or by direct skin-to-skin contact with the mother or father and then covering both parent and child. Prolonged bathing or prolonged medical exams should be avoided. Warming methods are usually most important at night.

Economics

There is a growing realization among aid groups that giving cash or cash vouchers instead of food is a cheaper, faster, and more efficient way to deliver help to the hungry, particularly in areas where food is available but unaffordable. The UN's World Food Program, the biggest non-governmental distributor of food, announced that it will begin distributing cash and vouchers instead of food in some areas, which Josette Sheeran, the WFP's executive director, described as a "revolution" in food aid. The aid agency Concern Worldwide is piloting a method through a mobile phone operator, Safaricom, which runs a money transfer program that allows cash to be sent from one part of the country to another.

However, for people in a drought living a long way from and with limited access to markets, delivering food may be the most appropriate way to help. Fred Cuny stated that "the chances of saving lives at the outset of a relief operation are greatly reduced when food is imported. By the time it arrives in the country and gets to people, many will have died." U.S. law, which requires buying food at home rather than where the hungry live, is inefficient because approximately half of what is spent goes for transport. Cuny further pointed out "studies of every recent famine have shown that food was available in-country — though not always in the immediate food deficit area" and "even though by local standards the prices are too high for the poor to purchase it, it would usually be cheaper for a donor to buy the hoarded food at the inflated price than to import it from abroad."

Ethiopia has been pioneering a program that has now become part of the World Bank's prescribed method for coping with a food crisis and had been seen by aid organizations as a model of how to best help hungry nations. Through the country's main food assistance program, the Productive Safety Net Program, Ethiopia has been giving rural residents who are chronically short of food, a chance to work for food or cash. Foreign aid organizations like the World Food Program were then able to buy food locally from surplus areas to distribute in areas with a shortage of food. Ethiopia been pioneering a program, and Brazil has established a recycling program for organic waste that benefits farmers, urban poor, and the city in general. City residents separate organic waste from their garbage, bag it, and then exchange it for fresh fruit and vegetables from local farmers. As a result, the country's waste is reduced and the urban poor get a steady supply of nutritious food.

Epidemiology

The figures provided in this section on epidemiology all refer to *undernutrition* even if the term malnutrition is used which, by definition, could also apply to too much nutrition.

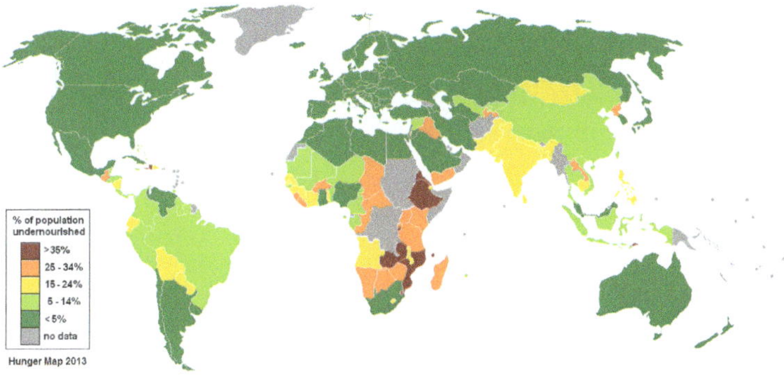

Percentage of population affected by undernutrition by country

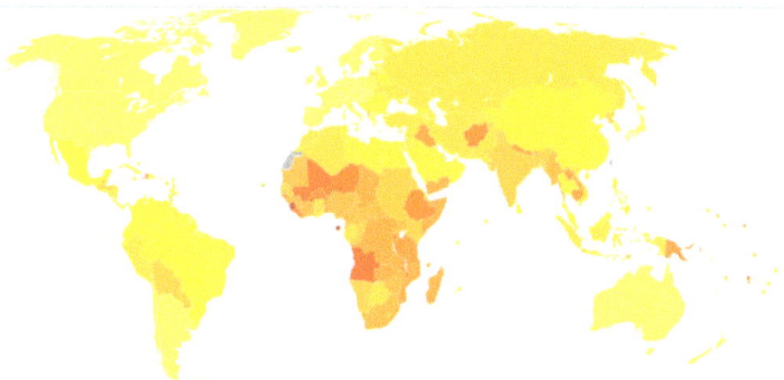

Disability-adjusted life year for nutritional deficiencies per 100,000 inhabitants in 2004. Nutritional deficiencies included: protein-energy malnutrition, iodine deficiency, vitamin A deficiency, and iron deficiency anaemia.

no data	1200-1400
<200	1400-1600
200-400	1600-1800
400-600	1800-2000
600-800	2000-2200
800-1000	>2200
1000-1200	

People Affected

There were 793 million undernourished people in the world in 2015. This was 216 million fewer people than in 1990 when it was 991 million undernourished people. This is despite the world's farmers producing enough food to feed around 12 billion people - almost double the current world population.

Malnutrition, as of 2010, was the cause of 1.4% of all disability adjusted life years.

Number of undernourished globally							
Year	**1970**	**1980**	**1990**	**1995**	**2005**	**2007/08**	**2014/16**
Number in millions			843	788	848	923	793
Percentage in the developing world	37%	28%	20%		16%	17%	13.5%

Mortality

Mortality due to malnutrition accounted for 58 percent of the total mortality in 2006: "In the world, approximately 62 million people, all causes of death combined, die each year. One in twelve people worldwide is malnourished and according to the Save the Children 2012 report, one in four of the world's children are chronically malnourished. In 2006, more than 36 million died of hunger or diseases due to deficiencies in micronutrients".

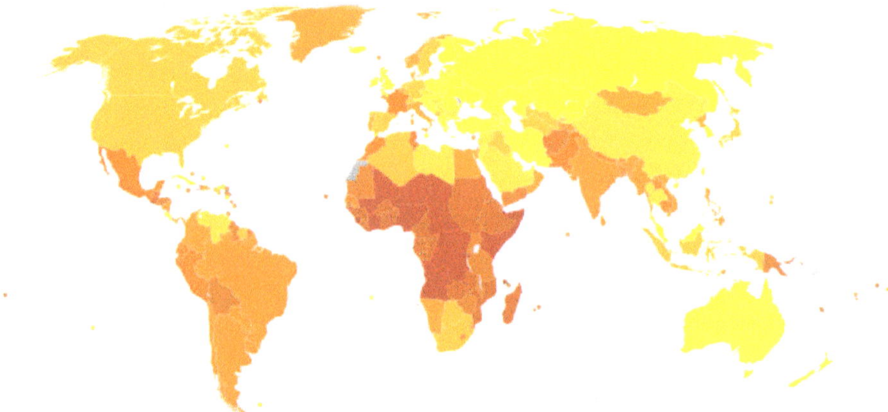

Deaths from nutritional deficiencies per million persons in 2012
0-4
5-8
9-13
14-23
24-34
35-56
57-91
92-220
221-365
366-1,207

In 2010 protein-energy malnutrition resulted in 600,000 deaths down from 883,000 deaths in 1990. Other nutritional deficiencies, which include iodine deficiency and iron deficiency anemia, result in another 84,000 deaths. In 2010 malnutrition caused about 1.5 million deaths in women and children.

According to the World Health Organization, malnutrition is the biggest contributor to child mortality, present in half of all cases. Six million children die of hunger every year. Underweight births and intrauterine growth restrictions cause 2.2 million child deaths a year. Poor or non-existent breastfeeding causes another 1.4 million. Other deficiencies, such as lack of vitamin A or zinc, for example, account for 1 million. Malnutrition in the first two years is irreversible. Malnourished children grow up with worse health and lower education achievement. Their own children tend to be smaller. Malnutrition was previously seen as something that exacerbates the problems of diseases as measles, pneumonia and diarrhea. But malnutrition actually causes diseases and can be fatal in its own right.

Society and Culture

Roughly $300 million of aid goes to basic nutrition each year, less than $2 for each child below two in the 20 worst affected countries. In contrast, HIV/AIDS, which causes fewer deaths than child malnutrition, received $2.2 billion—$67 per person with HIV in all countries.

The International Crops Research Institute for the Semi-Arid Tropics (ICRISAT), a member of the CGIAR consortium, partners with farmers, governments, researchers and NGOs to help farmers grow nutritious crops, such as chickpea, groundnut, pigeonpea, millet and sorghum. This helps their communities have more balanced diets and become more resilient to pests and drought. The Harnessing Opportunities for Productivity Enhancement of Sorghum and Millets in Sub-Saharan Africa and South Asia (HOPE) project, for example, is increasing yields of finger millet in Tanzania by encouraging farmers to grow improved varieties. Finger millet is very high in calcium, rich in iron and fiber, and has a better energy content than other cereals. These characteristics make it ideal for feeding to infants and the elderly.

Some organizations have begun working with teachers, policymakers, and managed food service contractors to mandate improved nutritional content and increased nutritional resources in school cafeterias from primary to university-level institutions. Health and nutrition have been proven to have close links with overall educational success.

The verb form is "malnourish"; "malnourishment" is sometimes used instead of "malnutrition."

Special Populations

Undernutrition is an important determinant of maternal and child health, accounting for more than a third of child deaths and more than 10 percent of the total global disease burden according to 2008 studies.

Children

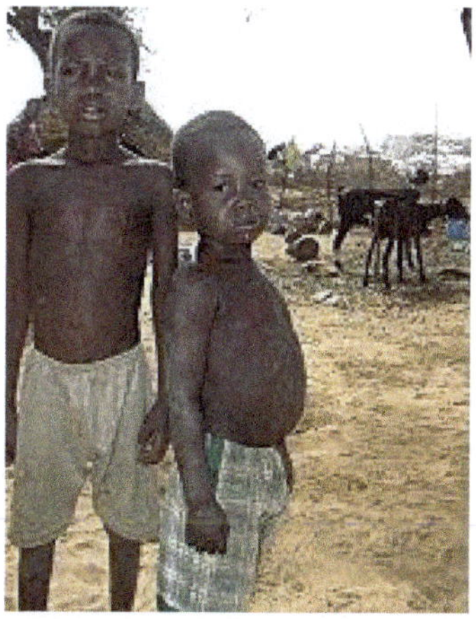

Malnourished children in Niger, during the 2005 famine.

The World Health Organization estimates that malnutrition accounts for 54 percent of child mortality worldwide, about 1 million children. Another estimate also by WHO states that childhood underweight is the cause for about 35% of all deaths of children under the age of five years worldwide.

As underweight children are more vulnerable to almost all infectious diseases, the *indirect* disease burden of malnutrition is estimated to be an order of magnitude higher than the disease burden of the *direct* effects of malnutrition. The combination of direct and indirect deaths from malnutrition caused by unsafe water, sanitation and hygiene (WASH) practices is estimated to lead to 860,000 deaths per year in children under five years of age.

Women

Gender

Researchers from the Centre for World Food Studies in 2003 found that the gap between levels of undernutrition in men and women is generally small, but that the gap varies from region to region and from country to country. These small-scale studies showed that female undernutrition prevalence rates exceeded male undernutrition prevalence rates in South/Southeast Asia and Latin America and were lower in Sub-Saharan Africa. Datasets for Ethiopia and Zimbabwe reported undernutrition rates between 1.5 and 2 times higher in men than in women; however, in India and Pakistan, datasets rates of undernutrition were 1.5-2 times higher in women than in men. Intra-country variation also occurs, with frequent high gaps between regional undernutrition rates. Gender inequality in nutrition in some countries such as India is present in all stages of life.

Studies on nutrition concerning gender bias within households look at patterns of food allocation, and one study from 2003 suggested that women often receive a lower share of food requirements than men. Gender discrimination, gender roles, and social norms affecting women can lead to early marriage and childbearing, close birth spacing, and undernutrition, all of which contribute to malnourished mothers.

Within the household, there may be differences in levels of malnutrition between men and women, and these differences have been shown to vary significantly from one region to another, with problem areas showing relative deprivation of women. Samples of 1000 women in India in 2008 demonstrated that malnutrition in women is associated with poverty, lack of development and awareness, and illiteracy. The same study showed that gender discrimination in households can prevent a woman's access to sufficient food and healthcare. How socialization affects the health of women in Bangladesh, Najma Rivzi explains in an article about a research program on this topic. In some cases, such as in parts of Kenya in 2006, rates of malnutrition in pregnant women were even higher than rates in children.

Women in some societies are traditionally given less food than men since men are perceived to have heavier workloads. Household chores and agricultural tasks can in fact be very arduous and require additional energy and nutrients; however, physical activity, which largely determines energy requirements, is difficult to estimate.

Physiology

Women have unique nutritional requirements, and in some cases need more nutrients than men; for example, women need twice as much calcium as men.

Pregnancy and Breastfeeding

During pregnancy and breastfeeding, women must ingest enough nutrients for themselves and their child, so they need significantly more protein and calories during these periods, as well as more vitamins and minerals (especially iron, iodine, calcium, folic acid, and vitamins A, C, and K). In 2001 the FAO of the UN reported that iron deficiency afflicted 43 percent of women in developing countries and increased the risk of death during childbirth. A 2008 review of interventions estimated that universal supplementation with calcium, iron, and folic acid during pregnancy could prevent 105,000 maternal deaths (23.6 percent of all maternal deaths).

Frequent pregnancies with short intervals between them and long periods of breastfeeding add an additional nutritional burden.

Educating Children

According to the FAO, women are often responsible for preparing food and have the chance to educate their children about beneficial food and health habits, giving mothers another chance to improve the nutrition of their children.

Elderly

Malnutrition and being underweight are more common in the elderly than in adults of other ages. If elderly people are healthy and active, the aging process alone does not usually cause malnutrition. However, changes in body composition, organ functions, adequate energy intake and ability to eat or access food are associated with aging, and may contribute to malnutrition. Sadness or depression can play a role, causing changes in appetite, digestion, energy level, weight, and well-being. A study on the relationship between malnutrition and other conditions in the elderly found that Malnutrition in the elderly can result from gastrointestinal and endocrine system disorders, loss of taste and smell, decreased appetite and inadequate dietary intake. Poor dental health, ill-fitting dentures, or chewing and swallowing problems can make eating difficult. As a result of these factors, malnutrition is seen to develop more easily in the elderly.

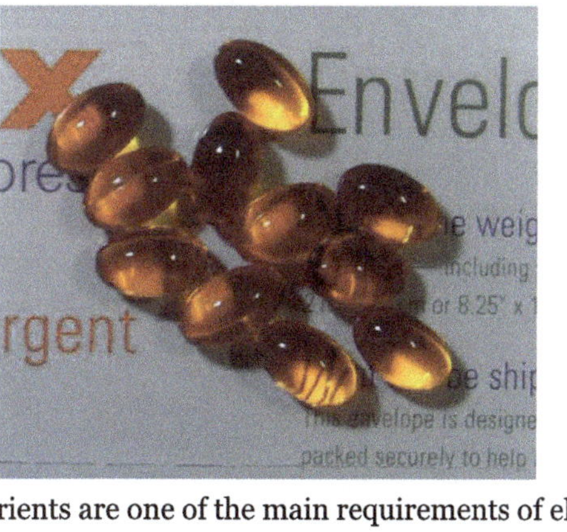

Essential nutrients are one of the main requirements of elderly care.

Rates of malnutrition tend to increase with age with less than 10 percent of the "young" elderly (up to age 75) malnourished, while 30 to 65 percent of the elderly in home care, long-term care facilities, or acute hospitals are malnourished. Many elderly people require assistance in eating, which may contribute to malnutrition. Because of this, one of the main requirements of elderly care is to provide an adequate diet and all essential nutrients.

In Australia malnutrition or risk of malnutrition occurs in 80 percent of elderly people presented to hospitals for admission. Malnutrition and weight loss can contribute to sarcopenia with loss of lean body mass and muscle function. Abdominal obesity or weight loss coupled with sarcopenia lead to immobility, skeletal disorders, insulin resistance, hypertension, atherosclerosis, and metabolic disorders. A paper from the *Journal of the American Dietetic Association* noted that routine nutrition screenings represent one way to detect and therefore decrease the prevalence of malnutrition in the elderly.

Obesity

Obesity is a medical condition in which excess body fat has accumulated to the extent that it may have a negative effect on health. People are generally considered obese when their body mass index (BMI), a measurement obtained by dividing a person's weight by the square of the person's height, is over 30 kg/m^2, with the range 25–30 kg/m^2 defined as overweight. Some East Asian countries use lower values. Obesity increases the likelihood of various diseases, particularly heart disease, type 2 diabetes, obstructive sleep apnea, certain types of cancer, and osteoarthritis.

Obesity is most commonly caused by a combination of excessive food intake, lack of physical activity, and genetic susceptibility. A few cases are caused primarily by genes, endocrine disorders, medications, or mental illness. Evidence to support the view that obese people eat little yet gain weight due to a slow metabolism is not generally supported. On average, obese people have a greater energy expenditure than their thin counterparts due to the energy required to maintain an increased body mass.

Obesity is mostly preventable through a combination of social changes and personal choices. Changes to diet and exercising are the main treatments. Diet quality can be improved by reducing the consumption of energy-dense foods, such as those high in fat and sugars, and by increasing the intake of dietary fiber. Medications may be taken, along with a suitable diet, to reduce appetite or decrease fat absorption. If diet, exercise, and medication are not effective, a gastric balloon or surgery may be performed to reduce stomach volume or bowel length, leading to feeling full earlier or a reduced ability to absorb nutrients from food.

Obesity is a leading preventable cause of death worldwide, with increasing rates in adults and children. In 2014, 600 million adults (13%) and 42 million children under the age of five were obese. Obesity is more common in women than men. Authorities view it as one of the most serious public health problems of the 21st century. Obesity is stigmatized in much of the modern world (particularly in the Western world), though it was seen as a symbol of wealth and fertility at other times in history and still is in some parts of the world. In 2013, the American Medical Association classified obesity as a disease.

Classification

Obesity is a medical condition in which excess body fat has accumulated to the extent that it may have an adverse effect on health. It is defined by body mass index (BMI) and further evaluated in terms of fat distribution via the waist–hip ratio and total cardiovascular risk factors. BMI is closely related to both percentage body fat and total body fat. In children, a healthy weight varies with age and sex. Obesity in children and adolescents is defined not as an absolute number but in relation to a historical normal group, such that obesity is a BMI greater than the 95th percentile. The reference data on which these percentiles were based date from 1963 to 1994, and thus have not been affected by the recent increases in weight. BMI is defined as the subject's weight divided by the square of their height and is calculated as follows.

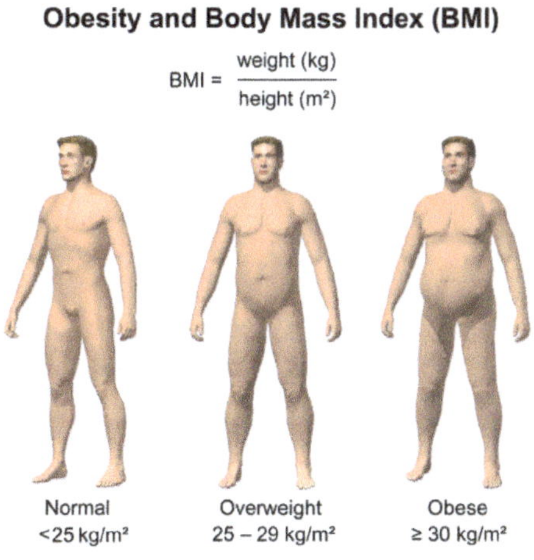

Obesity and BMI

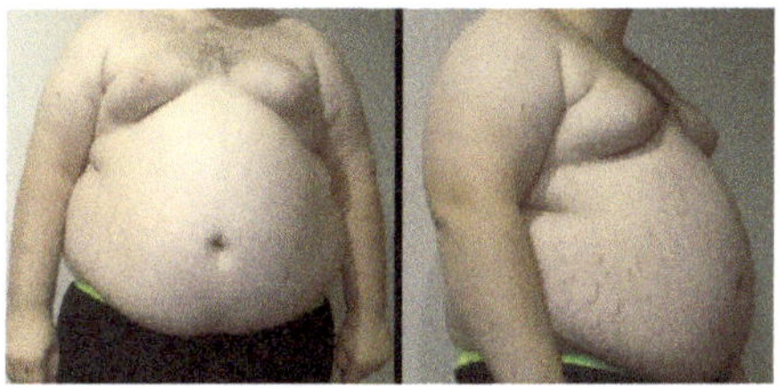

A "super obese" male with a BMI of 53 kg/m²: weight 182 kg (400 lb), height 185 cm (6 ft 1 in)

$$\text{BMI} = \frac{m}{h^2},$$

where *m* and *h* are the subject's weight and height respectively.

BMI is usually expressed in kilograms per square metre, resulting when weight is measured in kilograms and height in metres. To convert from pounds per square inch multiply by 703 (kg/m²)/(lb/sq in).

BMI (kg/m²)		Classification
from	up to	
	18.5	underweight
18.5	25.0	normal weight
25.0	30.0	overweight
30.0	35.0	class I obesity
35.0	40.0	class II obesity
40.0		class III obesity

The most commonly used definitions, established by the World Health Organization (WHO) in 1997 and published in 2000, provide the values listed in the table.

Some modifications to the WHO definitions have been made by particular bodies. The surgical literature breaks down "class III" obesity into further categories whose exact values are still disputed.

- Any BMI ≥ 35 or 40 kg/m² is *severe obesity.*
- A BMI of ≥ 35 kg/m² and experiencing obesity-related health conditions or ≥40–44.9 kg/m² is *morbid obesity.*
- A BMI of ≥ 45 or 50 kg/m² is *super obesity.*

As Asian populations develop negative health consequences at a lower BMI than Caucasians, some nations have redefined obesity; the Japanese have defined obesity as any BMI greater than 25 kg/m² while China uses a BMI of greater than 28 kg/m².

Effects on Health

Excessive body weight is associated with various diseases, particularly cardiovascular diseases, diabetes mellitus type 2, obstructive sleep apnea, certain types of cancer, osteoarthritis and asthma. As a result, obesity has been found to reduce life expectancy.

Mortality

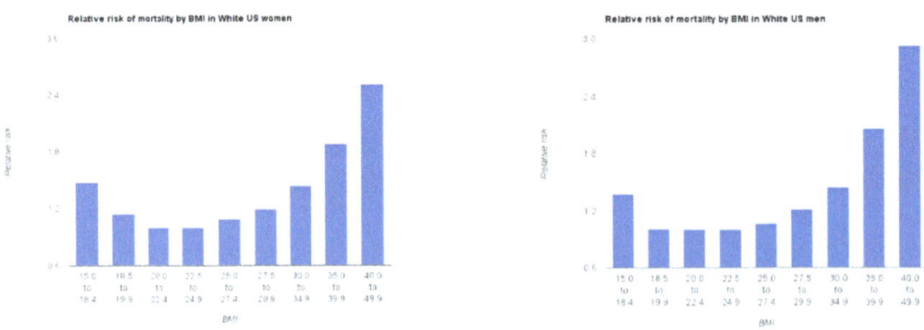

Relative risk of death over 10 years for white men (left) and women (right) who have never smoked in the United States by BMI.

Obesity is one of the leading preventable causes of death worldwide. A number of reviews have found that mortality risk is lowest at a BMI of 20–25 kg/m² in non-smokers and at 24–27 kg/m² in current smokers, with risk increasing along with changes in either direction. This appears to apply in at least four continents. In contrast, a 2013 review found that grade 1 obesity (BMI 30-35) was not associated with higher mortality than normal weight, and that overweight (BMI 25-30) was associated with "lower" mortality than was normal weight (BMI 18.5-25). Other evidence suggests that the association of BMI and waist circumference with mortality is U- or J-shaped, while the association between waist-to-hip ratio and waist-to-height ratio with mortality is more positive. In Asians the risk of negative health effects begins to increase between 22–25 kg/m². A BMI above 32 kg/m² has been associated with a doubled mortality rate among women over a 16-year period. In the United States obesity is estimated to cause 111,909 to 365,000 deaths per year, while 1 million (7.7%) of deaths in Europe are attributed to excess weight. On average, obesity reduces life expectancy by six to seven years, a BMI of 30–35 kg/m^2 reduces life expectancy by two to four years, while severe obesity (BMI > 40 kg/m^2) reduces life expectancy by ten years.

Morbidity

Obesity increases the risk of many physical and mental conditions. These comorbidities are most commonly shown in metabolic syndrome, a combination of medical disorders which includes: diabetes mellitus type 2, high blood pressure, high blood cholesterol, and high triglyceride levels.

Complications are either directly caused by obesity or indirectly related through mechanisms sharing a common cause such as a poor diet or a sedentary lifestyle. The strength of the link between obesity and specific conditions varies. One of the strongest is the link with type 2 diabetes. Excess body fat underlies 64% of cases of diabetes in men and 77% of cases in women.

Health consequences fall into two broad categories: those attributable to the effects of increased fat mass (such as osteoarthritis, obstructive sleep apnea, social stigmatization) and those due to the increased number of fat cells (diabetes, cancer, cardiovascular disease, non-alcoholic fatty liver disease). Increases in body fat alter the body's response to insulin, potentially leading to insulin resistance. Increased fat also creates a proinflammatory state, and a prothrombotic state.

Medical field	Condition	Medical field	Condition
Cardiology	• coronary heart disease: angina and myocardial infarction • congestive heart failure • high blood pressure • abnormal cholesterol levels • deep vein thrombosis and pulmonary embolism	Dermatology	• stretch marks • acanthosis nigricans • lymphedema • cellulitis • hirsutism • intertrigo
Endocrinology and Reproductive medicine	• diabetes mellitus • polycystic ovarian syndrome • menstrual disorders • infertility • complications during pregnancy • birth defects • intrauterine fetal death	Gastroenterology	• gastroesophageal reflux disease • fatty liver disease • cholelithiasis (gallstones)

Neurology	• stroke • meralgia paresthetica • migraines • carpal tunnel syndrome • dementia • idiopathic intracranial hypertension • multiple sclerosis	Oncology	• esophageal • colorectal • pancreatic • gallbladder, • endometrial • kidney • Leukemia • Hepatocellular carcinoma • malignant melanoma
Psychiatry	• depression in women • social stigmatization	Respirology	• obstructive sleep apnea • obesity hypoventilation syndrome • asthma • increased complications during general anaesthesia
Rheumatology and Orthopedics	• gout • poor mobility • osteoarthritis • low back pain	Urology and Nephrology	• erectile dysfunction • urinary incontinence • chronic renal failure • hypogonadism • buried penis

Survival Paradox

Although the negative health consequences of obesity in the general population are well supported by the available evidence, health outcomes in certain subgroups seem to be improved at an increased BMI, a phenomenon known as the obesity survival paradox. The paradox was first described in 1999 in overweight and obese people undergoing hemodialysis, and has subsequently been found in those with heart failure and peripheral artery disease (PAD).

In people with heart failure, those with a BMI between 30.0 and 34.9 had lower mortality than those with a normal weight. This has been attributed to the fact that people often lose weight as they become progressively more ill. Similar findings have been made in other types of heart disease. People with class I obesity and heart disease do not have greater rates of further heart problems than people of normal weight who also have heart disease. In people with greater degrees of obesity, however, the risk of further cardiovascular events is increased. Even after cardiac bypass surgery, no increase in mortality is seen in the overweight and obese. One study found that the improved survival could be explained by the more aggressive treatment obese people receive after a cardiac event. Another found that if one takes into account chronic obstructive pulmonary disease (COPD) in those with PAD, the benefit of obesity no longer exists.

Causes

At an individual level, a combination of excessive food energy intake and a lack of physical activity is thought to explain most cases of obesity. A limited number of cases are due primarily to genetics, medical reasons, or psychiatric illness. In contrast, increasing rates of obesity at a societal level are felt to be due to an easily accessible and palatable diet, increased reliance on cars, and mechanized manufacturing.

A 2006 review identified ten other possible contributors to the recent increase of obesity: (1) insufficient sleep, (2) endocrine disruptors (environmental pollutants that interfere with lipid metabolism), (3) decreased variability in ambient temperature, (4) decreased rates of smoking, because smoking suppresses appetite, (5) increased use of medications that can cause weight gain (e.g., atypical antipsychotics), (6) proportional increases in ethnic and age groups that tend to be heavier, (7) pregnancy at a later age (which may cause susceptibility to obesity in children), (8) epigenetic risk factors passed on generationally, (9) natural selection for higher BMI, and (10) assortative mating leading to increased concentration of obesity risk factors (this would increase the number of obese people by increasing population variance in weight). While there is substantial evidence supporting the influence of these mechanisms on the increased prevalence of obesity, the evidence is still inconclusive, and the authors state that these are probably less influential than the ones discussed in the previous paragraph.

Diet

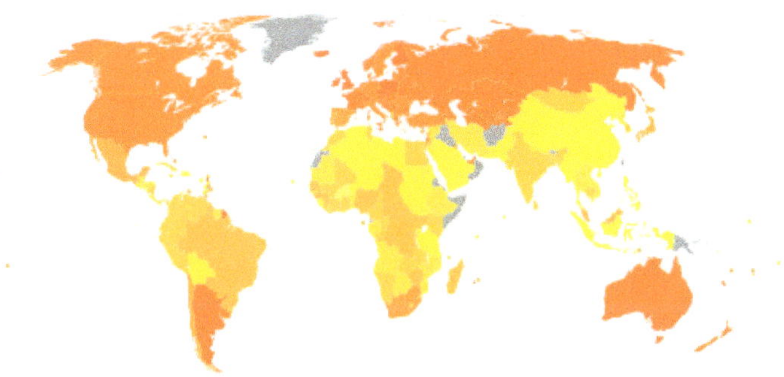

1961

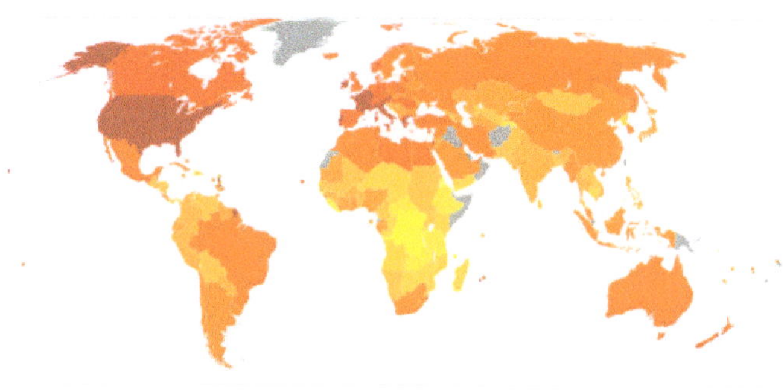

2001–03

Map of dietary energy availability per person per day in 1961 (left) and 2001–2003 (right) Calories per person per day (kilojoules per person per day)

no data
<1,600 (<6,700)
1,600–1,800 (6,700–7,500)
1,800–2,000 (7,500–8,400)
2,000–2,200 (8,400–9,200)
2,200–2,400 (9,200–10,000)
2,400–2,600 (10,000–10,900)
2,600–2,800 (10,900–11,700)
2,800–3,000 (11,700–12,600)
3,000–3,200 (12,600–13,400)
3,200–3,400 (13,400–14,200)
3,400–3,600 (14,200–15,100)
>3,600 (>15,100)

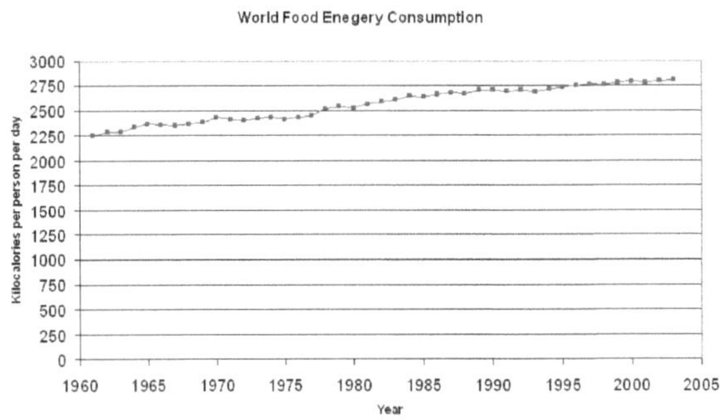

Average per capita energy consumption of the world from 1961 to 2002

Dietary energy supply per capita varies markedly between different regions and countries. It has also changed significantly over time. From the early 1970s to the late 1990s the average food energy available per person per day (the amount of food bought) increased in all parts of the world except Eastern Europe. The United States had the highest availability with 3,654 calories (15,290 kJ) per person in 1996. This increased further in 2003 to 3,754 calories (15,710 kJ). During the late 1990s Europeans had 3,394 calories (14,200 kJ) per person, in the developing areas of Asia there were 2,648 calories (11,080 kJ) per person, and in sub-Saharan Africa people had 2,176 calories (9,100 kJ) per person. Total food energy consumption has been found to be related to obesity.

The widespread availability of nutritional guidelines has done little to address the problems of overeating and poor dietary choice. From 1971 to 2000, obesity rates in the United States increased from 14.5% to 30.9%. During the same period, an increase occurred in the average amount of food energy consumed. For women, the average increase was 335 calories (1,400 kJ) per day (1,542 calories (6,450 kJ) in 1971 and 1,877 calories (7,850 kJ) in 2004), while for men the average increase was 168 calories (700 kJ) per day (2,450 calories (10,300 kJ) in 1971 and 2,618 calories (10,950 kJ) in 2004). Most of this extra food energy came from an increase in carbohydrate consumption rather than fat consumption. The primary sources of these extra carbohydrates are sweetened beverages, which now account for almost 25 percent of daily food energy in young adults in America, and potato chips. Consumption of sweetened drinks such as soft drinks, fruit drinks, iced tea, and energy and vitamin water drinks is believed to be contributing to the rising rates of obesity and to an increased risk of metabolic syndrome and type 2 diabetes.

As societies become increasingly reliant on energy-dense, big-portions, and fast-food meals, the association between fast-food consumption and obesity becomes more concerning. In the United States consumption of fast-food meals tripled and food energy intake from these meals quadrupled between 1977 and 1995.

Agricultural policy and techniques in the United States and Europe have led to lower food prices. In the United States, subsidization of corn, soy, wheat, and rice through the U.S. farm bill has made the main sources of processed food cheap compared to fruits and vegetables. Calorie count laws and nutrition facts labels attempt to steer people toward making healthier food choices, including awareness of how much food energy is being consumed.

Obese people consistently under-report their food consumption as compared to people of normal weight. This is supported both by tests of people carried out in a calorimeter room and by direct observation.

Sedentary Lifestyle

A sedentary lifestyle plays a significant role in obesity. Worldwide there has been a large shift towards less physically demanding work, and currently at least 30% of the world's population gets insufficient exercise. This is primarily due to increasing use of mechanized transportation and a greater prevalence of labor-saving technology in the home. In children, there appear to be declines in levels of physical activity due to less walking and physical education. World trends in active leisure time physical activity are less clear. The World Health Organization indicates people worldwide are taking up less active recreational pursuits, while a study from Finland found an increase and a study from the United States found leisure-time physical activity has not changed significantly.

In both children and adults, there is an association between television viewing time and the risk of obesity. A review found 63 of 73 studies (86%) showed an increased rate of childhood obesity with increased media exposure, with rates increasing proportionally to time spent watching television.

Genetics

Like many other medical conditions, obesity is the result of an interplay between genetic and environmental factors. Polymorphisms in various genes controlling appetite and metabolism predispose to obesity when sufficient food energy is present. As of 2006, more than 41 of these sites on the human genome have been linked to the development of obesity when a favorable environment is present. People with two copies of the FTO gene (fat mass and obesity associated gene) have been found on average to weigh 3–4 kg more and have a 1.67-fold greater risk of obesity compared with those without the risk allele. The differences in BMI between people that are due to genetics varies depending on the population examined from 6% to 85%.

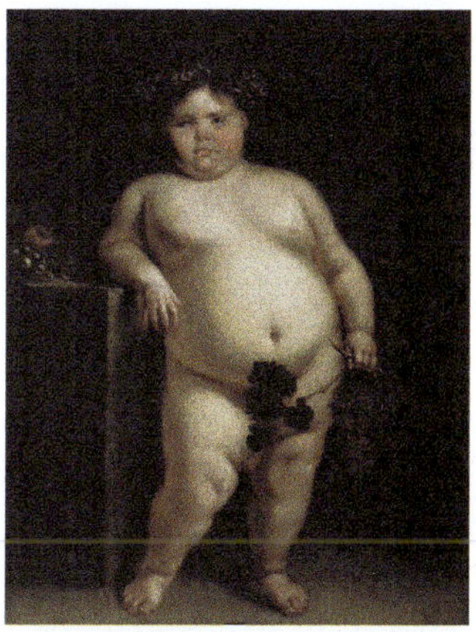

A 1680 painting by Juan Carreno de Miranda of a girl presumed to have Prader–Willi syndrome

Obesity is a major feature in several syndromes, such as Prader–Willi syndrome, Bardet–Biedl syndrome, Cohen syndrome, and MOMO syndrome. (The term "non-syndromic obesity" is sometimes used to exclude these conditions.) In people with early-onset severe obesity (defined by an onset before 10 years of age and body mass index over three standard deviations above normal), 7% harbor a single point DNA mutation.

Studies that have focused on inheritance patterns rather than on specific genes have found that 80% of the offspring of two obese parents were also obese, in contrast to less than 10% of the offspring of two parents who were of normal weight. Different people exposed to the same environment have different risks of obesity due to their underlying genetics.

The thrifty gene hypothesis postulates that, due to dietary scarcity during human evolution, people are prone to obesity. Their ability to take advantage of rare periods of abundance by storing energy as fat would be advantageous during times of varying food availability, and individuals with greater adipose reserves would be more likely to survive famine. This tendency to store fat, however, would be maladaptive in societies with stable food supplies. This theory has received various criticisms, and other evolutionarily-based theories such as the drifty gene hypothesis and the thrifty phenotype hypothesis have also been proposed.

Other Illnesses

Certain physical and mental illnesses and the pharmaceutical substances used to treat them can increase risk of obesity. Medical illnesses that increase obesity risk include several rare genetic syndromes (listed above) as well as some congenital or acquired conditions: hypothyroidism, Cushing's syndrome, growth hormone deficiency, and the eating disorders: binge eating disorder and night eating syndrome. However, obesity is not regarded as a psychiatric disorder, and therefore is not listed in the DSM-IVR as a psychiatric illness. The risk of overweight and obesity is higher in patients with psychiatric disorders than in persons without psychiatric disorders.

Certain medications may cause weight gain or changes in body composition; these include insulin, sulfonylureas, thiazolidinediones, atypical antipsychotics, antidepressants, steroids, certain anticonvulsants (phenytoin and valproate), pizotifen, and some forms of hormonal contraception.

Social Determinants

While genetic influences are important to understanding obesity, they cannot explain the current dramatic increase seen within specific countries or globally. Though it is accepted that energy consumption in excess of energy expenditure leads to obesity on an individual basis, the cause of the shifts in these two factors on the societal scale is much debated. There are a number of theories as to the cause but most believe it is a combination of various factors.

The correlation between social class and BMI varies globally. A review in 1989 found that in developed countries women of a high social class were less likely to be obese. No significant differences were seen among men of different social classes. In the developing world, women, men, and children from high social classes had greater rates of obesity. An update of this review carried out in 2007 found the same relationships, but they were weaker. The decrease in strength of correlation was felt to be due to the effects of globalization. Among developed countries, levels of adult obesity, and percentage of teenage children who are overweight, are correlated with income inequality. A similar relationship is seen among US states: more adults, even in higher social classes, are obese in more unequal states.

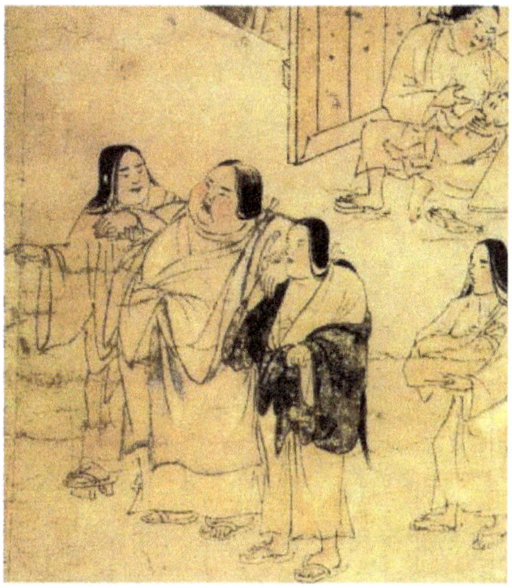

The disease scroll (Yamai no soshi, late 12th century) depicts a woman moneylender with obesity, considered a disease of the rich.

Many explanations have been put forth for associations between BMI and social class. It is thought that in developed countries, the wealthy are able to afford more nutritious food, they are under greater social pressure to remain slim, and have more opportunities along with greater expectations for physical fitness. In undeveloped countries the ability to afford food, high energy expenditure with physical labor, and cultural values favoring a larger body size are believed to contribute to the observed patterns. Attitudes toward body weight held by people in one's life may also play a role in obesity. A correlation in BMI changes over time has been found among friends, siblings, and spouses. Stress and perceived low social status appear to increase risk of obesity.

Smoking has a significant effect on an individual's weight. Those who quit smoking gain an average of 4.4 kilograms (9.7 lb) for men and 5.0 kilograms (11.0 lb) for women over ten years. However, changing rates of smoking have had little effect on the overall rates of obesity.

In the United States the number of children a person has is related to their risk of obesity. A woman's risk increases by 7% per child, while a man's risk increases by 4% per child. This could be partly explained by the fact that having dependent children decreases physical activity in Western parents.

In the developing world urbanization is playing a role in increasing rate of obesity. In China overall rates of obesity are below 5%; however, in some cities rates of obesity are greater than 20%.

Malnutrition in early life is believed to play a role in the rising rates of obesity in the developing world. Endocrine changes that occur during periods of malnutrition may promote the storage of fat once more food energy becomes available.

Consistent with cognitive epidemiological data, numerous studies confirm that obesity is associated with cognitive deficits. Whether obesity causes cognitive deficits, or vice versa is unclear at present.

Gut Bacteria

The study of the effect of infectious agents on metabolism is still in its early stages. Gut flora has been shown to differ between lean and obese humans. There is an indication that gut flora in obese and lean individuals can affect the metabolic potential. This apparent alteration of the metabolic potential is believed to confer a greater capacity to harvest energy contributing to obesity. Whether these differences are the direct cause or the result of obesity has yet to be determined unequivocally.

An association between viruses and obesity has been found in humans and several different animal species. The amount that these associations may have contributed to the rising rate of obesity is yet to be determined.

Pathophysiology

There are many possible pathophysiological mechanisms involved in the development and maintenance of obesity. This field of research had been almost unapproached until the leptin gene was discovered in 1994 by J. M. Friedman's laboratory. These investigators postulated that leptin was a satiety factor. In the ob/ob mouse, mutations in the leptin gene resulted in the obese phenotype opening the possibility of leptin therapy for human obesity. However, soon thereafter J. F. Caro's laboratory could not detect any mutations in the leptin gene in humans with obesity. On the contrary Leptin expression was increased proposing the possibility of Leptin-resistance in human obesity. Since this discovery, many other hormonal mechanisms have been elucidated that participate in the regulation of appetite and food intake, storage patterns of adipose tissue, and development of insulin resistance. Since leptin's discovery, ghrelin, insulin, orexin, PYY 3-36, cholecystokinin, adiponectin, as well as many other mediators have been studied. The adipokines are mediators produced by adipose tissue; their action is thought to modify many obesity-related diseases.

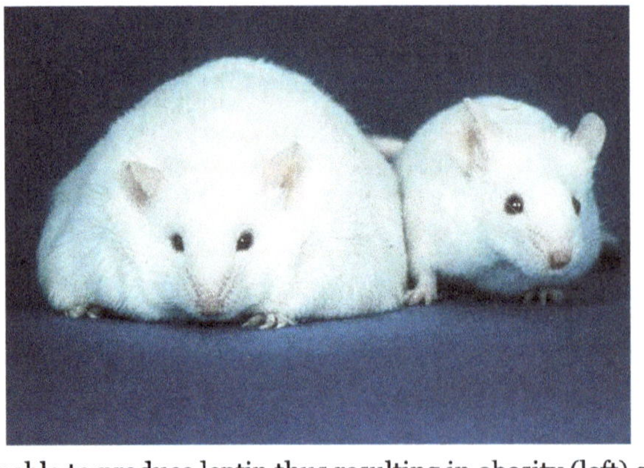

A comparison of a mouse unable to produce leptin thus resulting in obesity (left) and a normal mouse (right)

Leptin and ghrelin are considered to be complementary in their influence on appetite, with ghrelin produced by the stomach modulating short-term appetitive control (i.e. to eat when the stomach is empty and to stop when the stomach is stretched). Leptin is produced by adipose tissue to signal fat storage reserves in the body, and mediates long-term appetitive controls (i.e. to eat more when fat storages are low and less when fat storages are high). Although administration of leptin may be effective in a small subset of obese individuals who are leptin deficient, most obese individuals are thought to be leptin resistant and have been found to have high levels of leptin. This resistance is thought to explain in part why administration of leptin has not been shown to be effective in suppressing appetite in most obese people.

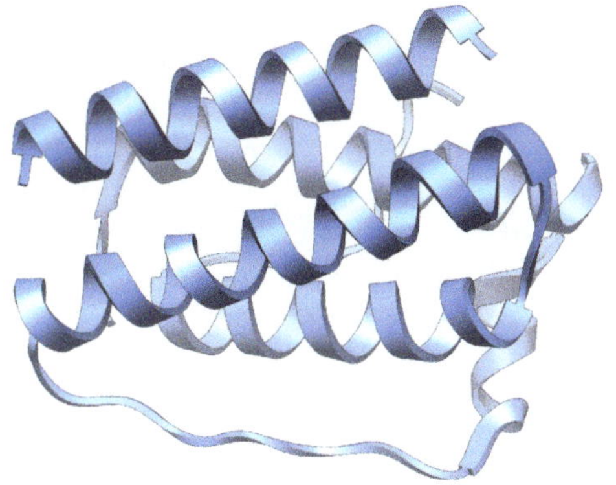

A graphic depiction of a leptin molecule

While leptin and ghrelin are produced peripherally, they control appetite through their actions on the central nervous system. In particular, they and other appetite-related hormones act on the hypothalamus, a region of the brain central to the regulation of food intake and energy expenditure. There are several circuits within the hypothalamus that contribute to its role in integrating appetite, the melanocortin pathway being the most well understood. The circuit begins with an area of the hypothalamus, the arcuate nucleus, that has outputs to the lateral hypothalamus (LH) and ventromedial hypothalamus (VMH), the brain's feeding and satiety centers, respectively.

The arcuate nucleus contains two distinct groups of neurons. The first group coexpresses neuropeptide Y (NPY) and agouti-related peptide (AgRP) and has stimulatory inputs to the LH and inhibitory inputs to the VMH. The second group coexpresses pro-opiomelanocortin (POMC) and cocaine- and amphetamine-regulated transcript (CART) and has stimulatory inputs to the VMH and inhibitory inputs to the LH. Consequently, NPY/AgRP neurons stimulate feeding and inhibit satiety, while POMC/CART neurons stimulate satiety and inhibit feeding. Both groups of arcuate nucleus neurons are regulated in part by leptin. Leptin inhibits the NPY/AgRP group while stimulating the POMC/CART group. Thus a deficiency in leptin signaling, either via leptin deficiency or leptin resistance, leads to overfeeding and may account for some genetic and acquired forms of obesity.

Public Health

The World Health Organization (WHO) predicts that overweight and obesity may soon replace more traditional public health concerns such as undernutrition and infectious diseases as the most significant cause of poor health. Obesity is a public health and policy problem because of its prevalence, costs, and health effects. The United States Preventive Services Task Force recommends screening for all adults followed by behavioral interventions in those who are obese. Public health efforts seek to understand and correct the environmental factors responsible for the increasing prevalence of obesity in the population. Solutions look at changing the factors that cause excess food energy consumption and inhibit physical activity. Efforts include federally reimbursed meal programs in schools, limiting direct junk food marketing to children, and decreasing access to sugar-sweetened beverages in schools. When constructing urban environments, efforts have been made to increase access to parks and to develop pedestrian routes.

Many countries and groups have published reports pertaining to obesity. In 1998, the first US Federal guidelines were published, titled "Clinical Guidelines on the Identification, Evaluation, and Treatment of Overweight and Obesity in Adults: The Evidence Report". In 2006 the Canadian Obesity Network published the "Canadian Clinical Practice Guidelines (CPG) on the Management and Prevention of Obesity in Adults and Children". This is a comprehensive evidence-based guideline to address the management and prevention of overweight and obesity in adults and children.

In 2004, the United Kingdom Royal College of Physicians, the Faculty of Public Health and the Royal College of Paediatrics and Child Health released the report "Storing up Problems", which highlighted the growing problem of obesity in the UK. The same year, the House of Commons Health Select Committee published its "most comprehensive inquiry [...] ever undertaken" into the impact of obesity on health and society in the UK and possible approaches to the problem. In 2006, the National Institute for Health and Clinical Excellence (NICE) issued a guideline on the diagnosis and management of obesity, as well as policy implications for non-healthcare organizations such as local councils. A 2007 report produced by Sir Derek Wanless for the King's Fund warned that unless further action was taken, obesity had the capacity to cripple the National Health Service financially.

Comprehensive approaches are being looked at to address the rising rates of obesity. The Obesity Policy Action (OPA) framework divides measure into 'upstream' policies, 'midstream' policies, 'downstream' policies. 'Upstream' policies look at changing society, 'midstream' policies try to alter individuals' behavior to prevent obesity, and 'downstream' policies try to treat currently afflicted people.

Management

The main treatment for obesity consists of dieting and physical exercise. Diet programs may produce weight loss over the short term, but maintaining this weight loss is frequently difficult and often requires making exercise and a lower food energy diet a permanent part of a person's lifestyle.

In the short-term low carbohydrate diets appear better than low fat diets for weight loss. In the long term; however, all types of low-carbohydrate and low-fat diets appear equally beneficial. A 2014 review found that the heart disease and diabetes risks associated with different diets appear to be similar. Promotion of the Mediterranean diets among the obese may lower the risk of heart disease. Decreased intake of sweet drinks is also related to weight-loss. Success rates of long-term weight loss maintenance with lifestyle changes are low, ranging from 2–20%. Dietary and lifestyle changes are effective in limiting excessive weight gain in pregnancy and improve outcomes for both the mother and the child. Intensive behavioral counseling is recommended in those who are both obese and have other risk factors for heart disease.

Three medications, orlistat, lorcaserin and a combination of phentermine and topiramate are currently available and have evidence for long term use. Weight loss with orlistat is modest, an average of 2.9 kg (6.4 lb) at 1 to 4 years. Its use is associated with high rates of gastrointestinal side effects and concerns have been raised about negative effects on the kidneys. The other two medications are available in the United States but not Europe. Lorcaserin results in an average 3.1 kg weight loss (3% of body weight) greater than placebo over a year; however, it may increase heart valve problems. A combination of phentermine and topiramate is also somewhat effective; however, it may be associated with heart problems. There is no information on how these drugs affect longer-term complications of obesity such as cardiovascular disease or death.

The most effective treatment for obesity is bariatric surgery. Surgery for severe obesity is associated with long-term weight loss, improvement in obesity related conditions, and decreased overall mortality. One study found a weight loss of between 14% and 25% (depending on the type of procedure performed) at 10 years, and a 29% reduction in all cause mortality when compared to standard weight loss measures. Complications occur in about 17% of cases and reoperation is needed in 7% of cases. Due to its cost and risks, researchers are searching for other effective yet less invasive treatments including devices that occupy space in the stomach.

Epidemiology

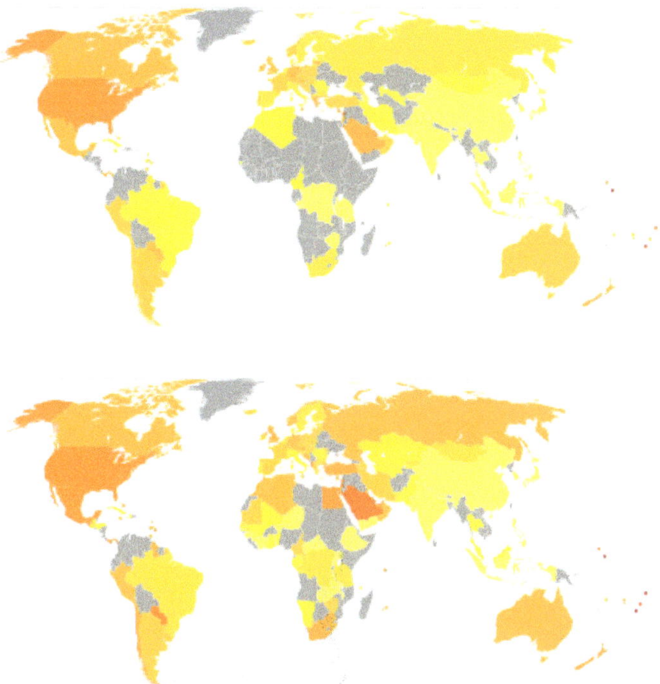

World obesity prevalence among males (left) and females (right).

<5%	15–20%	30–35%	45–50%
5–10%	20–25%	35–40%	50–55%
10–15%	25–30%	40–45%	>55%

In earlier historical periods obesity was rare, and achievable only by a small elite, although already recognised as a problem for health. But as prosperity increased in the Early Modern period, it affected increasingly larger groups of the population. In 1997 the WHO formally recognized obesity as a global epidemic. As of 2008 the WHO estimates that at least 500 million adults (greater than 10%) are obese, with higher rates among women than men. The rate of obesity also increases with age at least up to 50 or 60 years old and severe obesity in the United States, Australia, and Canada is increasing faster than the overall rate of obesity.

Once considered a problem only of high-income countries, obesity rates are rising worldwide and affecting both the developed and developing world. These increases have been felt most dramatically in urban settings. The only remaining region of the world where obesity is not common is sub-Saharan Africa.

History

Etymology

Obesity is from the Latin *obesitas*, which means "stout, fat, or plump". Ēsus is the past participle of *edere* (to eat), with *ob* (over) added to it. *The Oxford English Dictionary* documents its first usage in 1611 by Randle Cotgrave.

Historical Attitudes

Ancient Greek medicine recognizes obesity as a medical disorder, and records that the Ancient Egyptians saw it in the same way. Hippocrates wrote that "Corpulence is not only a disease itself, but the harbinger of others". The Indian surgeon Sushruta (6th century BCE) related obesity to diabetes and heart disorders. He recommended physical work to help cure it and its side effects. For most of human history mankind struggled with food scarcity. Obesity has thus historically been viewed as a sign of wealth and prosperity. It was common among high officials in Europe in the Middle Ages and the Renaissance as well as in Ancient East Asian civilizations. In the 17th century, English medical author Tobias Venner is credited with being one of the first to refer to the term as a societal disease in a published English language book.

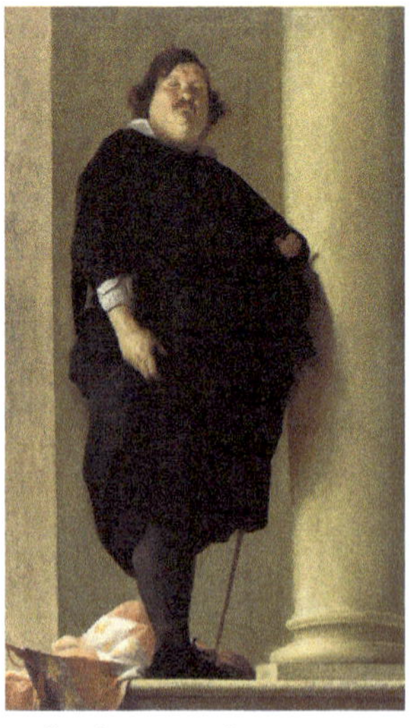

During the Middle Ages and the Renaissance obesity was often seen as a sign of wealth, and was relatively common among the elite: *The Tuscan General Alessandro del Borro*, attributed to Charles Mellin, 1645

With the onset of the industrial revolution it was realized that the military and economic might of nations were dependent on both the body size and strength of their soldiers and workers. Increasing the average body mass index from what is now considered underweight to what is now the normal range played a significant role in the development of industrialized societies. Height and weight thus both increased through the 19th century in the developed world. During the 20th century, as populations reached their genetic potential for height, weight began increasing much more than height, resulting in obesity. In the 1950s increasing wealth in the developed world decreased child mortality, but as body weight increased heart and kidney disease became more common. During this time period insurance companies realized the connection between weight and life expectancy and increased premiums for the obese.

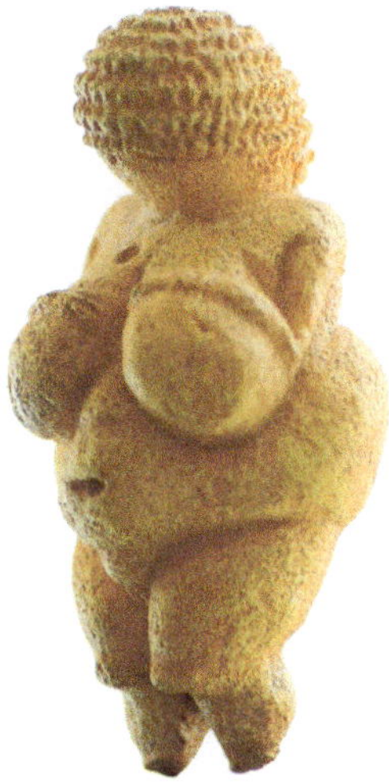

Venus of Willendorf created 24,000–22,000 BC

Many cultures throughout history have viewed obesity as the result of a character flaw. The *obesus* or fat character in Greek comedy was a glutton and figure of mockery. During Christian times food was viewed as a gateway to the sins of sloth and lust. In modern Western culture, excess weight is often regarded as unattractive, and obesity is commonly associated with various negative stereotypes. People of all ages can face social stigmatization, and may be targeted by bullies or shunned by their peers.

Public perceptions in Western society regarding healthy body weight differ from those regarding the weight that is considered ideal – and both have changed since the beginning of the 20th century. The weight that is viewed as an ideal has become lower since the 1920s. This is illustrated by the fact that the average height of Miss America pageant winners increased by 2% from 1922 to 1999, while their average weight decreased by 12%. On the other hand, people's views concerning healthy weight have changed in the opposite direction. In Britain the weight at which people considered themselves to be overweight was significantly higher in 2007 than in 1999. These changes are believed to be due to increasing rates of adiposity leading to increased acceptance of extra body fat as being normal.

Obesity is still seen as a sign of wealth and well-being in many parts of Africa. This has become particularly common since the HIV epidemic began.

The Arts

The first sculptural representations of the human body 20,000–35,000 years ago depict obese females. Some attribute the Venus figurines to the tendency to emphasize fertility while others feel they represent "fatness" in the people of the time. Corpulence is, however, absent in both Greek and Roman art, probably in keeping with their ideals regarding moderation. This continued through much of Christian European history, with only those of low socioeconomic status being depicted as obese.

During the Renaissance some of the upper class began flaunting their large size, as can be seen in portraits of Henry VIII of England and Alessandro del Borro. Rubens (1577–1640) regularly depicted full-bodied women in his pictures, from which derives the term Rubenesque. These women, however, still maintained the "hourglass" shape with its relationship to fertility. During the 19th century, views on obesity changed in the Western world. After centuries of obesity being synonymous with wealth and social status, slimness began to be seen as the desirable standard.

Society and Culture

Economic Impact

In addition to its health impacts, obesity leads to many problems including disadvantages in employment and increased business costs. These effects are felt by all levels of society from individuals, to corporations, to governments.

In 2005, the medical costs attributable to obesity in the US were an estimated $190.2 billion or 20.6% of all medical expenditures, while the cost of obesity in Canada was estimated at CA$2 billion in 1997 (2.4% of total health costs). The total annual direct cost of overweight and obesity in Australia in 2005 was A$21 billion. Overweight and obese Australians also received A$35.6 billion in government subsidies. The estimate range for annual expenditures on diet products is $40 billion to $100 billion in the US alone.

Obesity prevention programs have been found to reduce the cost of treating obesity-related disease. However, the longer people live, the more medical costs they incur. Researchers therefore conclude that reducing obesity may improve the public's health, but it is unlikely to reduce overall health spending.

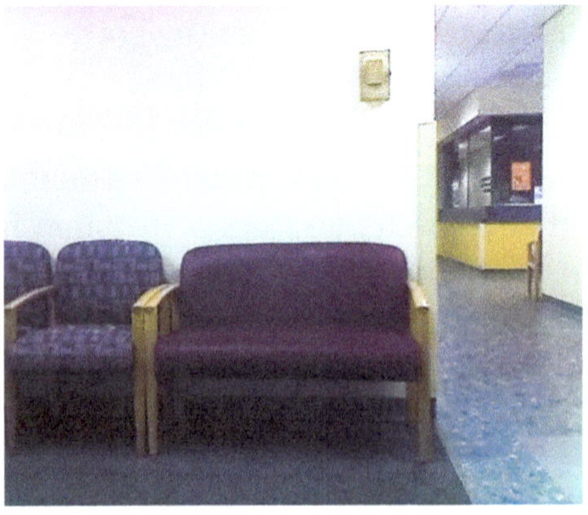

Services must accommodate obese people with specialist equipment such as much wider chairs.

Obesity can lead to social stigmatization and disadvantages in employment. When compared to their normal weight counterparts, obese workers on average have higher rates of absenteeism from work and take more disability leave, thus increasing costs for employers and decreasing productivity. A study examining Duke University employees found that people with a BMI over 40 kg/m^2 filed twice as many workers' compensation claims as those whose BMI was 18.5–24.9 kg/m^2. They also had more than 12 times as many lost work days. The most common injuries in this group were due to falls and lifting, thus affecting the lower extremities, wrists or hands, and backs. The Alabama State Employees' Insurance Board approved a controversial plan to charge obese workers

$25 a month for health insurance that would otherwise be free unless they take steps to lose weight and improve their health. These measures started in January 2010 and apply to those state workers whose BMI exceeds 35 kg/m^2 and who fail to make improvements in their health after one year.

Some research shows that obese people are less likely to be hired for a job and are less likely to be promoted. Obese people are also paid less than their non-obese counterparts for an equivalent job; obese women on average make 6% less and obese men make 3% less.

Specific industries, such as the airline, healthcare and food industries, have special concerns. Due to rising rates of obesity, airlines face higher fuel costs and pressures to increase seating width. In 2000, the extra weight of obese passengers cost airlines US$275 million. The healthcare industry has had to invest in special facilities for handling severely obese patients, including special lifting equipment and bariatric ambulances. Costs for restaurants are increased by litigation accusing them of causing obesity. In 2005 the US Congress discussed legislation to prevent civil lawsuits against the food industry in relation to obesity; however, it did not become law.

With the American Medical Association's 2013 classification of obesity as a chronic disease, it is thought that health insurance companies will more likely pay for obesity treatment, counseling and surgery, and the cost of research and development of fat treatment pills or gene therapy treatments should be more affordable if insurers help to subsidize their cost. The AMA classification is not legally binding, however, so health insurers still have the right to reject coverage for a treatment or procedure.

In 2014, The European Court of Justice ruled that morbid obesity is a disability. The Court argued that if an employee's obesity prevents him from "full and effective participation of that person in professional life on an equal basis with other workers", then it shall be considered a disability and that firing someone on such grounds is discriminatory.

Size Acceptance

The principal goal of the fat acceptance movement is to decrease discrimination against people who are overweight and obese. However, some in the movement are also attempting to challenge the established relationship between obesity and negative health outcomes.

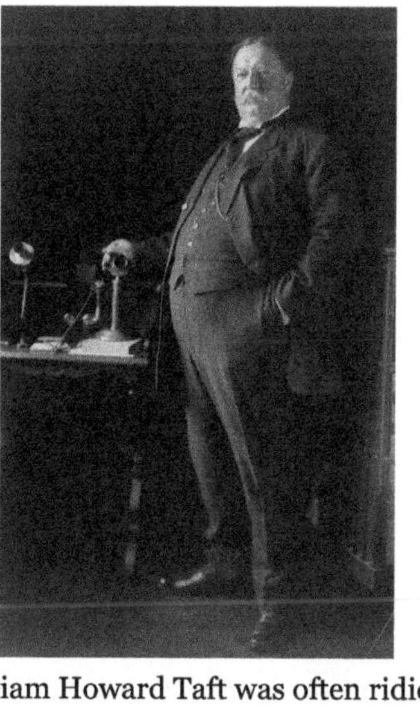

United States President William Howard Taft was often ridiculed for being overweight

A number of organizations exist that promote the acceptance of obesity. They have increased in prominence in the latter half of the 20th century. The US-based National Association to Advance Fat Acceptance (NAAFA) was formed in 1969 and describes itself as a civil rights organization dedicated to ending size discrimination.

The International Size Acceptance Association (ISAA) is a non-governmental organization (NGO) which was founded in 1997. It has more of a global orientation and describes its mission as promoting size acceptance and helping to end weight-based discrimination. These groups often argue for the recognition of obesity as a disability under the US Americans With Disabilities Act (ADA). The American legal system, however, has decided that the potential public health costs exceed the benefits of extending this anti-discrimination law to cover obesity.

Childhood Obesity

The healthy BMI range varies with the age and sex of the child. Obesity in children and adolescents is defined as a BMI greater than the 95th percentile. The reference data that these percentiles are based on is from 1963 to 1994 and thus has not been affected by the recent increases in rates of obesity. Childhood obesity has reached epidemic proportions in the 21st century, with rising rates in both the developed and developing world. Rates of obesity in Canadian boys have increased from 11% in the 1980s to over 30% in the 1990s, while during this same time period rates increased from 4 to 14% in Brazilian children.

As with obesity in adults, many factors contribute to the rising rates of childhood obesity. Changing diet and decreasing physical activity are believed to be the two most important causes for the recent increase in the incidence of child obesity. Because childhood obesity often persists into adulthood and is associated with numerous chronic illnesses, children who are obese are often tested for hypertension, diabetes, hyperlipidemia, and fatty liver. Treatments used in children are primarily lifestyle interventions and behavioral techniques, although efforts to increase activity in children have had little success. In the United States, medications are not FDA approved for use in this age group.

Other Animals

Obesity in pets is common in many countries. In the United States, 23–41% of dogs are overweight, and about 5.1% are obese. The rate of obesity in cats was slightly higher at 6.4%. In Australia the rate of obesity among dogs in a veterinary setting has been found to be 7.6%. The risk of obesity in dogs is related to whether or not their owners are obese; however, there is no similar correlation between cats and their owners.

References

- Fratamico PM (2005). Bayles DO, ed. Foodborne Pathogens: Microbiology and Molecular Biology. Caister Academic Press. ISBN 978-1-904455-00-4.
- Ljungh A, Wadstrom T, eds. (2009). Lactobacillus Molecular Biology: From Genomics to Probiotics. Caister Academic Press. ISBN 978-1-904455-41-7.
- Mayo, B (2010). van Sinderen, D, ed. Bifidobacteria: Genomics and Molecular Aspects. Caister Academic Press. ISBN 978-1-904455-68-4.

- Rehm BHA, ed. (2009). Microbial Production of Biopolymers and Polymer Precursors: Applications and Perspectives. Caister Academic Press. ISBN 978-1-904455-36-3.
- Remminghorst & Rehm (2009). "Microbial Production of Alginate: Biosynthesis and Applications". Microbial Production of Biopolymers and Polymer Precursors. Caister Academic Press. ISBN 978-1-904455-36-3.
- Shih & Wu (2009). "Biosynthesis and Application of Poly(gamma-glutamic acid)". Microbial Production of Biopolymers and Polymer Precursors. Caister Academic Press. ISBN 978-1-904455-36-3.
- Prentice, editor-in-chief, Benjamin Caballero ; editors, Lindsay Allen, Andrew (2005). Encyclopedia of human nutrition (2nd ed.). Amsterdam: Elsevier/Academic Press. p. 68. ISBN 9780080454283.
- Walker, [edited by] Christopher Duggan, John B. Watkins, W. Allan (2008). Nutrition in pediatrics: basic science, clinical application. Hamilton: BC Decker. pp. 127–141. ISBN 978-1-55009-361-2.
- Sen, Amartya Kumar (1981). Poverty and famines: An essay on entitlement and deprivation. Oxford University Press. ISBN 978-0-19-828463-5.
- Malthus, Thomas Robert; Appleman, Philip (1976). An essay on the principle of population: text, sources and background, criticism. Norton. ISBN 978-0-393-09202-8.
- Woodhouse R (2008). "Obesity in art: A brief overview". Front Horm Res. Frontiers of Hormone Research. 36: 271–86. doi:10.1159/000115370. ISBN 978-3-8055-8429-6. PMID 18230908.
- Wilkinson, Richard; Pickett, Kate (2009). The Spirit Level: Why More Equal Societies Almost Always Do Better. London: Allen Lane. pp. 91–101. ISBN 978-1-84614-039-6.
- Boulpaep, Emile L.; Boron, Walter F. (2003). Medical physiology: A cellular and molecular approach. Philadelphia: Saunders. p. 1227. ISBN 0-7216-3256-4.
- Loscalzo, Joseph; Fauci, Anthony S.; Braunwald, Eugene; Dennis L. Kasper; Hauser, Stephen L; Longo, Dan L. (2008). Harrison's principles of internal medicine. McGraw-Hill Medical. ISBN 0-07-146633-9.
- Satcher D (2001). The Surgeon General's Call to Action to Prevent and Decrease Overweight and Obesity. U.S. Dept. of Health and Human Services, Public Health Service, Office of Surgeon General. ISBN 978-0-16-051005-2.
- Theodore Mazzone; Giamila Fantuzzi (2006). Adipose Tissue And Adipokines in Health And Disease (Nutrition and Health). Totowa, NJ: Humana Press. p. 222. ISBN 1-58829-721-7.
- Fumento, Michael (1997). The Fat of the Land: Our Health Crisis and How Overweight Americans Can Help Themselves. Penguin (Non-Classics). p. 126. ISBN 0-14-026144-3.

Permissions

All chapters in this book are published with permission under the Creative Commons Attribution Share Alike License or equivalent. Every chapter published in this book has been scrutinized by our experts. Their significance has been extensively debated. The topics covered herein carry significant information for a comprehensive understanding. They may even be implemented as practical applications or may be referred to as a beginning point for further studies.

We would like to thank the editorial team for lending their expertise to make the book truly unique. They have played a crucial role in the development of this book. Without their invaluable contributions this book wouldn't have been possible. They have made vital efforts to compile up to date information on the varied aspects of this subject to make this book a valuable addition to the collection of many professionals and students.

This book was conceptualized with the vision of imparting up-to-date and integrated information in this field. To ensure the same, a matchless editorial board was set up. Every individual on the board went through rigorous rounds of assessment to prove their worth. After which they invested a large part of their time researching and compiling the most relevant data for our readers.

The editorial board has been involved in producing this book since its inception. They have spent rigorous hours researching and exploring the diverse topics which have resulted in the successful publishing of this book. They have passed on their knowledge of decades through this book. To expedite this challenging task, the publisher supported the team at every step. A small team of assistant editors was also appointed to further simplify the editing procedure and attain best results for the readers.

Apart from the editorial board, the designing team has also invested a significant amount of their time in understanding the subject and creating the most relevant covers. They scrutinized every image to scout for the most suitable representation of the subject and create an appropriate cover for the book.

The publishing team has been an ardent support to the editorial, designing and production team. Their endless efforts to recruit the best for this project, has resulted in the accomplishment of this book. They are a veteran in the field of academics and their pool of knowledge is as vast as their experience in printing. Their expertise and guidance has proved useful at every step. Their uncompromising quality standards have made this book an exceptional effort. Their encouragement from time to time has been an inspiration for everyone.

The publisher and the editorial board hope that this book will prove to be a valuable piece of knowledge for students, practitioners and scholars across the globe.

Index